HOW TO EAT TO BEAT DISEASE

ESSENTIAL GUIDE OF NUTRITION
TO SUPPORT YOUR BODY'S
NATURAL HEALING PROCESSES
AND PROMOTE OPTIMAL HEALTH

Copyright@2024

Adams Mumford

TABLE OF CONTENT

INTRODUCTION

The Power of Nutrition

Imagine having the potential to transform your health with the meals you consume each day. The alternatives you are making at the grocery shop, for your kitchen, and on the dining table can profoundly impact your ordinary properly being. Nutrition plays a pivotal position in preventing and dealing with many persistent illnesses, from heart disease to diabetes to cancer. By information and harnessing the electricity of vitamins, you may take control of your fitness and enhance your high quality of life.

THE SCIENCE BEHIND EATING TO BEAT DISEASE

Over the beyond few decades, scientific research has increasingly more highlighted the relationship among weight reduction plan and fitness. Numerous studies have shown that positive foods can assist prevent sickness, gradual down its progression, or even opposite harm. This e book is grounded in this evidence based studies, presenting you insights into how unique nutrients and nutritional styles can promote health and shield in opposition to contamination.

YOUR JOURNEY TO BETTER HEALTH

Welcome to "How to Eat to Beat Disease." This book is designed to be your comprehensive manual on the adventure to better fitness through vitamins. Whether you're looking to save you disorder, manage an current condition, or virtually beautify your common well being, you may discover practical advice, meal plans, and delicious recipes to assist your goals.

THE POWER OF NUTRITION

Transforming Health with Everyday Choices

Imagine a global where each meal you eat is a step towards better health. The meals you consume is more than simply gas in your body—it's a effective device that could save you disorder, decorate your mood, and increase your sturdiness. Each chew you take can either make a contribution to health or disorder, making nutrients one of the maximum great elements on your common well being.

THE IMPACT OF DIET ON HEALTH

Decades of research have proven that eating regimen plays a critical position within the prevention and control of many continual sicknesses. Heart disorder, diabetes, most cancers, or even cognitive decline are all stimulated via the meals we consume. By information the connection between food regimen and disorder, you can make informed alternatives that help your health desires.

Heart Disease: A food plan rich in end result, vegetables, complete grains, and lean proteins can substantially lessen the threat of heart ailment. These ingredients are high in important nutrients and low in unhealthy fats and cholesterol, supporting to preserve wholesome blood strain and levels of cholesterol.

Diabetes: Managing blood sugar degrees is crucial for preventing and controlling diabetes. Consuming lowglycemic meals inclusive of whole grains, legumes, and non starchy greens can assist regulate blood sugar and reduce insulin resistance.

Cancer: Certain ingredients incorporate photochemical that have been proven to reduce the threat of cancer. For instance, cruciferous veggies like broccoli and Brussels sprouts comprise compounds that help cleansing and inhibit the increase of cancer cells.

Cognitive Health: The mind requires a constant supply of vitamins to characteristic optimally. Omegathree fatty acids, antioxidants, and nutrients determined in ingredients like fish, berries, and leafy veggies can protect against cognitive decline and improve intellectual clarity.

THE SCIENCE BEHIND EATING TO BEAT DISEASE

Unveiling the Evidence

In current years, clinical research has supplied compelling proof that the ingredients we devour play a critical function in our fitness and toughness. By expertise the mechanisms thru which eating regimen impacts our bodies, we can make selections that aid disorder prevention and average properly being. This chapter delves into the clinical concepts underlying the idea of eating to beat disease.

Nutritional Biochemistry: The Foundation of Health

At the coronary heart of the relationship among diet and fitness is nutritional biochemistry—the observe of ways nutrients interact with the body on a molecular stage. Every cellular for your frame relies on a steady supply of nutrients to carry out its features. Vitamins, minerals, amino acids, and fatty acids are the building blocks of existence, permitting the whole thing from strength production to DNA restore.

Key Nutrients and Their Roles:

Vitamins and Minerals: Essential for numerous biochemical techniques, together with immune function, bone fitness, and metabolism.

Amino Acids: The constructing blocks of proteins, vital for tissue repair, enzyme production, and immune responses.

Fatty Acids: Important for cell membrane integrity, brain health, and anti inflammatory techniques.

Phytonutrients: Bioactive compounds discovered in plants that have antioxidant, anti inflammatory, and anticancer residences.

Inflammation and Oxidative Stress: The Disease Connection

Chronic infection and oxidative pressure are at the root of many persistent diseases. Inflammation is the body's response to harm or infection, but while it turns into persistent, it can damage tissues and organs. Oxidative pressure happens when there's an imbalance among unfastened radicals and antioxidants in the frame, leading to mobile harm.

Dietary Influences on Inflammation and Oxidative Stress:

Antioxidants: Compounds that neutralize unfastened radicals, preventing oxidative harm. Found in culmination, vegetables, nuts, and seeds.

Anti Inflammatory Foods: Include omega3 fatty acids (determined in fish and flax seeds), turmeric, and inexperienced tea.

ProInflammatory Foods: Processed meals high in sugar, trans fat, and delicate carbohydrates can boom infection.

The Gut Micro biome: A Central Player in Health

The intestine micro biome, which includes trillions of microorganisms, has emerged as a key player in health and sickness. These microorganisms resource in digestion, produce vital vitamins, and regulate the immune machine. A balanced gut microbiome is related to lower risks of continual illnesses, at the same time as dysbiosis (an imbalance) is connected to situations including obesity, diabetes, and autoimmune diseases.

Supporting a Healthy Gut Micro biome:

Prebiotics: Non digestible fibers that feed useful intestine micro organism. Found in garlic, onions, bananas, and entire grains.

Probiotics: Live beneficial bacteria observed in fermented meals like yogurt, kefir, and sauerkraut.

Diverse Diet: Consuming quite a few plant primarily based ingredients helps a numerous microbiome.

CHAPTER 1: UNDERSTANDING THE CONNECTION

BETWEEN DIET AND DISEASE

THE FUNDAMENTALS OF NUTRITION

Macro nutrients: Carbohydrates, proteins, and fats.

Macro nutrients: Carbohydrates, Proteins, and Fats

Macro nutrients are the vitamins that our bodies require in massive quantities for strength, growth, and bodily features. The three primary macro nutrients are carbohydrates, proteins, and fat. Each performs a awesome and critical function in preserving health and helping bodily techniques.

Carbohydrates: The Body's Main Energy Source

Function:

- Provide power: Carbohydrates are the frame's preferred supply of electricity. They are broken down into glucose, which fuels cell sports.

- Support mind function: The brain is predicated on glucose for electricity, making carbohydrates critical for cognitive function.

- Aid in digestion: Dietary fiber, a form of carbohydrate, promotes healthy digestion and prevents constipation.

Types of Carbohydrates:

1. Simple Carbohydrates: Quickly digested and absorbed, main to fast spikes in blood sugar. Found in fruits, milk, and sugary meals.

Examples: Glucose, fructose, sucrose.

2. Complex Carbohydrates: Consist of longer chains of sugar molecules, providing a extra sustained power release. Found in entire grains, legumes, and vegetables.

Examples: Starches, fiber.

Sources:

 Whole grains (brown rice, oats, quinoa)

 Vegetables (candy potatoes, broccoli, carrots)

 Fruits (apples, berries, oranges)

 Legumes (beans, lentils, chickpeas)

Health Benefits:

 Stabilize blood sugar tiers

 Provide sustained energy

 Support digestive fitness

 Proteins: Building Blocks of the Body

Function:

 Build and repair tissues: Proteins are vital for the growth and restore of tissues, including muscle mass, skin, and organs.

 Produce enzymes and hormones: Proteins are necessary for the manufacturing of enzymes and hormones that regulate various bodily capabilities.

Support immune characteristic: Proteins are crucial for the formation of antibodies and other additives of the immune machine. Micro nutrients: Vitamins and minerals.

 Micro nutrients: Vitamins and Minerals

Micro nutrients, which encompass vitamins and minerals, are vital for preserving health, helping bodily functions, and preventing illnesses. Although they are required in smaller amounts in comparison to macro nutrients, their effect on fitness is massive. This bankruptcy explores the roles of numerous nutrients and minerals and their importance in our eating regimen.

VITAMINS: ESSENTIAL ORGANIC COMPOUNDS

Vitamins are natural compounds which can be essential for metabolic approaches, immune feature, and overall fitness. They are categorized into two most important sorts: water soluble and fat soluble.

Water Soluble Vitamins: These nutrients dissolve in water and aren't saved within the frame, so that they want to be consumed regularly. They encompass the B nutrients and nutrition C.

1. Vitamin B Complex:

. B1 (Thiamine): Supports power metabolism and nerve characteristic.

Sources: Whole grains, pork, legumes.

B2 (Riboflavin): Important for power manufacturing and pores and skin health.

Sources: Dairy products, eggs, inexperienced leafy greens.

B3 (Niacin): Aids in DNA repair and strength metabolism.

Sources: Meat, fish, fowl, peanuts.

B5 (Pantothenic Acid): Essential for fatty acid metabolism.

Sources: Avocados, yogurt, candy potatoes.

B6 (Pyridoxine): Involved in amino acid metabolism and red blood cellular manufacturing.

Sources: Bananas, nuts, potatoes.

B7 (Biotin): Supports hair, pores and skin, and nail fitness.

Sources: Eggs, almonds, spinach.

B9 (Folate/Folic Acid): Crucial for DNA synthesis and cellular division.

Sources: Leafy greens, legumes, fortified grains.

B12 (Cobalamin): Necessary for nerve characteristic and red blood cellular formation.

Sources: Meat, fish, dairy products.

2. Vitamin C (Ascorbic Acid):

Role: Antioxidant that helps immune function, collagen synthesis, and wound recovery.

Sources: Citrus culmination, strawberries, bell peppers, broccoli.

Fat Soluble Vitamins: These vitamins are stored inside the frame's fatty tissues and liver, and include vitamins A, D, E, and K. The significance of hydration.

Micro nutrients: Vitamins and Minerals Micro nutrients, consisting of nutrients and minerals, are crucial for severa physiological functions. Unlike macro nutrients, they're required in smaller quantities however are vital for maintaining health, helping metabolic methods, and stopping illnesses.

VITAMINS: VITAL FOR HEALTH

Vitamins are natural compounds that play numerous roles inside the frame. They are classified into two businesses based totally on their solubility:

Fat Soluble Vitamins:

1. Vitamin A: Essential for vision, immune function, and pores and skin health.

Sources: Carrots, sweet potatoes, spinach, liver.

2. Vitamin D: Crucial for calcium absorption, bone fitness, and immune characteristic.

Sources: Sunlight, fatty fish, fortified dairy merchandise.

3. Vitamin E: Acts as an antioxidant, shielding cells from damage.

Sources: Nuts, seeds, spinach, broccoli.

4. Vitamin K: Important for blood clotting and bone health.

Sources: Leafy greens, broccoli, Brussels sprouts.

UNDERSTANDING INFLAMMATION

Inflammation is a critical immune response that helps the body combat off infections, heal accidents, and hold usual fitness. It involves the activation of immune cells, the release of signaling molecules, and elevated blood waft to the affected place.

Acute Inflammation:

Characteristics: Rapid onset, short period, localized to the web site of injury or infection.

Purpose: To do away with the initial motive of mobile injury, clean out damaged cells and tissues, and establish restore.

Examples: A reduce on the pores and skin, a sore throat from a chilly, or a sprained ankle.

CHRONIC INFLAMMATION:

Characteristics: Prolonged length, can final for months or years, often low grade and systemic.

Purpose: Unlike acute inflammation, persistent infection isn't always always beneficial and might end up a pathological condition.

Examples: Chronic inflammatory illnesses consisting of rheumatoid arthritis, inflammatory bowel ailment, and sort 2 diabetes.

Mechanisms of Chronic Inflammation
Chronic infection can arise from various factors, including chronic infections, extended exposure to irritants, autoimmune reactions, and lifestyle factors. It involves a complex interplay between immune cells, signaling molecules (cytokines), and biochemical pathways.

Key Players in Chronic Inflammation:

Immune Cells: Macrophages, lymphocytes, and neutrophils are concerned within the inflammatory response.

Cytokines: Signaling molecules consisting of interleukins, tumor necrosis factor (TNF), and interferons play roles in maintaining infection.

Reactive Oxygen Species (ROS): Molecules that may reason oxidative damage to cells and tissues.

INFLAMMATION AND DISEASE

Chronic irritation is related to the improvement and development of numerous sicknesses. It can cause damage to tissues and organs, disrupt everyday cell features, and contribute to various fitness situations.

CARDIOVASCULAR DISEASE:

Mechanism: Chronic irritation contributes to the improvement of atherosclerosis, the accumulation of fatty plaques inside the arteries. Inflammatory cells and cytokines sell plaque formation, main to narrowed and hardened arteries.

Consequences: Increased danger of heart attacks, strokes, and peripheral artery sickness.

DIABETES:

Mechanism: Inflammation plays a position in insulin resistance, a key factor in type 2 diabetes. Pro inflammatory cytokines interfere with insulin signaling pathways, main to expanded blood sugar stages.

Consequences: Poor blood glucose manipulate, headaches including neuropathy, retinopathy, and cardiovascular disease.

UNDERSTANDING THE GUT MICRO BIOME

The gut micro biome is a complicated network of trillions of microorganisms, along with bacteria, viruses, fungi, and different microbes, residing in the digestive tract. These microorganisms play a critical position in digestion, nutrient absorption, immune characteristic, and ordinary fitness. Maintaining a healthful intestine micro biome is critical for preventing illnesses and selling properly being.

HOW DIET INFLUENCES GUT HEALTH

Diet is one of the maximum full size elements influencing the composition and function of the intestine micro biome.

1. FiberRich Foods

Role: Dietary fiber, found in end result, vegetables, entire grains, and legumes, acts as a prebiotic, feeding useful intestine bacteria. These micro organism ferment fiber, generating quick chain fatty acids (SCFAs) like butyrate, which have anti inflammatory and protective outcomes on the gut lining.

Sources:

Fruits: Apples, berries, bananas

Vegetables: Broccoli, carrots, leafy greens

Whole grains: Oats, quinoa, brown rice

Legumes: Beans, lentils, chickpeas

Benefits:

Promotes the growth of useful bacteria

Enhances intestine motility and ordinary bowel moves

Reduces the threat of colorectal most cancers

2. Fermented Foods

Role: Fermented meals comprise stay beneficial micro organism (probiotics) which could colonize the intestine and decorate microbial range. Regular intake of fermented ingredients can help keep a balanced micro biome.

Sources:

- Yogurt
- Kefir
- Sauerkraut
- Kimchi
- Miso
- Kombucha

BENEFITS:

Supports digestive health

Strengthens the immune device

May reduce signs of gastrointestinal disorders like irritable bowel syndrome (IBS)

FOODS THAT SUPPORT A HEALTHY MICRO BIOME

Maintaining a numerous and balanced intestine micro biome is vital for general fitness.

FiberRich Foods

Dietary fiber is a important prebiotic that feeds useful gut bacteria, main to the production of quick chain fatty acids (SCFAs) like butyrate, which have anti inflammatory properties and aid gut health.

SOURCES:

Fruits: Apples, berries, bananas, pears, oranges

Vegetables: Broccoli, carrots, artichokes, leafy greens, Brussels sprouts

Whole Grains: Oats, quinoa, brown rice, barley, complete wheat

Legumes: Beans, lentils, chickpeas, peas

BENEFITS:

Promotes the boom of useful micro organism

Enhances intestine motility and ordinary bowel movements

Reduces the danger of colorectal cancer

FERMENTED FOODS

Fermented foods comprise live useful micro organism (probiotics) which can colonize the gut and decorate microbial variety. Regular consumption of fermented foods can help keep a balanced micro biome.

SOURCES:

Yogurt: Contains lines of Lactobacillus and

Kefir: A fermented milk drink rich in probiotics

Sauerkraut: Fermented cabbage containing lactic acid micro organism

Kimchi: A spicy fermented vegetable dish, normally cabbage and radishes

Miso: Fermented soybean paste used in soups and sauces

Kombucha: A fermented tea wealthy in probiotics

Tempeh: Fermented soy product high in protein and probiotics

BENEFITS:

Supports digestive health

Strengthens the immune system

May reduce symptoms of gastrointestinal issues like irritable bowel syndrome (IBS)

POLYPHENOLRICH FOODS

Polyphenols are plant compounds with antioxidant residences which might be metabolized by using intestine micro organism, selling the boom of beneficial microbes and inhibiting dangerous ones.

SOURCES:

Berries: Blueberries, strawberries, raspberries

Nuts and Seeds: Walnuts, almonds, flax seeds, chia seeds

Vegetables: Spinach, onions, artichokes

Tea and Coffee: Green tea, black tea, coffee

Dark Chocolate: Rich in flavonoid, a form of poly phenol

Red Wine: In moderation, carries resveratrol

BENEFITS:

Supports the boom of beneficial gut bacteria

Protects in opposition to oxidative strain and infection

May enhance gut barrier function

Omega3 Fatty AcidRich Foods

Omega three fatty acids have anti inflammatory properties and may definitely affect the composition of the intestine micro biome.

SOURCES:

Fatty Fish: Salmon, mackerel, sardines, trout

Chia Seeds: High in omega3 ALA (alphalinolenic acid)

Flax seeds: Another great source of ALA

Walnuts: Rich in omega three fats

CHAPTER 2: NUTRITIONAL STRATEGIES FOR PREVENTING AND MANAGING DISEASES

HEART HEALTH

UNDERSTANDING CARDIOVASCULAR DISEASES

Cardiovascular diseases (CVDs) encompass a number conditions that affect the heart and blood vessels. They are the main motive of dying globally, however many are preventable thru lifestyle changes and control of hazard factors. Understanding the sorts, causes, and preventive measures for cardiovascular illnesses is crucial for maintaining coronary heart fitness.

TYPES OF CARDIOVASCULAR
DISEASES

1. Coronary Artery Disease (CAD):

- Description: The maximum not unusual form of heart sickness, CAD happens when the coronary arteries that supply blood to the heart muscle become narrowed or blocked because of the buildup of plaque (atherosclerosis).

- Symptoms: Chest pain (angina), shortness of breath, fatigue, coronary heart assault.

2. Heart Attack (Myocardial Infarction):

- Description: Occurs when blood waft to a part of the coronary heart muscle is blocked, usually via a blood clot, causing harm to the heart muscle.

Symptoms: Severe chest pain, shortness of breath, nausea, lightheartedness, ache in the arm, neck, or jaw.

3. Heart Failure:

- Description: A condition in which the heart can't pump sufficient blood to fulfill the body's needs. It can end result from conditions that harm the coronary heart muscle, which includes CAD, excessive blood strain, and diabetes.
- Symptoms: Shortness of breath, fatigue, swollen legs, rapid or irregular heartbeat.

4. Arrhythmia:

- Description: Abnormal heart rhythms which could cause the heart to conquer too rapid, too slow, or irregularly.
- Symptoms: Palpitations, dizziness, fainting, shortness of breath.

5. Stroke:

- Description: Occurs when the blood deliver to a part of the mind is interrupted or decreased, depriving mind tissue of oxygen and nutrients.

- Symptoms: Sudden numbness or weak spot in the face, arm, or leg, confusion, hassle talking, vision issues, intense headache.

6. Peripheral Artery Disease (PAD):

- Description: A condition in which the arteries that deliver blood to the limbs come to be narrowed or blocked.

- Symptoms: Leg pain whilst taking walks, numbness or weak spot inside the legs, coldness in the decrease leg or foot.

7. Hypertension (High Blood Pressure):

- Description: A persistent circumstance in which the force of the blood in opposition to the artery walls is consistently too high, growing the risk of heart attack, stroke, and heart failure.

- Symptoms: Often asymptomatic, but can encompass headaches, shortness of breath, nosebleeds.

FOODS THAT SUPPORT HEART
HEALTH

A coronary heart wholesome eating regimen
is vital for preventing cardiovascular
illnesses and promoting overall nicely being.
Incorporating certain meals into your each
day weight reduction plan can assist
improve levels of cholesterol, lessen blood
strain, decrease irritation, and support
coronary heart feature.

1. Fruits and Vegetables
Fruits and veggies are rich in nutrients,
minerals, fiber, and antioxidants, which
might be critical for coronary heart fitness.
EXAMPLES:

Berries: Blueberries, strawberries, and
raspberries are excessive in antioxidants like
anthocyanins, which reduce inflammation
and oxidative strain.

Leafy Greens: Spinach, kale, and Swiss chard are wealthy in nutrients, minerals, and nitrates that help lower blood strain.

Citrus Fruits: Oranges, grapefruits, and lemons are high in diet C and flavonoid, which improve cholesterol levels and reduce coronary heart ailment chance.

Cruciferous Vegetables: Broccoli, cauliflower, and Brussels sprouts are excessive in fiber and antioxidants that guard against cardiovascular sickness.

2. Whole Grains

Whole grains offer vital nutrients and fiber that assist hold healthy cholesterol levels and decrease the danger of heart ailment. Examples:

Oats: Contain beta glucan, a soluble fiber that lowers LDL cholesterol levels.

Quinoa: High in protein, fiber, and various nutrients and minerals.

Brown Rice: A precise source of magnesium, which helps adjust heart rhythm.

Whole Wheat: Provides fiber and nutrients that help heart health.

3. Nuts and Seeds

Nuts and seeds are wealthy in healthful fats, fiber, and protein, which might be beneficial for heart fitness.

Examples:

Walnuts: High in omega three fatty acids, which lessen inflammation and lower the threat of coronary heart sickness.

Almonds: Contain monounsaturated fat, fiber, and antioxidants that improve cholesterol levels.

Flax seeds: Rich in omega3 fatty acids and lignans, that have coronary heart shielding homes.

Chia Seeds: High in fiber and omegathree fatty acids, promoting heart fitness.

4. Fatty Fish

Fatty fish are amazing resources of omega3 fatty acids, that have severa coronary heart advantages.

Examples:

Salmon: Rich in omega3 fatty acids, which reduce triglycerides, lower blood pressure, and decrease the risk of arrhythmias.

Mackerel: High in omega3s and vitamin D, assisting coronary heart fitness.

Sardines: Provide omega3s and also are a good source of calcium and vitamin D.

Trout: Contains omega3 fatty acids and antioxidants.

DIABETES PREVENTION AND MANAGEMENT

Diabetes is a persistent condition characterized by using excessive blood sugar ranges. Effective prevention and control of diabetes involve a mixture of lifestyle changes, nutritional adjustments, and, whilst necessary, medication.

UNDERSTANDING DIABETES

Types of Diabetes:

Type 1 Diabetes: An autoimmune situation in which the body assaults insulin generating cells inside the pancreas. It generally develops in early life or youth.

Type 2 Diabetes: A circumstance in which the frame becomes immune to insulin or doesn't produce sufficient insulin. It is greater commonplace and often related to lifestyle elements.

Gestational Diabetes: Develops for the duration of being pregnant and typically disappears after childbirth however will increase the danger of growing type 2 diabetes later.

Risk Factors

Non Modifiable Risk Factors:

Genetics: Family records of diabetes increases hazard.

Age: Risk increases with age, specifically after 45.

Ethnicity: Certain ethnic organizations (e.G., African American, Hispanic, Native American, Asian) have a higher danger.

MODIFIABLE RISK FACTORS:

- Overweight and Obesity: Excess body fats, in particular around the stomach, increases insulin resistance.

- Sedentary Lifestyle: Lack of physical interest contributes to weight advantage and insulin resistance.

- Unhealthy Diet: High intake of sugary, processed ingredients and low consumption of fiberrich ingredients boom threat.

- Smoking: Increases the danger of type 2 diabetes and headaches.

PREVENTION STRATEGIES

1. Healthy Eating:

- Balanced Diet: Include lots of culmination, greens, complete grains, lean proteins, and healthy fat.

- Reduce Sugar and Refined Carbs: Limit sugary beverages, desserts, and delicate grains.

- Increase Fiber Intake: Foods excessive in fiber, such as complete grains, legumes, culmination, and veggies, help control blood sugar tiers.

- Choose Healthy Fats: Opt for assets of unsaturated fat like olive oil, nuts, and avocados at the same time as restricting saturated and trans fats.

2. Regular Physical Activity:

- Aim for at the least 150 minutes of mild intensity cardio hobby or seventy five minutes of energetic pastime in line with week.

Include strength training sports at least twice every week..

CANCER PREVENTION

Cancer prevention entails a combination of lifestyle alternatives, dietary behavior, and regular screenings. By making knowledgeable selections, people can substantially reduce their hazard of developing cancer.

1. Healthy Diet

A balanced eating regimen rich in vitamins can lower the hazard of cancer. Key nutritional tips consist of:

Eat a Variety of Fruits and Vegetables: These foods are high in vitamins, minerals, fiber, and antioxidants, which assist protect towards cancer.

Examples: Berries, leafy greens, cruciferous vegetables (like broccoli and cauliflower), and citrus fruits.

Choose Whole Grains Over Refined Grains:
Whole grains provide greater fiber and
vitamins.

Examples: Brown rice, quinoa, complete
wheat, oats.

Limit Processed and Red Meats: These had
been linked to an extended hazard of
colorectal most cancers.

- Recommendations: Opt for lean meats,
  poultry, fish, or plant based totally
  proteins like beans and lentils.

- Reduce Sugar and Refined Carbs: High
  sugar intake can cause obesity, that's a
  hazard factor for plenty cancers.

- Recommendations: Limit sugary
  liquids, desserts, and snacks.

- Incorporate Healthy Fats: Choose
  unsaturated fats over saturated and trans
  fats.

Examples: Olive oil, nuts, seeds, avocados,
fatty fish.

2. Regular Physical Activity

Regular exercise helps keep a healthy weight and decreases the hazard of diverse cancers, inclusive of breast, colon, and endometrial cancers.

Recommendations: Aim for as a minimum one hundred fifty mins of mild intensity or 75 minutes of full of life depth exercise every week. Include electricity education physical activities at the least twice every week.

3. Maintain a Healthy Weight

Obesity is related to an improved threat of numerous cancers, together with breast, prostate, lung, colon, and kidney most cancers.

Recommendations: Combine a wholesome weight loss plan with regular bodily pastime to reap and hold a wholesome weight.

CHAPTER 3: BRAIN HEALTH

THE CONNECTION AMONG EATING REGIMEN AND COGNITIVE FEATURE.

FOODS THAT BOOST BRAIN HEALTH

A diet wealthy in particular vitamins can support brain function, decorate memory, enhance temper, and decrease the threat of neurodegenerative illnesses.

1. Fatty Fish

Fatty fish are high in omega three fatty acids, which are important for mind health.

Examples:

Salmon

Mackerel

Sardines

Trout

Benefits:

Omega3s construct cellular membranes inside the brain and enhance neuron characteristic.

They reduce infection and oxidative pressure, lowering the risk of Alzheimer's sickness.

2. Blueberries

Blueberries are packed with antioxidants, consisting of flavonoid.

Benefits:

Antioxidants help reduce oxidative stress and irritation inside the mind.

They enhance communique between brain cells and can delay brain growing older.

3. Turmeric

Turmeric carries curcumin, a compound with strong anti inflammatory and antioxidant blessings.

BENEFITS:

Curcumin can pass the blood brain barrier and has been shown to enhance reminiscence and stimulate the production of mind derived neurotrophic element (BDNF), a increase hormone that functions in mind characteristic.

It may also assist clean amyloid plaques, which might be related to Alzheimer's ailment.

MEAL PLANS FOR COGNITIVE SUPPORT

A food regimen rich in precise vitamins can appreciably decorate cognitive characteristic, reminiscence, and average brain health.

Day 1

Breakfast:

Spinach and Mushroom Omelet: Made with 2 eggs, a handful of spinach, and sliced mushrooms. Serve with a side of whole grain toast.

Blueberry Smoothie: Blend 1 cup of blueberries, 1 banana, a handful of spinach,

1 cup of almond milk, and a tablespoon of chia seeds.

Lunch:

Quinoa Salad: Combine cooked quinoa, cherry tomatoes, cucumber, red onion, feta cheese, and a handful of sparkling parsley. Drizzle with olive oil and lemon juice.

Apple Slices: Serve with almond butter.

Dinner:

Grilled Salmon: Serve with a side of steamed broccoli and brown rice.

Mixed Green Salad: Toss collectively combined veggies, walnuts, dried cranberries, and a balsamic vinaigrette.

Snacks:

Greek Yogurt: Top with honey and a handful of walnuts.

Carrot Sticks: Serve with hummus.

Day 2

Breakfast:

Overnight Oats: Combine rolled oats, almond milk, chia seeds, and a teaspoon of honey. Refrigerate in a single day. In the morning, top with sparkling berries and a sprinkle of flax seeds.

Green Tea: A cup of inexperienced tea for its antioxidant properties.

Lunch:

Turkey and Avocado Wrap: Whole grain tortilla filled with sliced turkey breast, avocado, lettuce, and tomato.

Orange Slices: For a boost of nutrition C.

Dinner:

Baked Chicken Breast: Season with rosemary and garlic, and bake. Serve with candy potato mash and sauteed kale.

Quinoa Pilaf: Cooked with vegetable broth, diced carrots, peas, and a hint of turmeric.

Snacks:

Almonds: A handful of raw almonds.

Dark Chocolate: One or small squares of darkish chocolate (70% cocoa or better).

Day 3

Breakfast:

Whole Grain Avocado Toast: Top complete grain toast with mashed avocado, a sprinkle of chia seeds, and a poached egg.

Berry Parfait: Layer Greek yogurt with combined berries and granola.

Lunch:

Lentil Soup: Made with lentils, carrots, celery, onions, and tomatoes. Season with cumin and turmeric.

Side Salad: Mixed greens with a mild olive oil and lemon dressing.

Dinner:

Stir Fried Tofu and Vegetables: Tofu, bell peppers, broccoli, snap peas, and carrots stir fried in a mild soy sauce and ginger.

Brown Rice: As a side.

Snacks:

Apple Slices: With a handful of walnuts.

Cottage Cheese: With pineapple chunks.

Day 4

Breakfast:

Chia Pudding: Combine chia seeds, almond milk, and a hint of vanilla. Refrigerate in a single day. Top with sparkling mango slices within the morning.

Herbal Tea: Such as chamomile or peppermint.

Lunch:

Grilled Chicken Salad: Grilled hen breast on a mattress of blended vegetables, cherry tomatoes, cucumber, and pink onion. Drizzle with a lemon tahini dressing.

Whole Grain Crackers: Serve with hummus.

Dinner:

Baked Cod: Seasoned with lemon, garlic, and herbs. Serve with roasted Brussels sprouts and quinoa.

Spinach Salad: Spinach, strawberries, goat cheese, and pecans with a balsamic vinaigrette.

Snacks:

Mixed Nuts: A handful of combined nuts.

Celery Sticks: With almond butter.

Day 5

Breakfast:

Banana and Walnut Porridge: Oatmeal cooked with almond milk, topped with sliced banana, walnuts, and a drizzle of honey.

Green Smoothie: Blend spinach, kale, green apple, cucumber, and a dash of coconut water.

Lunch:

Mediterranean Chickpea Salad: Chickpeas, diced cucumber, tomatoes, purple onion, olives, and feta cheese, tossed with olive oil and lemon juice.

Whole Grain Pita: Serve with tzatziki.

Dinner:

Vegetable Stir Fry: Broccoli, bell peppers, snap peas, and carrots stir fried with tofu in a mild soy sauce and ginger.

Brown Rice: As a aspect.

Snacks:

Greek Yogurt: With a handful of berries.

Carrot and Cucumber Sticks: With hummus.

Day 6

Breakfast:

Smoothie Bowl: Blend frozen berries, banana, and a touch of almond milk till thick. Top with granola, chia seeds, and sliced fruit.

Herbal Tea: Such as chamomile or peppermint.

Lunch:

Quinoa and Black Bean Bowl: Cooked quinoa, black beans, corn, avocado, and salsa.

Orange Slices: For a boost of vitamin C.

Dinner:

 Baked Salmon: Season with dill and lemon, and serve with a side of steamed asparagus and quinoa.

 Mixed Green Salad: Tossed with olive oil and balsamic vinegar.

Snacks:

 Almonds: A handful of raw almonds.

 Dark Chocolate: One or small squares of darkish chocolate (70% cocoa or higher).

 Day 7

Breakfast:

 Whole Grain Pancakes: Made with whole grain flour, crowned with clean berries and a drizzle of maple syrup.

 Green Tea: A cup of green tea for its antioxidant residences.

Lunch:

 Turkey and Avocado Wrap: Whole grain tortilla full of sliced turkey breast, avocado, lettuce, and tomato.

Apple Slices: For a lift of fiber.

Dinner:

Baked Chicken Breast: Seasoned with rosemary and garlic, served with sweet potato mash and sauteed kale.

Quinoa Pilaf: Cooked with vegetable broth, diced carrots, peas, and a touch of turmeric.

Snacks:

Mixed Nuts: A handful of combined nuts.

Cottage Cheese: With pineapple chunks.

UNDERSTANDING AUTOIMMUNE DISEASES

Autoimmune sicknesses arise whilst the frame's immune device mistakenly assaults its very own tissues and organs. These sicknesses can have an effect on numerous elements of the body, leading to a range of symptoms and complications.

Understanding autoimmune diseases includes knowing their types, causes, danger factors, signs and symptoms, and management techniques.

WHAT ARE AUTOIMMUNE DISEASES?

Autoimmune diseases are conditions wherein the immune machine, designed to shield the body from infections and sicknesses, erroneously targets and attacks wholesome cells. This immune response can reason infection, tissue damage, and disorder in affected organs.

TYPES OF AUTOIMMUNE DISEASES

There are over 80 known autoimmune sicknesses, inclusive of:

1. Rheumatoid Arthritis (RA):

- Description: A persistent inflammatory disease affecting joints, inflicting ache, swelling, and stiffness.
- Symptoms: Joint pain, swelling, fatigue, and deformity.

2. Systemic Lupus Erythematosus (SLE):

- Description: A systemic condition that may affect pores and skin, joints, kidneys, brain, and different organs.
- Symptoms: Fatigue, joint pain, rash, fever, and kidney problems.

3. Type 1 Diabetes:

- Description: The immune device attacks insulin generating cells in the pancreas, leading to excessive blood sugar tiers.
- Symptoms: Increased thirst, common urination, fatigue, and weight loss.

4. Multiple Sclerosis (MS):

- Description: A disorder where the immune gadget attacks the protecting masking of nerves (myelin), inflicting communication troubles among the brain and the relaxation of the frame.

Symptoms: Numbness, weakness, balance issues, and cognitive difficulties.

5. Inflammatory Bowel Disease (IBD):

- Description: Includes conditions like Crohn's disorder and ulcerative colitis, which cause continual infection of the digestive tract.
- Symptoms: Abdominal ache, diarrhea, weight loss, and fatigue.

6. Psoriasis:

Description: An autoimmune pores and skin circumstance that reasons speedy skin cell turnover, leading to pink, scaly patches.

Symptoms: Red patches of skin with silvery scales, itching, and ache.

7. Graves' Disease:

Description: The immune system assaults the thyroid gland, causing it to supply too much thyroid hormone (hyperthyroidism).

Symptoms: Weight loss, speedy heartbeat, nervousness, and irritability.

CHAPTER 4: BONE AND JOINT HEALTH

THE ROLE OF FOOD REGIMEN IN BONE DENSITY AND JOINT HEALTH.

CALCIUM, VITAMIN D, AND OTHER ESSENTIAL NUTRIENTS

Calcium and diet D are vital for preserving bone fitness, however numerous different vitamins additionally play crucial roles in ordinary health and health.

1. Calcium

Function:

Bone Health: Essential for the development and renovation of strong bones and teeth.

Muscle Function: Plays a position in muscle contraction.

Nerve Transmission: Vital for transmitting nerve impulses.

Blood Clotting: Necessary for the blood clotting method.

Sources:

Dairy Products: Milk, cheese, yogurt.

Leafy Greens: Kale, bok choy, collard veggies.

Fortified Foods: Some plant based milks, orange juice, and cereals.

Nuts and Seeds: Almonds, chia seeds, sesame seeds.

Fish: Sardines and salmon with bones.

Recommended Intake:

Adults: 1,000 mg according to day (1,2 hundred mg for ladies over 50 and men over 70).

2. Vitamin D

Function:

- Calcium Absorption: Enhances the absorption of calcium from the digestive tract.
- Bone Health: Supports bone formation and preservation.
- Immune Function: Plays a role in immune system law.

Sources:

- Sunlight: The frame produces vitamin D when uncovered to sunlight.
- Fatty Fish: Salmon, mackerel, sardines.
- Fortified Foods: Fortified milk, orange juice, and cereals.

Egg Yolks: Contains small amounts of nutrition D.

Mushrooms: Some types like maitake and shiitake are precise sources.

Recommended Intake:

Adults: 600 IU (15 mcg) per day (800 IU or 20 mcg for adults over 70).

3. Vitamin K

Function:

Blood Clotting: Essential for the synthesis of clotting elements.

Bone Health: Contributes to bone mineralization and strength.

Sources:

Leafy Greens: Kale, spinach, broccoli.

Cruciferous Vegetables: Brussels sprouts, cabbage.

Fermented Foods: Natto (a fermented soybean product).

Recommended Intake:

Adults: 90 mcg in keeping with day for ladies, one hundred twenty mcg for guys.

4. Magnesium

FUNCTION:

Bone Health: Plays a position in bone formation and maintenance.

Muscle and Nerve Function: Essential for muscle contraction and nerve feature.

Energy Production: Involved in over three hundred biochemical reactions in the frame.

Sources:

Nuts and Seeds: Almonds, pumpkin seeds, sunflower seeds.

Whole Grains: Brown rice, quinoa, whole wheat.

Leafy Greens: Spinach, Swiss chard.

Legumes: Black beans, lentils.

RECOMMENDED INTAKE:

Adults: 310320 mg consistent with day for women, 400420 mg for guys.

CHAPTER 5: PRACTICAL APPLICATIONS

BUILDING A HEALTHY PLATE

PRINCIPLES OF BALANCED CONSUMING.

Balanced consuming is key to retaining normal fitness, ensuring the body receives the vitamins it wishes, and helping numerous bodily functions.

1. Variety

Include Different Food Groups: Aim to consume a whole lot of foods from all meals organizations—culmination, greens, grains, proteins, and dairy or alternatives—to make certain you get a extensive variety of vitamins.

Colorful Plates: Incorporate a variety of colourful end result and greens to advantage from special vitamins, minerals, and antioxidants.

2. Moderation

Portion Control: Be conscious of component sizes to avoid overeating and to help control weight.

Limit High Calorie, Low Nutrient Foods: Reduce intake of meals excessive in brought sugars, saturated fats, and refined grains. Enjoy those ingredients once in a while as opposed to frequently.

3. Proportionality

Balance Macro nutrients: Ensure your weight loss program consists of suitable proportions of carbohydrates, proteins, and fat. Generally, goal for a balanced plate with approximately half of veggies and culmination, a quarter protein, and a quarter whole grains.

Focus on Healthy Fats: Choose unsaturated fats (e.G., olive oil, avocados) over saturated and trans fat.

4. Nutrient Density

Choose Nutrient Rich Foods: Opt for foods that provide the most vitamins in line with calorie, consisting of leafy greens, complete grains, and lean proteins.

Minimize Empty Calories: Avoid food and drinks that provide energy without huge nutritional price, inclusive of sugary sodas and candies.

5. Hydration

Drink Plenty of Water: Aim for as a minimum eight cups (2 liters) of water an afternoon, and alter based on pastime level, weather, and person desires.

Limit Sugary Drinks: Reduce consumption of sugary liquids like sodas and fruit juices.

6. Meal Timing

Regular Meals: Eat normal food and snacks at some stage in the day to maintain electricity degrees and prevent overeating.

Balanced Breakfast: Start the day with a balanced breakfast to boost metabolism and set a tremendous tone for the day.

7. Mindful Eating

Listen to Your Body: Eat whilst you're hungry and prevent when you're complete. Pay interest to hunger cues and emotional triggers for ingesting.

Savor Your Food: Eat slowly and experience your meals to improve digestion and pride.

8. Whole Foods

Minimize Processed Foods: Focus on entire, unprocessed ingredients like clean fruits and veggies, whole grains, and lean proteins.

Read Labels: Be privy to delivered sugars, bad fat, and immoderate sodium in packaged meals.

PORTION CONTROL AND MINDFUL EATING

Portion control and mindful consuming are essential strategies for preserving a healthful diet, managing weight, and enhancing normal well being.

PORTION CONTROL

Definition:

Portion manipulate includes dealing with the quantity of food you devour at every meal or snack. It enables in regulating calorie intake and ensures which you're ingesting suitable amounts of vitamins.

STRATEGIES FOR PORTION CONTROL:

1. Use Smaller Plates and Bowls:

- Smaller dishes could make quantities look large, assisting you feel satisfied with less meals.

2. Measure Serving Sizes:

● Use measuring cups or a kitchen scale to gauge proper portions, in particular for high calorie ingredients.

3. Read Nutrition Labels:

● Pay interest to serving sizes on nutrients labels to understand how plenty constitutes a unmarried serving.

4. Avoid Eating from the Package:

● Serve your food on a plate in place of consuming at once from applications or packing containers to assist with element manage.

5. Be Aware of Portion Sizes:

Familiarize your self with well known component sizes for exclusive food groups (e.G., a serving of meat is ready the size of a deck of playing cards).

6. Focus on Nutrient Dense Foods:

Choose foods that offer vital vitamins with fewer energy. For instance, culmination, vegetables, and lean proteins are nutrient dense.

7. Balance Your Plate:

- Aim for a balanced plate with appropriate quantities of vegetables, lean proteins, complete grains, and healthful fat.

8. Plan Your Meals:

- Prepare and element food earlier to keep away from overeating and make wholesome selections more convenient.

MINDFUL EATING

Definition:

Mindful eating is the practice of paying full interest to the eating revel in, consisting of the flavor, texture, and sensations of food. It additionally entails being attentive to starvation and fullness cues to guide ingesting conduct.

Principles of Mindful Eating:

1. Eat Without Distractions:

● Avoid eating even as watching TV, working, or the use of electronic devices. Focus on the meal and the ingesting manner.

2. Chew Thoroughly:

● Take the time to chunk each bite thoroughly, that can aid digestion and assist you have fun with the flavors of your meals.

3. Pay Attention to Hunger Cues:

● Eat when you're in reality hungry and forestall when you're effortlessly complete. Avoid ingesting out of boredom or strain.

4. Savor Your Food:

● Enjoy the flavors, textures, and aromas of your meals. Take small bites and enjoy each one to growth pleasure.

5. Listen to Your Body:

- Be attuned to how unique meals make you experience bodily and emotionally. Choose meals that nourish and satisfy.

6. Practice Gratitude:

- Appreciate the food you have, and acknowledge the effort that went into preparing it. Gratitude can enhance your ingesting experience.

7. Avoid Rush:

- Take your time throughout food. Eating slowly permits you to apprehend while you're complete and might prevent overeating.

8. Portion Awareness:

- Be conscious of element sizes and the way they align along with your hunger and fullness cues.

9. Reflect on Your Eating Habits:

- Regularly determine your consuming patterns and make modifications to align with conscious eating practices.

BENEFITS OF PORTION CONTROL AND MINDFUL EATING

Improved Digestion: Chewing meals very well and eating slowly can aid in digestion and nutrient absorption.

Better Weight Management: Portion manipulate enables regulate calorie intake, while mindful eating can prevent overeating and emotional consuming.

Enhanced Enjoyment of Food: Mindful consuming promotes a greater appreciation of meals and ingesting experiences.

Increased Satisfaction: By paying attention to starvation and fullness cues, you are more likely to sense satisfied with appropriate portion sizes.

CREATING NUTRIENT DENSE MEALS

Nutrient dense food provide a excessive quantity of vital nutrients in line with calorie, assisting you gain most useful health at the same time as managing calorie intake.

1. Focus on Whole Foods

- Fruits and Vegetables: Choose a variety of colorful culmination and greens to maximize nutrients, minerals, and antioxidants.

Examples: Spinach, berries, bell peppers, candy potatoes.

- Whole Grains: Opt for whole grains over refined grains to get extra fiber, nutrients, and minerals.

- Examples: Quinoa, brown rice, oats, whole wheat.

- Lean Proteins: Select lean protein sources to provide important amino acids with out excessive saturated fat.

Examples: Chicken breast, tofu, lentils, beans, fish.

Healthy Fats: Incorporate resources of unsaturated fats for coronary heart fitness and nutrient absorption.

Examples: Avocados, nuts, seeds, olive oil.

2. Balance Macro nutrients

Carbohydrates: Include complicated carbohydrates which can be rich in fiber and vitamins.

- Sources: Whole grains, legumes, veggies.
- Proteins: Aim for a whole lot of protein sources to ensure you get all vital amino acids.
- Sources: Lean meats, fish, dairy, legumes, nuts.
- Fats: Choose healthful fat and avoid trans fat and excessive saturated fat.

Sources: Olive oil, avocados, nuts, seeds.

3. Incorporate Super foods

Leafy Greens: Rich in nutrients A, C, K, and folate.

Examples: Kale, spinach, Swiss chard.

Berries: High in antioxidants and vitamins.

Examples: Blueberries, strawberries, raspberries.

Nuts and Seeds: Provide healthful fat, protein, and essential minerals.

Examples: Chia seeds, flax seeds, almonds.

Fatty Fish: Source of omega3 fatty acids.

Examples: Salmon, mackerel, sardines.

4. Add Herbs and Spices

Flavor Enhancement: Use herbs and spices to decorate flavor without brought calories or sodium.

Examples: Turmeric, ginger, garlic, basil.

Health Benefits: Many herbs and spices have anti inflammatory and antioxidant properties.

Examples: Cinnamon, rosemary, thyme.

5. Portion Control

Balanced Plates: Use the "plate technique" to balance quantities of veggies, proteins, and grains.

Half Plate: Vegetables and fruits.

Quarter Plate: Lean proteins.

Quarter Plate: Whole grains or starchy greens.

Avoid Overeating: Be aware of portion sizes to maintain calorie stability and avoid excessive consumption.

6. Meal Planning and Preparation

Plan Ahead: Create meal plans that encompass quite a few nutrient dense foods.

Example: A week's worth of breakfast, lunch, and dinner ideas.

Prep in Advance: Cook and put together food in batches to make wholesome eating greater convenient.

Examples: Prechop veggies, prepare dinner grains in bulk.

7. Incorporate Diverse Ingredients

Variety: Use numerous foods to make sure a large spectrum of vitamins.

Example: Combine specific types of veggies and proteins in a stir fry.

Experiment: Try new recipes and ingredients to keep food exciting and nutritious.

Examples: Add quinoa to salads, use cauliflower rice.

Example Nutrient Dense Meals

1. Breakfast:

Smoothie Bowl: Blend spinach, berries, banana, and Greek yogurt. Top with chia seeds and a handful of nuts.

2. Lunch:

Quinoa Salad: Mix cooked quinoa with chickpeas, cherry tomatoes, cucumbers, avocado, and a lemon tahini dressing.

3. Dinner:

Grilled Salmon: Serve with a aspect of roasted candy potatoes and steamed broccoli. Add a squeeze of lemon for taste.

4. Snack:

Apple Slices with Almond Butter: Provides a mix of healthy fats, protein, and fiber.

A Golden World

Lauren Working

A Golden World

*How the Americas
Transformed
Renaissance England*

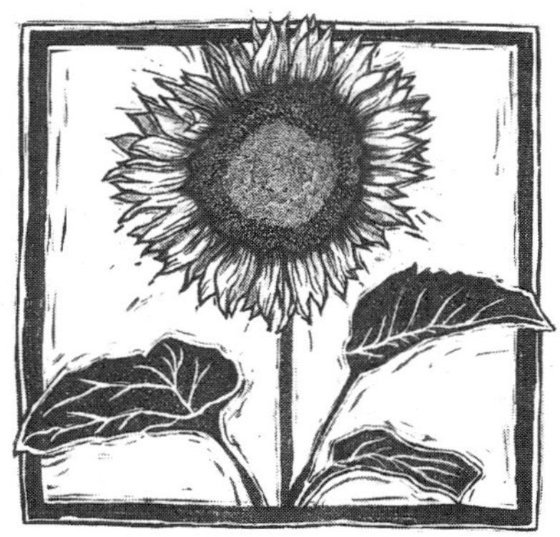

faber

In this book, original early modern spelling and punctuation have been retained, except to distinguish between 'u' and 'v', and 'i' and 'j' (for example, 'mvskrat' appears as 'muskrat'). Where a name is spelled multiple ways in the records (for example, 'Ralegh', 'Raleigh', 'Rawleigh'), its most recurrent form is used (with the exception of introducing readers to the more familiar 'Raleigh' spelling on the book jacket). The dates have been adjusted according to modern conventions, with a new year beginning on 1 January rather than 25 March.

First published in 2026
by Faber & Faber Limited
The Bindery, 51 Hatton Garden
London EC1N 8HN

Typeset by Typo•glyphix, Burton-on-Trent, DE14 3HE
Printed and bound by CPI Group (UK) Ltd, Croydon, CR0 4YY

A CIP record for this book
is available from the British Library

ISBN 978–0–571–39383–1

Printed and bound in the UK on FSC® certified paper in line with our continuing commitment to ethical business practices, sustainability and the environment.
For further information see faber.co.uk/environmental-policy

Our authorised representative in the EU for product safety is
Easy Access System Europe, Mustamäe tee 50, 10621 Tallinn, Estonia
gpsr.requests@easproject.com

2 4 6 8 10 9 7 5 3 1

Golde is our fate,
Which all our actes doth fashion and create.
George Chapman, 'De Guiana' (1596)

We also occupied, reclaimed the Old World.
Glicéria Tupinambá (2023)

Contents

Prologue

Between Sunflower and Brushstroke

The flower lived as a blaze, bright and yellow like sustaining mother corn. Algonquian hands laid its seeds into the soil, cultivating the sunflower alongside squash, beans, and maize. Rain and rivers from the region's many waterways nourished it. The flower grew to be taller than humans. Marvelling at its height, one English observer compared the sunflower to a marigold that had reached outlandish proportions, its surface spanning the size of an outstretched hand. This plant, he wrote, turned its golden face to the sun, following its movements from east to west and back again.

In the early 1630s, a celebrated artist at the English court painted *Self-Portrait with a Sunflower*. The plant was far from any Indigenous environment: it appeared, radiant and rare, in a composition with Anthony van Dyck himself. The artist's right hand points to the flower, his finger barely grazing a curving petal. A gold chain, perhaps given to him by the king himself, wraps around his other hand. In the drama and fluidity of Van Dyck's brushstrokes, everything is connected. Cloud and shirtsleeve, chain and flower, all playing a part in this expression of baroque elegance. The gentleman's loyalty to the monarch, Charles I, is suggested by the devotion and fealty that sunflowers symbolised, ever turning towards the sun.

In the sixteenth and early seventeenth centuries, people, plants, animals, and artefacts from the Americas entered English art and literature for the first time. Transatlantic exchanges made it possible for an Antwerp-born artist in London to come face to face with an

American plant, first cultivated by peoples living thousands of miles away. Yet traditional approaches to a painting like Van Dyck's *Self-Portrait with a Sunflower* position the fashionable Cavalier figure as the sole protagonist. We are less likely to place the sunflower, and its life in Algonquian or Nahua homelands, within English history.

For a long time, treasure ships and the feats of flamboyant privateers have held centre stage in stories of the Renaissance, even as other travels and details lie in plain sight, like the sunflower in Van Dyck's composition. The dominant way of thinking about transatlantic travel has focused on the English going out and leaving their mark on the world, not the Americas coming in. Entire stories – about the earliest beginnings of English territorial expansion to other continents, and Indigenous presences and resistance to the imperial project – have been left out.

Yet, at every turn, Indigenous labour and expertise are there when we look for them. Copper-gold alloy figures made by Arawakan metallurgists came to sit on English tables, carried in the same cargoes as glimmering bars of silver looted from Spanish treasure ships. Barrels of crushed insects from Central America, gathered by workers in striped cottons, furnished the English with a dye that saturated the velvet curtains of a king's bedchamber. In herbals and travel books, sunflowers often accompanied other American flora, such as evergreen cacao, prickly pear cactuses, and tobacco. These plants connected readers to communities who lived on Caribbean shorelines, or carved canoes from trees in northern woodlands.

A Golden World is a story of why materials and artefacts from the Americas matter to English history. It is an invitation to look for woven macaw feathers and the fruits of plantation industries in so much of what seems to define the golden age of the Tudors and Stuarts. Although colonialism, Indigenous knowledge, and English culture have often been viewed separately, bringing them together can transform the way we understand the art and politics of Shakespeare's day. Travelling objects help to illuminate the contributions of Andean miners and goldsmiths, African pearl divers, and Algonquian cultivators to the Renaissance as we know it.

A flower grows taller than humans, capturing the admiration of a painter. But the story of its migrations is wilder and darker than any artist's fancy.

Introduction

From Golden Age to Golden World

In 1595, the Virgin Queen received at court an Indigenous prince from South America. His bow and arrows hung over one shoulder, possibly decorated with the jewel-toned feathers of tropical birds. An accompanying interpreter informed the court that this 'Indian youth' – hailing from 'what those in Europe call the West Indies, and near the fountain of the Amazon' – desired nothing more than to meet the world-renowned monarch, Elizabeth I. Admiration for the queen, the prince assured her, extended across the Atlantic.

Such a traveller may have been accustomed to sailing on a raft, made from trunks of the balsa tree, or in a canoe made from hollowed-out wood. Although he had entered into the dazzling heart of the Tudor court, appearing in the company of courtiers in lustrous brocade, he lived by senses other than sight. As the interpreter informed Elizabeth, the prince was blind, undertaking the arduous voyage out of his belief in an ancient prophecy:

> *Seated between the old world and the new,*
> *A land there is no other land may touch,*
> *Where reigns a Queen of peace and honour true;*
> *Stories or fables do describe no such.*

The oracle had foretold that an alliance with a powerful nation from across the seas would restore the prince's sight and help his father to overthrow the Spanish conquistadors who had invaded his territories. The queen, after all, had calmed her own warlike nation of knights, creating a peaceful land that had entered a golden age through the flourishing of literature: 'No age hath ever wit refined so far.' And so the prince had crossed the Atlantic to find this famed island that sat between Europe and America, pendent like a jewel, hoping to see the prophecy fulfilled.

Or so the story went. Little is known about this performance – found in a short, page-long script, and sponsored by the queen's favourite, the Earl of Essex – but there is a good chance it was enacted for Elizabeth as a post-supper entertainment in late 1595, months after the courtier Walter Ralegh had returned from his first voyage to Guiana, the land of many waters, in what is now Venezuela and Guyana. Perhaps Ralegh returned from an entertainment like this one, tipsy from spiced wine, and worked on the manuscript that would become *The Discoverie of the Large, Rich, and Bewtiful Empyre of Guiana*, printed in 1596. All the dreams that animate Ralegh's *Discoverie* are there in the play: breaking Spanish strongholds in America; alliances with Indigenous rulers, facilitated by their deference to English power; and depictions of the queen as the magnetic force behind these alliances, binding white European and Indigenous Americans together through her love and grace. Ralegh may even have played the character himself, bursting into the hall as the prince, desperate for Elizabeth's favour. The whole performance was characteristic of the Elizabethans' love of layered conceits and cryptic wordplay. Blindness, arrows, a speech professing ardent devotion – Ralegh may have been playing an Arawakan, but he was also Cupid, scrambling back to the embrace of the goddess of love.

Ralegh's long obsession with South America – he would return over twenty years later, in 1617 – tends to be remembered as a mark of his eccentricity. Because his character is so extravagant, the colonial ideas that underpinned his voyaging can also seem out of the ordinary. Few wealthy Elizabethans, after all, were willing to sell parts of their estates to conduct risky journeys to Indigenous lands. Ralegh's gold fever, however, was shared by many of his contemporaries. Martin Frobisher's mid-1570s voyages to the North Atlantic in search of a north-west passage to China fuelled English hopes of 'discovering' large stores of wealth across the ocean, gripping politicians, poets, and travellers alike. The humanist statesman Thomas More had used gold and transatlantic travel to satirise Tudor greed in *Utopia* (1516), his scathing denunciation of princely wealth; but Protestant courtiers in the reign of Elizabeth would have viewed More's stance as somewhat old-fashioned. 'Golde is our Fate,' the poet George Chapman wrote in his endorsement of Ralegh's 1595 voyage, 'Which all our actes doth fashion and create.'[2]

The art and literature of Shakespeare's time are rich with allusions to the promise and emptiness of precious metals. References to gold and silver glistened in the phrases of inky manuscripts and in the margins of printed books. Since these metals came from deep in the ground, writers spoke of them either as natural bounty (the earth as a womb, yielding parts of herself for the advancement of humankind) or as plunder, involving ruthless exploitation and extraction. Aesthetically, gold signalled beauty, even divinity. Poets compared their mistresses' tresses to spun gold, and golden light to spiritual truth. Alchemists conducted feverish investigations into how base matter might be transmuted into fine metal. These projects were endlessly parodied, but humanists considered alchemy to be an art and a science, one that could be harnessed in service of the commonwealth. For every sermon against the corrosive effects of gold, there were fervent defences of its importance, even necessity, in maintaining social relations and national security. The surge of innovation, whether in metalwork or literary technique, has contributed to our own enduring sense of the Tudors as inhabiting a golden age marked by unprecedented style – the 'high astounding terms' of Christopher Marlowe's thundering plays, the glitter of jewels pinned onto velvet. But, even in Elizabethan times, metaphors about glittering cultural accomplishment mingled with discussions of wealth and capital.

When Elizabethan poets and statesmen wrote about precious metals, America was never far away. Reports on silver and gold mines proliferated in accounts about Florida and Peru. A visitor to one of London's print shops could emerge clutching poetry collections or devotional treatises, but also books about the silver veins running through the mining town of Potosí in the Viceroyalty of Peru (in present-day Bolivia). Poems hailed Francis Drake as England's Ulysses, a hero whose journeys in the Americas to intercept Spanish silver distribution surpassed the adventures in Homer's *Odyssey*. Early colonial projects in North America were equally driven by hopes for mineral wealth. In 1606, the poet Michael Drayton penned an ode to English colonisation in Virginia, where pearls and gold would entice voyagers as much as honour and fame.

In Tudor and Stuart literature, the 'Indias of spice and mine' located spices in Asia and metals in the Americas. In reality, the circulation of goods was a vast global affair. Ancient trade routes and new Atlantic passages brought an array of commodities to England through a series of interrelated networks of traffic and exchange. For centuries, Portuguese merchants had circulated gold from Africa, and Venetian traders carried gold alongside spices, silk, and furs across the Ottoman Empire and to the Black Sea. There were already long-established mines in the Harz mountains of Germany. In 1606, a vein of silver found in Scotland brought a flurry of experienced miners to West Lothian from Cornwall and Germany. Yet the sheer amount of silver found in Potosí following the Spanish invasion and occupation of South America was unprecedented. Though trade networks connected Europe and the Americas to regions in the Indian and Pacific oceans, such as West Africa and Japan, the flow of silver from South America profoundly changed the English imagination. Metaphors of spice-rich India and golden America influenced one author, then another, until they became convention. 'The West sends gold,' the poet John Donne wrote, the 'East sends hither her deliciousness.'[3]

Literary fancies aside, England had a cash problem. Costly wars in Ireland and Continental Europe led Tudor monarchs to seek new sources of revenue. Henry VIII sanctioned a drop in gold and silver standards, allowing sterling silver to be mixed with increasing amounts of copper. The purity of coins plummeted, significantly depreciating English currency. England's primary export, wool, dominated other trades and made merchants and landowners wealthy, but conflict and economic dearth, at home and abroad, could disrupt the trade. As the population increased, authorities looked to diversify the economy through a range of smaller-scale industries, which allowed poorer members of society to sustain their families while producing regionally specific manufactures and wares. In the midst of this, the bullion from Spanish treasure ships captured in Elizabeth's reign presented at least a temporary solution to economic pressures. Silver from Mexico and Peru was melted and stamped in London's Royal Mint. It appeared, too, in the form of glistening objects that were used for sacred and secular expressions of magnificence and virtue. Bars of silver became an important asset for the fledgling East India Company, enabling it to trade in silver for highly coveted manufactures, such as calicoes and silks.

When seeking to endorse a plantation in North America in the mid-1580s, the poet Philip Sidney appealed less to religion or honour than to courtiers' desire for precious metals. The very word *gold*, a close friend wrote of Sidney's preparations, was generally enough 'to make men venture that which they have, in hope to grow rich by that which they have not'.[4] In 1577, before he became known as one of the most prominent and beloved poets of his age, the young Sidney had written an enthusiastic letter to his mentor about the privateer Martin Frobisher. Sidney recounted that a crew member had picked up a piece of glittering rock on Frobisher's voyage to the northern part of North America, near Greenland. Frobisher had initially dismissed the object, believing the crew to be too far north to find gold. After further investigation, Frobisher had brought significant amounts of the ore to London for testing. 'The ore shows sure signs', Sidney pressed, 'that the island is so metal-rich as far to surpass the regions of Peru.'[5]

Sidney's mentor, the French Protestant reformer and diplomat Hubert Languet, wrote a lengthy and stern reply to his protege. Gold could dangerously entice, he wrote, leading the covetous follower to mortal peril. Quoting the classical Roman poet Virgil, Languet warned Sidney that 'hunger for gold will creep into your soul'.[6] Sidney's ardour risked individual corruption, but it had wider implications, too, binding the poet's desire to the foolhardy fate of a whole nation. Languet's warning rings like a prophecy: 'I am very much afraid that England, seduced by desire for gold, will throw itself upon those islands recently discovered by Frobisher.'[7] Eight years and a spirited treatise on poetry later, Sidney attempted to join Drake on his voyage to the West Indies, but his plans were foiled by Elizabeth, who ordered her brash courtier back to Whitehall.

As Languet insinuated, this desire for gold actually ran *against* Renaissance notions of the Golden Age. In Greek mythology, the Golden Age was celebrated as a time of natural abundance, harmony, and peace. The wise councillor Gonzalo looks for precisely this idyll when he is washed onto the unnamed island in Shakespeare's *The Tempest* (1611). When he dreams of 'plantation of this isle', his vision of the land is influenced by classical pastoral, where its inhabitants live in a state of innocence and plenty.[8] There is no 'use of metal', no need for trade, extraction, or political mechanisms of control such as magistrates or monarchical power, for the earth yields what is necessary and delightful. Gonzalo rejects industry and extraction – the very things colonialism depended on to maximise its profits – in favour of living off the land, never taking more than needed. This vision stood in stark contrast to the rising figure of the 'projector', a Jacobean schemer alternately portrayed as a ruthless opportunist or eccentric dreamer, ever in search of 'farfetched constructions' and plans 'to enrich men, or to make them great'.[9]

Even those merchants who encouraged trade acknowledged that the violence and greed underpinning colonial ventures ran counter to pastoral perfection. 'The Golden Age, so much celebrated by ancient Writers,' the merchant Walter Hamond wrote, 'was not so called, from the Estimation or predomination that Gold had in the Heart of men . . . But from the Contempt thereof, so that we must needs confesse that it had beene happy for us, if Gold had never beene knowne.'[10] Nestled in a rather extravagant 1616 poem against tobacco is a pointed, if brief, condemnation of colonial desire. We must question, Samuel Daniel wrote, 'Whether Discoverie of *America*, / That *New-found World*, have yielded to our Ould / More Hurt or Good'. It would have been better, he concluded, 'that onely Good men to their Coast had come, / Or, that the Evill had still staid at home'.[11]

In *Metamorphoses*, a text that influenced countless poems and paintings in the Renaissance, the Roman poet Ovid chronicled just how far humankind had fallen from its golden beginnings. Humans now lived in the brutal age of iron. New technologies and arts, including navigation, warfare, and mining, had rendered Europeans so rapacious and conflict-ridden that they had imperilled the human race and broken their harmonious relationship with the land. 'I think that more properly this age should be called the golden world,' one Jacobean civil servant wrote, 'because gold bears so much sway. The former age was called the golden world of innocence . . . [but we] enter even into the bowels of the earth and go hunting after riches even to the place of the damned.'[12] Far from containing any of the values of the Golden Age, this golden world was an idolatrous one. It wasn't paradise, but hell. Worse – to go scavenging after riches was to damn *others*, sending them into the depths of the earth to produce a bit of silver for the dining table.

Footsteps and Floating Cities

And yet they went. Monarchs signed charters with a flourish. Trading companies gathered the necessary capital to send ships and agents across seas. Elite and merchant women donated money to fund ships, provisions, and schools. Sailors from many parts of the world enlisted or were pressed into service. The English were adamant that their methods of colonisation differed from those of their Catholic rivals, the Spanish and Portuguese. The warlike conquistadors, Protestant writers insisted, had enriched themselves through immense cruelty and bloodshed. You couldn't walk through the streets of Seville or Lisbon, with their new cathedrals and glittering altarpieces, without thinking about the tyranny of the Iberian Empire and its baroque efflorescence. Meanwhile, Protestant patrons and projectors commissioned translations of Spanish intelligence about the Americas, relying on the geopolitical material it contained, and downplayed the atrocities that their own countrymen were currently unleashing against the Gaelic Irish under the banner of English civility. Prominent government officials received pensions from the King of Spain for their diplomatic services, so that those Iberian luxuries so criticised in Elizabethan polemic nevertheless made their way into English stately homes.

As calling it the New World suggests, there was something about the unfamiliarity of the Americas that excited Europeans of the time, even when the Americas were not, of course, new at all. Colonialism is marked by encounter, not discovery.[13] In *The Tempest*, Prospero reminds his daughter Miranda that her 'brave new world' was merely 'new to thee.'[14] Yet the fact that the Greeks and Romans, so revered by humanists, had remained ignorant of what Europeans called the fourth part of the world stirred the writing of the time with a sense of urgency and opportunism. The establishment of the new Tudor dynasty in 1485, and Henry VIII's decision to break with Rome and declare himself head of Church and state in 1534, had fuelled English nationalism and sparked Atlantic competition. By the 1580s, the courtier Fulke Greville later recalled, there was no 'greater possibility of improving merit, wealth, & friends' than through Atlantic involvement.[15]

Many English proponents of colonialism viewed Atlantic plantation as a part of a larger whole, integral to their hopes of building a Protestant empire that would enable them to reach the dizzying wealth held by eastern powers. In visual culture and dramatic performance, America was often personified as the young newcomer in the company of Europe, Asia, and Africa. For centuries, the English had met with Jewish communities and Muslim rulers through intellectual exchange, trade, and war. They wrote of the sumptuous silks and calicoes to be acquired by trade with Mughal India, expressed awe at the military strength of the Ottomans, and scribbled chronicles and histories of eastern rulers and diverse religious communities. Tales of captured English sailors serving as galley slaves in the Mediterranean – or, worse, of rogue English pirates 'turning Turk' and converting to Islam – were printed in London and adapted into stage productions. One of the diplomatic consequences of the Reformation was that direct alliances with Muslim powers, always prohibited by the Catholic Church, suddenly lay open to English rulers, who began sending ambassadors and merchants to the Ottoman, Mughal, and Persian Safavid courts.[16] As merchants established trades with the West Coast of Africa, restless fortune-seekers, like Anthony Shirley and his brothers Robert and Thomas, travelled to Persia and became embroiled in diplomatic affairs that stretched across continents. In 1600, a North African ambassador, Abd al-Wahid bin Mas'ud bin Mohammed Anun, resided in London and gained an audience with Queen Elizabeth.

As cartographers produced new atlases awash in the greens and blues of unfamiliar landmasses and waterways, the 'Occidental Indies' began to upend old balances of power. The Americas were incorporated into European fantasies and worldviews while simultaneously forcing a drastic recalibration of global relations. The East India Company was established in 1600, but it was still in its infancy in the final years of Queen Elizabeth's reign (1558–1603), and even into the reign of James VI and I (1603–1625). The Company conducted regular journeys to Asia but had not yet grown into the powerful merchant corporation and military entity it would later become. The search for deposits of precious metals to enable global trade became the prime motivation for Atlantic voyaging and the development of English colonial projects. Failed settlements in Guiana, in Roanoke (an island off the coast of North Carolina), and in Sagadahoc (Maine) paved the way for longer-term colonial settlements in the Chesapeake (Virginia and Maryland), Newfoundland, Bermuda, New England, and parts of the Caribbean, all by the 1630s.

The successful establishments of colonial settlements in Ireland and the Americas, starting with Jamestown in 1607, made land acquisition and territorial occupation – settler colonialism – a part of English statecraft, endorsed by the Crown but initially managed by joint-stock companies. Atlantic joint-stock companies followed in the wake of the East India Company's beginnings, their councils governed by many of the same merchants and financiers. The formation of the Virginia Company/Plymouth Company (1606), the Somers Isles/Bermuda Company (1615), the short-lived Amazon Company (1619), and the Massachusetts Bay Company (1628) made council chambers and private homes in London arenas for lively debate and fierce disagreements about colonial governance and control.

Jamestown's founding came only four years after the Scottish King James VI became James I of England. This incorporated the Atlantic world and American colonies into the history of what James called 'Great Britain' from its very beginnings. Since James liked to draw comparisons between himself and Phoebus/Apollo, god of light and the sun, subjects wrote celebratory poems that likened the king's authority to the light-giving blaze of refined metals, reflecting his majesty onto his subjects even as he enriched and expanded his dominions into the Atlantic.

Even before they colonised parts of North America, the English had encountered empires in the Americas – just not their own. They collected Aztec/Mexica codices that recounted expansive Mesoamerican polities and their tribute systems. They sought inroads into Peru, on the hunt for Incan riches they believed to be hidden in tropical forests. They met with Arawak- and Carib-speaking groups, such as the Lokono and Kalina in Guiana, who told them about their political histories and ways of life. English travellers also witnessed life in and beyond the colonial towns and plantations of the Iberian Empire. One Elizabethan sailor laboured in a sugar mill in Brazil and learned Tupi dialects; another worked in Central American silver mines. An English priest taught Latin in a convent school in Mexico. In their raids on Spanish treasure ships and in their service under European patrons and masters, these travellers moved through multicultural settlements. They worked alongside Indigenous and African craftspeople, some marrying African-descended people. It was to trade with Iberian merchants and colonial administrators in South America and the Caribbean that the English undertook their first slaving voyages to the West Coast of Africa under John Hawkins and his cousin Francis Drake in the 1560s.

For much of the Elizabethan era, English politicians were content with intercepting Spanish and Portuguese bullion from the Americas to fill their coffers at home. But as James I pursued peace with Spain and settler-colonial projects in North America took off, councillors, merchants, and planters found a need for a steady workforce. Settlers and colonial administrators soon relied on African as well as indentured European labour. By the 1610s, first in Bermuda and then Virginia, colonial patrons such as Robert Rich, second Earl of Warwick, sent African people to English colonies, recognising and relying on their knowledge of botany and pearl diving. As demand for plantation goods grew, so did the need for labour, leading the English to incorporate Africans and enslaved labour more concertedly into their colonial designs as the seventeenth century progressed. Long before the legal codification of slavery in the 1660s, ideas about skin colour and blackness framed moral judgements about the worth and nature of other peoples and bodies.[17] Even as blackness became increasingly racialised, African and African-descended individuals in England lived diverse lives as artisans, navigators, divers, diplomats, and servants. A number of them, such as those captured by English pirates, or those living in the households of Iberian merchants, had been enslaved in the Americas before making another voyage back across the Atlantic.

How did these conditions and environments influence the lives of those who never travelled beyond England's shores? For a long time, the assumption was that they didn't – that a history of colonialism was a history of other places. In a 1594 performance at the Inns of Court, young lawyers and law students imagined their navy extending like a 'huge floating City', serving to 'eternize your Name, and leave deep Foot-steps of your Power in the World'.[18] In many ways, their fantasy succeeded. The stories of those who sought to leave deep footsteps in the world – privateers such as Frobisher and Drake, or hardy military men such as John Smith – are endlessly retold. Colonialism is an elsewhere, happening in swamplands and so-called wildernesses, conveniently disconnected from royal castles or parliamentary debates. The inhabitants of the Americas remain on the margins of domestic history, deemed irrelevant to English life. But those huge floating cities remind us that the paths we can follow into the past are cut with endless migrations and uprootings, and the footsteps of many.

Hurricanes on the Thames

Taking objects as its starting point, *A Golden World* traces the tangible imprints that Indigenous peoples across the Americas made on Tudor and Stuart society through the things Londoners wore, consumed, and collected. Travelling objects can upend old assumptions about the one-way influence of transatlantic encounters. They remind us that, even as the English drew lines on a map and claimed to export their civil ideas to the 'savage' parts of the world, a steady flow of people, flora, fauna, and artefacts from the Americas was also coming *in*, engendering all kinds of small- and large-scale transformations. There were macaws and kayaks in mansions on the Thames. People of all social classes smoked tobacco cultivated in the West Indies, or stored the plants in kitchens to make infusions for the relief of bodily afflictions. One colonist in New England wrote about the premium that

London tobacco sellers placed on the green and black stone pipes and moulds made by the Wampanoag people, 'much desired . . . for their rarity, strength, handsomenesse, and coolnesse'.[19] Indigenous words appear in unexpected places, including a speech in *King Lear*. When the raging king welcomes an impending storm, he calls for 'hurricanoes, [to] spout / Till you have drench't our steeples'.[20] 'Hurricane' (*hurakan*) is a Taíno loanword, which the English could read about in translations of Spanish colonial accounts – a tantalising hint at the kind of knowledge about the Americas that Shakespeare had at his disposal.

In this way, this book is a travel account in reverse. It is a guide that searches for Atlantic markers in a sprawling city that had become England's largest urban centre. London was a bustling, multilingual, fast-expanding port town. It was also a site of colonial encounters, both real and imagined. A small watercolour drawing of a feathered Algonquian man in fringed deerskin, standing in St James's Park, survives in the friendship book of a European traveller. By the 1610s, one writer advised that putting a picture of a 'Blackamoore, or a Virginia-man' in front of a tavern or tobacco shop would attract more customers than a traditional pub sign. Theatres, churches, and booksellers' stalls became gathering places to discuss 'your ships at Sea, / To bring you Gold and Stone from rich Peru'.[21] Sixteenth-century cucurbit (squash) seeds found at the Globe and Rose theatres suggest that audience members might have munched on a spiced pumpkin snack from the Americas while watching the plays of Marlowe and Shakespeare.

The chapters that follow cover roughly the first half-century of English colonial efforts in the Americas. They observe a loosely chronological order, starting with Frobisher's search for a north-west passage across the Atlantic from 1576, and ending with some of the plants and plantation industries that beguiled writers, artists, and

Puritan patrons in the 1620s and 1630s. There are forays into the lives of earlier Tudors, such as Henry VIII or Mary I, and into the fortunes of shipwrecked mariners. Within the book's broader arc of Tudor to Stuart, of small colonial outposts to large-scale plantations, each chapter follows its own micronarrative. There are circulations and returns, like a maze in a Renaissance garden, the objects steering us down history's hidden, criss-crossing paths. A mountain in Colombia leads to the court of Elizabeth I and then to a later queen's turtle-shaped clock, studded with emeralds to resemble a shell. A gleaming gold stage prop in Whitehall, designed by the celebrated architect Inigo Jones, leads to a Nauset man named Epanow reuniting with his kin.

Over the course of this half-century, English attitudes towards Indigenous material culture remained mixed. The opening chapters on Inuit sealskin or Mesoamerican codices give a sense of how Elizabethan travellers and colonial promoters reconciled their gold-and-silver fever with a curiosity, even admiration, for Indigenous ways of life. The focus on particular objects offers a way into the varying impressions, interests, and aims of those who handled them. In the uncertain moments of initial encounter, the English often operated from positions of weakness and vulnerability, seeking to gather firsthand knowledge about Native peoples while lacking a coherent strategy for achieving settlement. In the 1580s and 1590s, gentlemen travellers such as Walter Ralegh or the mathematician Thomas Hariot – hoping for an Anglo-Peruvian alliance against the Spanish, or for assistance from the Croatan against other groups in Roanoke – sought firsthand experience of Indigenous languages and political processes.

The English were at war with Spain in these last decades of the sixteenth century. Control of the Atlantic world was at stake, and they made use of the Black Legend to foster alliances with Indigenous nations against this common enemy. Lacking any military or political power in the Americas, Elizabethan courtiers and patrons focused on the diplomatic language of friendship and love, set against the atrocities of Spanish violence and Catholic dominion. This propagated a particular aesthetic about Indigenous peoples and environments in and around the Tudor court. Watercolour drawings of flying fish and cobs of maize circulated alongside the exquisite miniatures characteristic of European court painting. Aspirations for alliances with Native groups help to make sense of that entertainment staged for Elizabeth in 1595, where an Amazonian prince became a manifestation of Cupid, personifying love. Displayed with tapestries and paintings of classical myths were portraits of an Inuk man or an Algonquian spiritual healer – images of individuals that gave no indication of the trail of destruction and disruption that the English often left in their wake.

As the English began to form colonial settlements in the early seventeenth century, travellers, politicians, and propagandists found themselves in a bind. Exhibiting too much admiration for the cultures of the Americas risked undoing a colonial project that hinged on the supposed need to 'civilise' and convert others. As their colonial projects grew more ambitious, undergirded by escalating conflict with European states and Native nations (including the First Anglo-Powhatan War of 1609–14, attacks against the Kalinago in St Kitts in the 1620s, and the Pequot War of 1636–8), English attitudes towards Indigenous groups, resources, and belongings began to change. Acknowledging Indigenous sovereignty became less beneficial as hopes receded of finding stores of gold guarded by potential regional allies, and an attention to settlement and industry took hold. A 1623 publication urged the king to 'possess as much as you can of those Heathen Countries', not only to propagate Protestantism but to affix 'a golden world to the Crowne of England', enriching the state 'by the Indian treasures'.

Land – 'that huge tract [north of Florida], whose infinitenesse is such, as no mortall tongue can expresse' – would grant the English 'free accesse to the *Indies*, either to traffique or plant'.[22]

Lustrous materials and beautifully made artefacts from the Americas were used to project status and sophistication – not by identifying with Indigenous value systems or expertise, but by showcasing English people's access to, and involvement in, colonial affairs. Rare pieces of Native handiwork, such as featherwork or deerskin garments decorated with shells or porcupine quills, retained their connection to the Americas as a form of exoticism or wonder; or were given new associations. They might be repurposed in theatrical performances, or kept by godly women and men as material reminders of God's call to convert the nations of the earth. Pearls, dyes, tropical fruits, and even live animals began to be seen as evidence of English imperial successes, over both Indigenous peoples and European rivals.

Alongside a host of travellers, agents, projectors, and poets, *A Golden World* features a range of recurring players. Wealthy patrons, who had the means to sign charters, commission portraits, and consolidate overseas interests in the halls of political power, are vital to understanding how colonialism became a matter of high politics and culture in the Renaissance, especially Elizabeth I; James I and his wife, Anna of Denmark; and Charles and Henrietta Maria, his French queen. Courtiers and favourites, such as Ralegh, or George Villiers, Duke of Buckingham, served as important taste-makers through their involvement in Atlantic affairs. There is the wit, and compassion, of the poet John Donne, who used metaphors of gold mines in his love poetry and who features as the interlocutor in a modern Caribbean poet's verses about plantation slavery. Van Dyck's splashy paintings helped to create a recognisable Stuart aesthetic for royals and aristocrats in this burgeoning imperial moment. Then there are the many Indigenous peoples whom the English met as the result of their schemes and projects, particularly Arawak and Kalinago groups in South America and the Caribbean; the Tupi peoples of Brazil; and many Algonquian nations along the north-eastern coast of Turtle Island, or in North America, from the Powhatan to the Wampanoag. Beaver, maize, and sunflower are protagonists, too. They appear in ink and daubs of paint, climbing the scrolls of Renaissance drawings and bookplates. They serve as guides through the gilded world of projectors and patrons who both relied on Native peoples' offerings and denied them agency.

Although early English colonialism is often associated with 'Virginia' – lands that stretched from the Carolina Outer Banks to what would become New England – South America and the greater Caribbean gripped the imagination of many travellers, merchants, and politicians. The inclusion of places such as Florida, Brazil, and Providence Island in this book are a powerful reminder of this tropical dream. Silver and parrot or hummingbird feathers beguiled Tudors long before Chesapeake tobacco. Later, the Caribbean sugar boom, which began in the mid-seventeenth century on islands including Jamaica and Barbados, would become a major catalyst for making England a slave society. The schemes of early Stuart privateers, merchants, and aristocratic patrons helped set a presence and a precedent.

By the time of Charles I's rule (1625–49), a Catholic colony in Maryland and a Puritan settlement off the coast of Central America both played important roles in supplying English people's demand for American goods. The hope for gold mines, so prevalent in Elizabethan and Jacobean writings about empire, began to be replaced by a focus on industrious planting. Merchants wrote economic treatises that outlined the shortcomings of large-scale metal extraction, using Spain as an example of how relying on silver hampered diversification, causing eventual decline. Still, golden fancies lingered. When sending guavas, cinnamon bark, and a cactus to his son in 1631, the Barbados colonist Henry Colt affixed a hasty note next to his signature: 'You shall heer shortly of a mine of gold at St Christophers. I pray God it be soe.'[23]

Objects and Islands of Living Memories

Tudor and Stuart history is preserved in all kinds of writing – court documents, diaries and letters, inventories, travel books, plays, merchants' ledgers, and parish records. What does this history look like when Indigenous voices are brought in alongside them? When beavers, featherwork, and emeralds become sources, and Indigenous storytellers are also their interpreters? The troves of shipwrecked colonial-era emeralds found on the ocean floor are, as Indigenous groups in Colombia and Bolivia have maintained, like little islands, preserving histories in the fragments of the past.[24] A gemstone might be offered as a Tudor love token, or spark a poetic reflection on the transience of worldly goods, but it also holds ancestral memories for the people it was taken from.

Why do these multiple perspectives matter? One reason is simply because the golden world of early modern London cannot be disentangled from English projects in the Americas. The transatlantic encounters sparked by colonialism make Indigenous peoples and lands a part of the development of English culture. Ignoring this perpetuates the centuries-old 'logic of elimination, [of] effacing and erasing Indigenous experience.'[25] There are elements of traditional, tribally protected knowledge that non-Indigenous people cannot, and should not, access; but these limitations are different from the purposeful occlusion or misrepresentation of Indigenous peoples that accompanied the development of empire over the centuries.

The colonial project was, in its very nature, about exporting English civil society abroad, not welcoming Indigenous ways of life at home. Citing – not speaking *for* – Indigenous communities serves to build their knowledge and ways of seeing into histories of encounter.[26]

Even with the generosity of Indigenous knowledge-holders who have shared details of their societies and beliefs with outsiders, significant challenges stand in the way of recovering Indigenous presences and influences in Elizabethan England.[27] Much of this goes back to those state documents, and to how colonial encounters were recorded and preserved. Indigenous copper-and-gold alloys from South America were categorised as 'idols' by Protestant authorities. Sometimes, they were melted down to test the purity of their metals, the anthropomorphic shapes disappearing in a surge of hot liquid. Often, Black and Indigenous sailors, servants, and go-betweens were rechristened, or remain unnamed in the colonial record. In 1605, the shipwrecked English on the Caribbean island of St Lucia relied on the help of an 'Indian Captaine called *Anthonie*', his name likely given to him by his former enslavers, the Spanish. We don't know the name of the African man who died of a caiman attack when travelling with Ralegh to the Amazon in the mid-1590s. The life of this 'very proper yo[u]ng fellow' is recorded only for his sensational death.[28]

With women, the silences can be greater still. Tracing the lives of Indigenous, African, and African-descended women who came to England from across the Atlantic in the wake of enslavement and territorial warfare brings its own limitations and frustrations. Writing with and against archival documents, drawing multiple sources together, can produce a wide portfolio of information to help piece fragments together. But a paucity of evidence remains a real challenge for studying women, and women of colour in particular.[29] Karenne Wood (Monacan) expressed frustration at the way that colonial archives force Indigenous women into certain representations, trapping them in stereotypes because so little of their lives can be recovered. The 'mainstream stories of our people are deeply flawed but [we are] unable to find more authentic accounts, usually because American Indians remain voiceless or were deliberately silenced'.[30] Since, Wood writes, there is slightly more evidence about the life of a woman such as Matoaka, also known as Pocahontas, she comes to represent or stand in for a whole spectrum of Indigenous women.

In the midst of these silences in English writings, artefacts are important archival fragments. Given the near-total erasure of Native peoples from English history – and working against the 'logic of elimination' – tracing kayaks or Mexica mirrors in Renaissance shops and libraries can be a way of acknowledging Indigenous presences in Tudor and Stuart life. Though widely described in English sources, these belongings also contain lives, codes, and meanings of their own. In the mid-seventeenth century, an Englishwoman named Virginia Ferrar received an Algonquian basket and an assortment of terracotta tobacco pipes, along with pearls, roots, animal skins, and a live turtle from North America. Virginia came from a family of merchants; her father had named her after those lands Matoaka came from, and she may have viewed these gifts as evidence of the beauty and fertility of a region she had taken a personal interest in. But the basket and pipes that travelled from the Chesapeake to Cambridgeshire are also evidence of Algonquian expertise in England. We cannot know the name of the basket's maker, but it brings the knowledge and labour of Native women into England through birchbark, husks, and sweetgrasses.

Such artefacts – or cultural belongings, a term that moves away from considering materials as inactive forces – embody what the Anishinaabe writer Gerald Vizenor calls 'survivance', a term that conveys 'an active sense of presence, [and] the continuance of Native stories'.[31] These stories renounce victimisation and bring out the vitality and ongoing flourishing of Indigenous peoples. A turkey-feather mantle in a Renaissance cabinet is not an inert collector's item but a form of memory-keeping and power, holding narratives that can only be unlocked by tribal songs and the knowledge of community ancestors. Recognising this sheds light on sixteenth-century history and also makes clear that colonialism is not a thing of the past. Indigenous resistance to dispossession and exploitation, of land and resources, is ongoing.

When we begin to think about the makers and lands connected to travelling things, the material record becomes an entry point into entwined histories that are as much about Algonquian elders and weavers as Virginia Company merchants and their daughters. The resins in apothecary shops that smelled of lemons and jasmine flowers 'from *Carthagena*, by the Natives called *Tolu*', are evidence of Indigenous hands at work, the balsam safely transported into the realm in gourds according to Native practices. Seeds, as Megan Peiser (Choctaw) writes, are archives, living containers of Indigenous knowledge that hold stories, ancestral histories, and sacred covenants.[32]

During his long imprisonment in the Tower, Ralegh experimented with plants from the Americas, possibly with the assistance of two Indigenous men known as Harry and Leonard. Atlantic plants became ingredients in Ralegh's cordials and salves, mixed with elder-flower, thistle, rose, and copious amounts of sugar, before being packaged as 'Great Cordial' and 'Balsam of Guiana' and administered to friends and patrons. But the Indigenous knowledge that lay behind the uses of plants was still there. Later apothecaries recognised that some of the plant knowledge contained in Ralegh's cordial had been gleaned viva voce, in conversation, 'from the Inhabitants of the American Islands'.[33] Sometimes, Indigenous contributions are more visible in English writings than we might first imagine.

A different perspective can shift what we see in Tudor images, too. An Elizabethan engraving of figures wearing sealskin or caribou parkas looks different when we consider the Inuit women who made many of the garments that came to England from Nunavut in the Arctic Archipelago. Suddenly, this image is not just a piece of Renaissance mannerist art, but evidence of a confluence of European and Native style. *A Golden World* begins and ends with the Indigenous women who can bring new views of the Renaissance and how we remember it.

In 1622, John Donne lamented how quickly gentlemen rushed to a newly docked ship, not to ask 'how many *Indians* were converted to *Christ*', but to scramble to get their hands on Atlantic drugs and dyes.[34] While material connections encourage a greater attention to Native action and sovereignty, they equally invite considerations of how colonial extraction and wealth influenced European culture and politics.[35] The volume of transatlantic materials that entered England undercuts much of the lofty rhetoric that policy-makers adopted around the benefits of overseas intervention, or about the urgency of saving souls. In a line, Donne exposed the hypocrisy of those whose pious professions were just wind, fanning the sails of merchant cargoes. Again and again, the English professed that their golden world would be one of friendly, mutually beneficial exchange. But their yearning for objects – and, increasingly, for the lands they came from – exposed just how far their own ideas about ownership and possession stood in the way of these ambitions. As they set baroque pearls into jewellery and distilled syrups from tropical gums, many consumers failed to understand, much less value, the lives, skills, and environments that ignited their fantasies in the first place.

What if there were a way of relishing the gilded prose and exuberant drama of Renaissance culture *without* relegating the history of colonialism and the Indigenous presence to the shadows? What if bringing these together actually yielded something more rewarding, more compelling? Tracing cargoes of Atlantic pearls to Tudor portraits, or feathered headdresses to debauched Whitehall masques, is a tale of consumption and empire-making, but it is also an exercise in telling a different kind of history. For too long, the romance and daring associated with the English going out into Indigenous spaces has obscured so many other tales of migration and transfer. The sources in this book reveal that there is never just one way of telling a story. There are, as the seventeenth-century author Margaret Cavendish whimsically envisaged, many worlds in a single earring. The pendant dangling from your ear might contain flooding rivers and golden fancies, earthquakes and gardens, catastrophe and joy. Bringing together manuscripts and literature, paintings, clothing, flora and fauna, gemstones, and archaeological remains, *A Golden World* pieces together a view of the past where Muzo and Muisca emeralds, an Inuit mother and child in sealskin, and Algonquian words written and spoken in London are as much a part of Tudor and Stuart history as sonnets and timber-frame houses.

Sealskin Parkas and
a Yellow Jerkin

A blue line made from soot and seal oil, poked by a needle made of bone, marks the woman's face. Then there's the ink of the artist, who drew these lines somewhere in London. He has dotted Arnaq's chin and forehead with blue markings and bordered her face with a fur hood. A baby, known to us as Nutaaq, peers out from her *amauti,* a parka specially designed for a woman to carry, protect, feed, and bond with her infant. Some of her tattoos may have been inscribed onto her body to mark this baby's momentous entry into the world.

Blue is the colour of Arnaq's homelands. In the spring, on the *sinaaq,* or floe edge, chunks of melting ice break and spread towards the Arctic Sea. Narwhals, seals, and birds gather noisily at the shoreline. Clouds are reflected in the crystalline water, so that whales breaking the surface seem to be spinning in the sky. The turquoises and cobalts are more saturated, more immersive, than the most shimmering ultramarine draping a Madonna in a quattrocento painting. The Inuktitut word *upringaaq,* spring or early summer, translates into 'which is surprised – or surprising – at first', perhaps alluding to the thawing conditions of the landscape after three seasons of ice. In the Arctic environment of the North Atlantic, as one English traveller reported, the 'ayre is very subtile, piercing and searching'. Summer days were so long and full of light that members of the crew could read and write late into the evening without needing to light a candle.[1]

The seals who swam along the floe edge were central to Inuit life. Arnaq, an Inuk woman from the Qikiqtaaluk region of Nunavut in what is now Canada, grew up close to seals and their furs. They were used, with the skins of other animals, to make houses, kayaks, and clothing. The Arctic *amauti* was one of many garments crafted by women. The process of scraping, wetting, and rescraping seal and caribou skins was arduous work. After removing the tissues, the skin needed to be moistened, then scraped and gently stretched, to give the surface a refined texture. Afterwards, the skin was ready for sewing and decoration. Garments were carefully constructed to fit each individual. Timings were essential: to prevent damage or roughness, every step had to be completed when the skins were in just the right condition. Once they were made, clothes needed to be carefully maintained and kept free of dampness to prevent decay and brittleness. The skin of baby seals worked well for slippers, but might be too fragile for outdoor boots. Around eight skins were needed to make a hunter's spring and summer parka and trousers. Multiple skins went into making boots and mitts.[2] Infants wore the soft skin of young animals captured and killed in the summers, when their furs were especially smooth and light.

Sealskin clothes were among some of the earliest known Indigenous cultural belongings to arrive in Tudor England. Between 1501 and 1502, three men from 'the Newe ffounde Ile land' arrived at Henry VII's court, dressed in 'beastes skinnes'. They had been 'brought' to the city, 'kept' by the king, words that suggest they had been taken by force. At least two of the men were spotted in Westminster Palace two years later, not in sealskin or caribou, but in English dress.[3] Nothing more is known of these three Native travellers, some of the first to arrive on English shores. Their brief years in London were to be much longer sojourns than those of the next known Arctic travellers, who arrived in England as the result of a sea captain's obsession with finding gold. In all these instances, Inuit parkas travelled to England on the bodies of captives.

Arnaq and her baby were two of the four known Inuit who were forcibly brought to London between 1576 and 1577, on the first and second voyages undertaken by the privateer Martin Frobisher to what would later be named Baffin Island. Although Frobisher travelled to the North Atlantic in search of a north-west passage to 'Cathay', or China, the most immediately lucrative aspect of his journey was the gold he believed he had found in the region. The voyage captivated the poet Philip Sidney, whose family had invested in the venture. In 1577, Sidney wrote about the rumours that Frobisher's 'ore shows sure signs that the island is so metal-rich as to far surpass the regions of Peru'.[4]

Frobisher's search for a new route to Asia, which quickly turned into a desperate hunt for gold, failed to reap the rewards he had hoped for. The English dug two mines on Kodlunarn Island. By Frobisher's third journey in 1578, it was becoming clear that the shiny, cubic crystals of black ore were worthless. All four captives, meanwhile, were brought to England under violent conditions and died within weeks of leaving their homelands.

What does the history of Frobisher's high-profile voyages look like if we put seals and seamstresses at its heart – materials and knowledge-carriers that have rarely been considered in accounts of his travels? Scraped seal fur, stitches of caribou and narwhal sinew, and the skilled hands of women lay behind much of the distinct visuals of Inuit craft and creativity that filtered into Renaissance art. The abilities and knowledge of these women are key to understanding a narrative that otherwise risks being dominated by the likes of Frobisher.

The short-lived ventures of the late 1570s brought a proliferation of artistic renderings depicting the captives and key patrons of the project. Paintings and drawings of the kidnapped Inuit were commissioned from skilled artists in the aftermath of Frobisher's first two voyages, circulating to various patrons and stakeholders including Queen Elizabeth herself. The drawings survive, but the paintings were lost, consumed in a late seventeenth-century fire that destroyed all of Tudor Whitehall and its treasures. From a series of over a dozen full-length images that had been made to commemorate the voyage, Frobisher's is the only portrait that survives. The Native subjects of these artworks died so soon after landing in England that Cornelis Ketel, the artist commissioned by the so-called (but never officially chartered) Cathay Company, might not even have painted them from life. Yet a desire to see and touch Inuit material culture persisted for decades. Beyond paint and paper, items like lustrous sealskin and translucent parkas and kayaks made from animal gut also travelled to English shores.

To stare at Frobisher is to stare down the barrel of a gun. One of the first things you notice when you look at Cornelis Ketel's large portrait of the privateer, now hanging in Oxford's Bodleian Library, is the polished wheel-lock pistol in his hand, poised to shoot. The other is the lustrous ochre yellow of his jerkin (a sleeveless jacket), breeches, and hose. He almost appears to radiate gold, as if illuminated by the imaginary treasure he so desperately sought. He is ready to do the dirty work of conquest. Along with the pistol in his right hand, his left wrist balances on the hilt of his sword. A bosun's whistle for calling attention hangs around his neck. The handle of a dagger just peeps from the back of his tailored waist, nudging the viewer towards the globe on the table behind him. But Frobisher is also presenting himself as a person of distinction. He wears the pleated, layered ruff fashionable among courtiers in the 1570s. There are matching cuffs, in addition to the frilled edging of his rippling sleeves – swathes of glossy fabrics that double back on themselves, making sure we know he can afford them in extravagance.

The portrait was commissioned in the aftermath of Frobisher's first voyage, when the privateer was keen to drum up support for his ventures. Frobisher's associate was the seasoned seafarer and merchant Michael Lok, the appointed Governor of the Cathay Company. Drawing on an extensive network of agents and wealthy patrons, Lok and Frobisher had secured a patent for two small ships, the *Gabriel* and *Michael*, to journey in search of an alternative route to Asia via the Atlantic. Finding the means of establishing trade directly with China, and with the Ottomans, Safavids, and Mughals, would allow the English to cut out their dependence on European merchants altogether, enabling them to access luxuries such as dyes and silks without competition, for unrivalled profit. Given this aim, pursuing the possibility of gold was a dangerous distraction. Within weeks of Frobisher's first arrival on Baffin Island in the summer of 1576, English relations with the Inuit had gone from guarded to violent. The mysterious disappearance of five members of the crew led to retaliation, and to the capture of the first Inuk man.

Frobisher's first voyage was hardly a raging success, but English interests were piqued. His portrait was a visual embodiment of the hopes and accolades that supporters lavished on the venture in print. In 1578, the chronicler George Best, who accompanied Frobisher on his second and third voyages, opened his account with a portrait of Frobisher in armour and a ruff, inscribed with a rather stilted celebratory poem that began: 'The noble flames that glowd in his stout brest / Could ne're be quencht.'

Frobisher's actions were connected to the glory of the nation as a whole. Best hoped that his discourse would showcase 'the great industrie of our present age, and the invincible mindes of our English nation, who have never lefte anye worthy thing unattempted, nor anye parte almoste of the whole world unsearched.'5 Echoing Sidney's hopes that the Arctic might be England's Peru, Best believed that the 'golde Ore in these new Discoveries' would make the North Atlantic what the South had been 'for the Spaniarde or Portingale'.[6]

The arrival of the Inuk man in England caused something of a sensation, according to Michael Lok, who reported that, when Frobisher and his crew arrived in London in the *Gabriel* in October 1576, they were 'joyfully received with the great Admiration of the People, bringing with them their strange man & his Bote, which was such a wonder unto th[e] whole City, & to the rest of the Realm that heard of it, as seemed never to have happened the like great matter to any mans knowledge'. News of his arrival spread quickly. In a letter dated 10 October 1576 – one day after Frobisher docked in London – one Thomas Wood sent a letter to a friend, offering him artichoke 'slips' or cuttings from his garden, some lemons, and a little map of the world. The letter ended with news that Frobisher had returned from his journey in search of Cathay, and that the crew had brought back 'a man of the Country', taken by force.[7] Somewhere in the countryside, the recipient of a letter from London might sit in their kitchen with some citrus fruits and artichoke scraps, reading the latest news about Frobisher's journey and the captive who had come into the realm as a result. This is how quickly large-scale colonial endeavours could be assimilated into the fabric of day-to-day life. English gardens and the North Atlantic came together in a folded piece of paper. Perhaps Wood's correspondent spread the world map in front of him, searching for the place of the Inuk man's origins.

Back in London, while Lok sent pieces of the black ore to assayers, Ketel was instructed to paint a pair of portraits of the Inuk man, one in his own fur garments and another in English apparel, in addition to a bust portrait of the man's head and shoulders. Each full-length portrait cost £5. This was a standard amount to charge for a portrait of a non-royal; but, taken together, the number of paintings commissioned by Company investors became a means of showcasing the prestige of their Arctic ventures. Along with the dozen or so paintings of key patrons and even Frobisher's ship, these hung as prominent displays, telling a story of cross-cultural encounter and English navigational power to all those who passed them. Ketel then produced copies of his paintings of the Inuk man to send to Elizabeth I. These were soon hanging in Hampton Court Palace, alongside sumptuous tapestries and royal treasures. Ketel would go on to paint Arnaq and Nutaaq for the collection, too.[8]

It's hard to hold these two things together, the capture and the paintings. Despite the immense curiosity that people showed towards the Inuk man, we don't even know his name. When he died in London only a few days later, records show that he had been terribly ill. Payments were made to an apothecary and servants to tend to him and change his bedding. The English prepared him for burial, and paid for a wax death mask to be made, 'to make his mould in pictur'.[9] Death masks were not uncommon for high-ranking Tudor individuals, including monarchs. Using wax to create a mould of a person's face could then form the basis for more accurate portraits of the recently deceased. The death mask suggests that Ketel's lifelike images of the Inuk man were carried out in the wake of his death.

When Frobisher set out on his second voyage to Baffin Island in 1577, he was backed by a number of prominent courtiers, including the queen and her eccentric astrologer, John Dee. The crew gathered samples from several islands in the region, and eventually settled on Kodlunarn Island, renamed Countess of Warwick Island. In addition to a large quantity of mined ore, the English returned with three new captives, and material belongings including a kayak. First, a man they called Kalicho. Shortly after, in a different attack, they captured Arnaq. A member of the crew shot at her, initially thinking she was a man. The bullet pierced her baby's arm. Once on board the ship, Arnaq refused the surgeon's salves, preferring to dress Nutaaq's wounds herself. It was there that she was first introduced to Kalicho. Having 'got a woman captive for the comforte of our man', the crew watched as the two gradually became accustomed to each other's presence. At first, they beheld each other 'withoute speeche or worde uttered, with greate change of coloure and countenance, as though it seemed, the greefe and disdeyne of their captivitie' had taken away their desire to speak. Over the course of the voyage, Kalicho and Arnaq seem to have become friends, singing and speaking together, 'so that (I thinke) the one would hardly have lived, without the comfort of the other'.[10]

When they arrived in Bristol, the Lord Mayor organised a reception, and Kalicho used his kayak to hunt ducks in the River Avon. Several years before, in 1574, Elizabeth had visited the city in the aftermath of a new Anglo-Spanish agreement that became known as the Treaty of Bristol. To commemorate the renewed trading opportunities between England and Spain, Bristol authorities had spent significant amounts of money preparing entertainments for the royal visit, and renovating public spaces to give them a bit more polish. The gates, schools, and churches that Elizabeth would encounter during her progress had been painted, plastered, and gilded. Although the speeches and mock battles were more ephemeral markers of the occasion, Kalicho and Arnaq might have passed the royal and civic coats of arms that had been constructed, which remained displayed outside the Guildhall.

In many ways, the Inuit found themselves in Bristol as an indirect result of this treaty, which had come at a time of escalating friction. Issues of international law, and possible war, were at stake. Drake and Hawkins had been raiding Spanish ships in the West Indies, and Philip II still sought retribution for an incident from 1568, when the queen and her ministers had seized five Spanish ships laden with gold in the English Channel. Having promised to stop attacking

Spanish treasure ships, the queen now sought to locate alternative sources of bullion. Frobisher's search for gold in the North Atlantic, far from Spanish-occupied waters, was an attempt to do just this. Baffin Island might be England's Peru; but, just as importantly, it was unclaimed by other European princes.

The Inuit were not in Bristol for long. Within a month, Kalicho was dead, possibly as a result of the broken ribs and other injuries he had sustained during his capture. Arnaq died a week later. Nutaaq did not survive long without his mother. Attempts were made to rush him to London to meet the queen, but he died within eight days. Elizabeth never saw the little Inuk whose arrival on English shores, far from the floe edge, had been so entangled with Anglo-Spanish diplomacy.

In the months that followed, various tests on the metals were carried out, yielding uncertain results and disagreements between the various assayers about the quality of the ore. With the captives dead and the ore sitting in the laboratories of metallurgists, Frobisher began preparations for his third journey, amassing a large fleet of fifteen ships to carry the ore he planned to bring back. The Arctic winter, with its heavy snowfall, storms, and icebergs, would begin in early autumn and could last eight or nine months; Frobisher only had a short window of time to excavate the metals he wanted. In the early autumn of 1578, he returned with vast quantities of mineral ore. In the end, none of it had any value. Investors never recovered their funds. The death of the four Inuit hung over the English enterprises. The people in the Arctic, Best reported, 'are nowe become so warye, and so circumspecte, by reason of their former losses, that by no means can we apprehend any of them.'[11]

Even as Frobisher's hopes for gold dissolved, artists in London and on the Continent continued to paint the Inuit in their parkas. Images in albums and costume books replicated individuals who were no longer there. Their portraits remained on display at Hampton Court. In 1599, some two decades after Frobisher's third voyage, the Swiss traveller Thomas Platter was delighted to receive a tour of the palace. In his diary, he described the inner apartments, full of tapestries so vivid that the figures in them seemed to come alive. In the very first room, Platter came face to face with the portraits of Kalicho, Arnaq, and Nutaaq. Even as he admired the lively qualities of the paintings, Platter knew the story of dispossession that lay behind them. They had, Platter noted, been captured by Frobisher during his voyage to America, and brought back to England alive.[12]

The full-length portraits of Kalicho and Arnaq in their own clothes were displayed prominently in the royal palace. They brought Arctic customs and fashions distinctly into view, perhaps fuelling ongoing interests in sealskin material culture. English captains were credited with bringing kayaks back to England, 'covered over with Seale skins artificially dressed' and stretched over 'little ribs of Timber'. For sixpence, visitors to the collector and botanist John Tradescant's 'Ark' in Lambeth could view the 'picture of an Indian with his Bow and Dart, taken . . . [in the year 15]76', and possibly also the original kayak of the first Inuk taken captive. Among other plant specimens and artefacts from around the globe, Tradescant had also acquired a crinkled gut parka (a 'match-coat from Greenland of the Intrails of Fishes') and fur boots, as well as 'shooes to walk on Snow without sinking'.[13]

Travellers who accompanied Frobisher on the search for a northwest passage, or Henry Hudson and James Hall in the early 1600s, expressed fascination with Inuit craft. Alongside natural marvels such as 'a kind of Horne which we doe suppose to be a Unicornes Horne' (likely narwhal) and a 'gr[e]at scull of Whales', the English repeatedly acknowledged and admired the labour and skill of Inuit clothing and kayak design. Sewn skins, fashioned into hooded parkas, as well as soft hose and pocket-like additions, were 'very softe and souple'. On Henry Hudson's voyage in 1610, sailors travelled through the region's icy waters, past snow-capped mountains that reminded onlookers of 'sugar-loaves'. Here, local craftspeople hunted foxes and seals and produced 'very well drest' skins. Their homes were full of coats made of seals and birds, the fur and feathers turned inwards for more warmth in the winter months. Sails made from guts were deemed exquisite in their lightness and durability.[14]

The men who wrote these accounts of their travels lived in an era of making, a time when people secured their livelihoods with the work of their hands. Throughout the Middle Ages and the Renaissance, tailors and weavers, rope-makers and ironmongers, referred to their crafts as 'mysteries'. Craft itself had a distinct relationship with divine creation. God had told Moses that he had equipped Bezalel with the Holy Spirit and 'with all kinds of skills – to make artistic designs for work in gold, silver, and bronze, to cut and set stones, to work in wood, and to engage in all kinds of crafts'.[15] When early English travellers encountered Indigenous craft, they often appraised what they saw through their appreciation for human manipulation or reworking of nature's materials. Something 'artful' or 'artificially' made referred to the technical side of construction and creation, casting Inuit craft in a positive light. The frequent mention of 'artificial' or well-dressed skins recognised the manual labour that went into preparing and working animal materials. George Best noticed details like the stitching of sealskin. He marvelled at Inuit garments made of feathers. They were skilfully sewn, he told his readers, compelling crew members to bring some with them to England.

The recurring mention of kayaks suggests that the English were particularly interested, and not a little provoked, by these Inuit belongings. They were drawn to the skilled ways that Inuit women and men traversed the waterways of their homelands. Perhaps the sailors who had grown up in Plymouth or Bristol saw parallels between the swift-moving kayaks and their own experiences of growing up on the coast back home. There might have been traces of envy, or competition, in watching those technical masterpieces cutting through the water. The transatlantic voyages that the English celebrated as demonstrations of their expanding maritime power exposed their vulnerabilities. Surviving storms and other dangers in the open sea was one thing, but they possessed little knowledge about the conditions and microclimates of the places they reached on the other side.

English observers marvelled at Inuit speed and mobility. One traveller wrote that the Inuit could navigate the waters far more expertly with a single oar than the English could with ten.[16] Rowers were so swift that it was 'almost incredible: for no ship in the World is able to keepe way with them'. When the interlopers arrived, Inuit skill was deployed as a matter of resistance. Nestled in frames of driftwood and whalebone covered in dried and scraped skins, the Inuit could elude the threatening presence of the figures arriving in the big ships, coming in search of a precious metal that wasn't there. Though the English captured the Inuit in paintings, drawings, and travel accounts, those same people fought the desire to be seen, categorised, and observed.

The English did not stay in the Arctic for long enough to truly understand Inuit culture. But when they touched fur clothing, and viewed the expert sewing of guts and skins, they gained a glimpse of the Inuit women and men who lay behind those parkas, tents, and kayaks that travellers and collectors coveted. Days of labour lay beneath every garment. Nerves from specific animals, such as bearded seals or caribou, were used for different purposes. Seamstresses scraped the skins with their *ulu*, the semilunar or curved knife used to prepare skins. It was not gold or silver that counted as their riches, the traveller Dionyse Settle wrote in 1577, but houses and kayaks made from skins, and the ancestral knowledge that enabled community members to rework and fashion this material into garments. Inuit artists and elders speak about the care and labour that went into traditional ways of preparing sealskin garments, and still do. As Inuit women tell us, the seal 'provides us with our identity. It is through sharing and having a seal communion that we regain our strength.'[17]

Techniques of garment construction give us clues, beyond European-drawn images, of what the Inuit wore when they were captured. Women wore high, wide boots and stockings that were different from those of men. The soles of Inuit boots covered the bottom and sides of the foot, shaped to its contours with fine pleating. If Nutaaq had been premature, he might have been nestled in a seal bladder or sac of caribou skin for additional warmth in the weeks after his birth. He might then have been placed, naked, in Arnaq's *amauti*, slowly growing into garments made from caribou fawn or birds, then caribou or fox. Nutaaq did not live long enough to grow into the clothing that typically clad a two- or three-year-old – an *atajuq*, a hooded garment of light caribou skin, slit in the back, often with accompanying mittens. Mothers carried their babies in their *amauti*, with no material to separate them, for several years, allowing the woman to care for the baby in a secure and warm environment, and helping bonds to develop between child and mother.[18] This innovative garment is what we see in all the images of Arnaq. While she carried on the difficult work of caring for Nutaaq during the uncertain voyage across the Atlantic, the baby peered at the world around him from against his mother's skin.

Women's skills with needles also lay behind Arnaq's facial tattoos. Dionyse Settle observed that it was women who marked their faces, laying a 'darke azurine' colour on their chin, cheeks, forehead, and wrists. Vivid blue has particular resonance in Inuit art, standing for sea, sky, and ice. We cannot know what Arnaq's tattoos meant, or how accurately Tudor artists rendered them, but we cannot ignore them. Tattoos were highly personal, allowing an Inuk woman to inscribe her body with her achievements or her place in her community, each line or dot connecting her to other people and stories. Tattoos could be related to birth and fertility, to welcoming a new baby into the world. Blue lines connected women to their daughters and sons, and to parents and other kin.

Ten years before Arnaq arrived in Bristol, a woodcut printed in Nuremberg in 1567 described the twenty-year-old Inuk woman who had been brought to Antwerp after being captured by the French. Initially, her captors had tried to separate her from her seven-year-old child, but she offered such fierce resistance that the sailors relented. A caption that described her appearance commented on her sealskin clothes, and how the 'paint marks she has on her face are completely blue, like sky blue . . . [and] cannot be taken off again . . . these marks are made with the juice of a kind of plant, which grows there in the country.'[19]

Perhaps Arnaq's tattoos afforded her a sense of home, of resilience, in the midst of her disorienting loss. Whatever life events her marks signalled, they proclaimed her and her people's story to those English strangers who gathered around her and spoke in a language she did not understand. Like sealskin, her tattoos materially connected her to her own environment, to the seals and narwhals congregating on the floe edge.[20]

Frobisher's ventures laid the groundwork for subsequent voyages to the Arctic, but no experiments or alchemical transformations could turn his ore to gold. Sidney's letter to the French reformer Hubert Languet, conveying the enthralling possibilities of the gold rumoured to have been found, captures something of the buzz and excitement that lay behind many Elizabethans' feverish expectations for colonial expansion. At that very moment, Sidney's father, Sir Henry, was brutally suppressing Gaelic forces in Ulster, laying claims to Irish lands in the name of the English Crown. Sidney had briefly joined his father there in the summer of 1576. The sparkle of precious metals further west may have appeared more enticing to the budding courtier than the prospect of military service closer to home.

Yet Sidney's mentor issued a stern rebuke. Languet told his protege that he feared that England, seduced by the desire for gold, would lose sight of what mattered. Virtue would be left by the wayside, like an abandoned mine.

Languet's response drew on a well-established humanist critique of luxury, but he was also tapping into moral and political conversations about wealth and colonialism that were rife in 1560s and 1570s England. While Kalicho navigated his kayak in view of the citizens of Bristol in the years following the new Anglo-Spanish treaty, and campaigns were carried out in Ireland at huge expense to the Crown, politicians, merchants, and investors were hotly debating the best means of bringing vast amounts of wealth into the realm. The merchant Thomas Gresham, who had built a lucrative career serving as one of the queen's financial agents in Europe, raised the necessary funds to build the Royal Exchange, a large public place for merchants to conduct their business and encourage trade.

Gresham had spent a lot of time in Antwerp, a prosperous and cosmopolitan city whose economic ambitions were visible in its architecture and artisans' workshops. The Bourse, with its galleries, arches, and towers, had become a leading centre for trade among European merchants. Antwerp's goldsmiths were unrivalled, creating the glittering objects that decorated the courts of the Tudors and Medicis. In 1571, Elizabeth feasted with Gresham and officially unveiled the Exchange to the sound of trumpets. The large neoclassical building became a fashionable place for Elizabethans to shop for global goods. But it was also a clear statement about England's commercial ambitions: a grand, imposing centre of commerce modelled on the great civic buildings of Italy, bringing together merchants under the banner of royalty.

In advising the impressionable young poet to steer clear of Frobisher's golden fancies, Sidney's mentor advised him to think about more suitable and virtuous models for colonialism. Rather than plunder and money-grabbing ventures, he wrote, the English should consider plantation and agricultural settlement. Leave the flashy gold for the privateers and merchants, he seemed to say. An attraction to raw bullion was unbefitting for the pious and morally minded courtier, who should be thinking about models of expansion that involved sustained land management and concerns for the common good. Even Dionyse Settle, who travelled with Frobisher, commented on the foolhardy way the crew risked their lives for gold. 'Behold the glorie of man,' he scoffed, who condemned riches at night, and in the morning devised how to satisfy greedy appetites. 'The stones of this supposed continent with America, be altogether sparkled, and glister in the Sunne like Gold: so likewise doth the sande in the bright water, yet they verifie the olde Proverbe: *All is not golde that glistereth*.'[21] Frobisher's burnished yellow jerkin and hose proclaimed a wealth that was built on illusion.

Beneath England's budding imperial imagination and the false lustre of all those tonnes of ore, subject to countless fruitless tests in London, the sealskin remains. Women's craft, the history of their being and their kin, lay behind the parkas that were brought to England in the same ships that carried the fool's gold. Copy after copy, renderings of these garments found their way into different media.

The Allegory of America was probably etched sometime in the 1590s by Philip Galle, based on an earlier drawing by Marcus Gheeraerts the Elder. At first glance, the engraving is all fantasy. As the title suggests, it is a visual representation that signals something larger and more abstract. It is a pastiche of European ways of seeing the Americas, arranged in all the strange exuberance of the mannerist style. Feathered garments, draped cloths of printed cotton, and perched parrots jostle for space among classicised and grotesque figures; scrolls and tassels; flowers and clusters of fruit. But there they are, Kalicho in the lower left (combined with representations of the earlier Inuk man), and Arnaq and Nutaaq on the right. Gheeraerts had lived in London in the 1570s, a witness to the excitement of Frobisher's initial voyage.

In the engraving, Nutaaq peers out from his mother's *amauti*. The man holds a bow, but also his oar, signalling his readiness to move swiftly through Arctic waters in his kayak, or beyond the gaze of the viewer. His hood snugly circles his face, leaving little room for the frosty air to penetrate. Arnaq's hood is larger, made to accommodate the movements of her baby, who remains secured with the string she wears around her middle. In the particularities of their boots and parkas; in the technology of Arnaq's *amauti*, perfected by women over the centuries to facilitate carrying a child; and in the stitches and lustrousness of the fur, we can see many hands at work: generations of women and their labour, informing the aesthetics of Renaissance mannerism. The image of the Inuit mother and child would even come to appear on a small windowpane of stained glass at the statesman Francis Bacon's residence in Herefordshire.

Even as Elizabethans turned to the Atlantic in their hopes of sourcing imperial wealth, and Frobisher piled his ships with pyrite, it was the physical presence of the Inuit and the things they made that endured. As Frobisher's tarnished and dented scraps lay discarded in London workshops and shipyards, engravers etched the textures and materials of Inuit life into copperplates, pressing and replicating these images for wider audiences. Years before the English had been to Roanoke or the Chesapeake, they were already learning that what one sought and what one found were rarely the same thing.

Florida and Roanoke
in Watercolour

Oyster shells lay scattered around the artist like the remnants of a debauched banquet. These shells, alongside brittle skulls and tobacco pipes, would come to appear in still life paintings as emblems of wantonness and vanity. But for this Elizabethan painter, shells were a tool, holding mixtures made from crushed minerals, plants, and insects, bound together with gum arabic sourced from the Saharan acacia tree. Sweeping the pigment across the shell's interior, the artist could see whether his paint had reached the right consistency, or whether it needed to be revived by adding more water. The whole process was alchemical: stones and animals gathered from faraway places were crushed into powder in a grinding stone. Lead and sulphur were exposed to fumes to create hues of yellow and white.[1] Shellfish and blossoms were ground and pressed beyond recognition, only to be resurrected on the page, lending their colours to a velvet doublet, or a plantain.

Such was the work of the limner, whose water-based renderings of colourful flowers, fruits, and portraits served to bring 'home with us from the farthest part of the world in our bosomes, whatever is rare and worthy the observance'.[2] Limning was a 'gentle art', as the era's most celebrated miniaturist, Nicholas Hilliard, wrote in his treatise on the subject. It stood apart from other forms of painting, neither requiring the time and effort needed to produce larger, oil-based paintings, nor turning the gentleman or gentlewoman into an artisan – someone whose painting was considered manual labour. Unlike the decorative painting used in courtly and civic pageantry – stages and props, barges, furniture – the limner shared a professional ancestry with the illuminator of medieval manuscripts, literally giving light to a subject by using jewel-bright colours and gold and silver leaf.[3]

The ships that carried steel and linens to the Americas, and brought back silver coins, fragrant barks, and potatoes (akin to sweet potatoes today), also carried artists across the Atlantic. In 1585, John White packed up his pigments into paper envelopes and boxes, locking them in a chest or pocket desk, and accompanied the wave of colonists who went to Ossomocomuck, the large coastal region of the Carolina Outer Banks. He travelled under the command of Ralph Lane, a veteran of English colonisation in Ireland at a time when the English were also establishing a colony in Munster. It was seven years after Frobisher's third Arctic voyage. White may have caught the attention of his patron, Walter Ralegh, with his drawings of the Inuit Arnaq, Nutaaq, and Kalicho, and perhaps even accompanied Frobisher to Nunavut.

Roanoke was the first English colony in the Americas, but it was a short-lived one. The settlement was abandoned within several years of its founding, becoming known as the 'lost colony'. Despite the failure of the Roanoke project, White's watercolours survive – exquisite portraits of Carolina Algonquians, from a child on their mother's back to an elder in a winter garment. Some dance, others move in and out of dwellings or eat together, adorned in copper, beads, pearls, and deerskins. Held at the British Museum, these watercolours have been viewed as remarkable snapshots of Algonquian ways of life, and as one of the museum's greatest treasures.[4] But how accurate are these images? And what can they tell us about how Elizabethans chose to depict Indigenous peoples in the earliest moments of colonial expansion?

In the mid-1580s, English colonial promoters were throwing all they could into making North American colonisation a part of

Tudor statecraft. Ralegh and his associates scouted writers and artists whose treatises, travel diaries, and paintings about the Americas might serve the Protestant cause in the Atlantic. Elizabeth's secretary Francis Walsingham sent the geographer Richard Hakluyt to Paris to make 'diligent inquirie of such things as might yield any light unto our westerne discoveries in America'.[5] During this time, Hakluyt wrote *A Discourse of Western Planting*, a treatise that drew on domestic and European economic and religious troubles to make a case for Atlantic plantation.

In addition to the urgency of claiming lands before other European princes might, these promoters knew that they had to allure and beguile – to make people feel that giving up money, or time, or even their lives, was a worthwhile endeavour. As White painted figures fishing in their canoes and farming sunflowers and maize, Ralegh commissioned an artist named Jacques Le Moyne de Morgues to prepare 'the Florida illustrations' of the Timucua people whom the painter had met during his brief travels to Florida two decades before, in 1564. Le Moyne was a celebrated botanical illustrator who had fled France as a Protestant refugee in the aftermath of the bloody St Bartholomew's Day massacre of 1572, eventually settling in Blackfriars near the north bank of the Thames. Little is known of Le Moyne's life in London, but it is unsurprising that Ralegh took an interest in this talented artist, who had firsthand experience of life in North America.

The limner, working with his or her water-based paints, created elegant renderings of plants, animals, and people, in meticulous compositions that could be as small as a playing card. Watercolours today are thin, transparent mixtures, but such paints only came to be used in the eighteenth century. Tudor and Stuart watercolour mixtures were thicker and more opaque. Nonetheless, the work of the limner was different from that of the large-scale painter, whose subject might include mythical goddesses, or biblical scenes of motherly adoration and pious sacrifice. Full-sized court portraits begin to look almost pathological compared with the pared-back intimacy of the limner's work. 'A hand or eye / By Hilliard drawn is worth an history / By a worse painter made,' the poet John Donne wrote in 1597.[6]

It's hard not to approach the work of a masterful limner like Nicholas Hilliard without a little bit of reverence, as if beholding something mystical. Set in precious stones and metals, miniatures became jewels themselves, fastened onto clothing, worn close to the body like a secular relic that invited devotion to a lover, or a queen. There is something almost holy in the endeavour of capturing the likeness of a person, or, for other watercolourists, a long-stemmed iris. In narrowing in on the subject's *aliveness,* on their being there, in that moment, on their having existed at all. Forget the noise around you, the religious divisions, the hate speeches, the gossip about who slept with whom and who is getting promoted and who gave their last, disgraced speech in the House of Commons. For a moment, today or in 1585, you're simply locking your gaze on the quiet existence of a human, or a leaf, or a parrot, who had once dwelled on this earth, their skins vulnerable to light and air and heat.

In Hilliard's world, men in loose linen shirts and diamond crosses languish in the flames of desire. Aristocratic soldiers in embroidered shirts cradle Italian-made armour. Women in pearlescent quilted dresses clutch at the silky gauze of their sail-like veils. As the son of a goldsmith, Hilliard knew how to work with precious metals. He and White both incorporated real gold and silver into their works, rather than imitating them with less costly materials. Like illuminated manuscripts, powdered gold and silver speckled the highly saturated pigments, bathing their subject in an entrancing brightness. Most of the traces of gold have disappeared from White's watercolours of the Americas, but technical analysis suggests silver had been used widely on the scales of fish, on drawings that were captioned with their Algonquian names, and on the jewellery worn by a young girl and the Elizabethan doll she clutches.[7]

The Algonquians of the Carolina Sounds were accustomed to foreigners and visitors. When White arrived in the summer of 1585, in the middle of the growing season, various groups including the Roanoke had already met the English in the first supply the year before. Oral accounts circulated of the Secota's meeting with Europeans decades earlier, when they rescued some castaways, possibly Spanish, on Ocracoke Island.[8] Walking through its marshlands and coastal plains, White could have found the shells he needed to mix his pigments in. The forests and grasses provided hickories, walnuts, persimmons, and blackberries. Indigenous women with extensive knowledge of the region's bushes, vines, and berries collected and prepared foods, sharing their environment with turkeys and bears, swans (*woanogusso*, White noted above his drawing of one such bird), and white trout (*ribuckon*).[9]

White's portraits of Algonquian life mapped the artist's courtly sensibilities onto Ossomocomuck. The artist painted men and women wearing beads and shells, signals of their high status. He acknowledged the value of copper to political and spiritual authority. His wealthier subjects wore it in their bodily adornments, and feathers knotted into their hair. The status of the goods they wore often derived from the fact that they had been imported through trade networks: copper from far up the Roanoke River and ultimately towards the Great Lakes, red dye from puccoon roots grown in the sand hills of South Carolina, and pearls, which could be found in nearby freshwater oysters, but were most plentiful in the eastern river pearl mussel further north.[10]

The watercolours of artists like Hilliard or White were undeniably accomplished, but how accurate were they? The Akwesasne Mohawk scholar Scott Manning Stevens has warned that viewing these images as straightforward representations of Indigenous life is misleading: 'There's very little to be learned about Native culture from that visual representation, but there's a lot to be learned about how Europeans think about that Native culture.'[11] While miniaturists and limners were praised for their works of realism, they also viewed themselves as artists, creating images that bore a complicated relationship to reality. If White's drawings are unparalleled pieces of Renaissance art, they cannot also be straightforward documents of Algonquian society.

For one, the images hardly convey the rivalries and uneasy interactions between the English and various groups in and around Roanoke Island. There is a risk of regarding the figures on the page as some kind of timeless portrayal of Indigenous life, without recognising that their cultures and politics were ever-shifting, never static. The settlers in Ossomocomuck met with the Croatan, Roanoke, Pomeioke, Aquascogoc, Secota, Weapemeoc, Chesapeake, and Chowanoke, and their diplomatic strategies and manoeuvres were heavily shaped by each of these groups' different responses to their presence. Some, like the Croatans, remained friendly with the English. Others resisted their presence from the beginning, and others still shifted their policies or switched alliances as the months went on.[12]

White's paintings and the graphite sketches underneath convey a sense of immediacy, as if drawn on the spot. Yet there is no evidence that he painted the album illustrations *in situ*. He likely conducted a series of sketches, capturing details of faces or clothing from close observation, using these to produce the finished product months later in England. Spain's attempted invasion with the 1588 Armada put English settler-colonial efforts in America on hold. When he returned to Roanoke in 1590, he found the colony abandoned. Its colonists, including his daughter Eleanor and his three-year-old grandchild, Virginia, had vanished. Buried in the soil were some of his belongings, possibly even some of these initial sketches. Among the five hidden chests he found, 'three were my owne,' White recalled, 'and about the place many of my things spoyled and broken, and my books torne from the covers, the frames of some of my pictures and Mappes rotten and spoyled with rayne'.[13]

When White came to make his portfolio for the colony's backers, his abilities were shaped by Continental artistic theory and Italian mannerism. As Hilliard had written in his treatise on limning, 'perfection is to imitate the face of mankind', in 'likeness' but also in the 'best graces and countenance'. White's adherence to Renaissance art theory is evident in the graceful movements and expressions of the men, women, and children he drew. In spite of their seeming naturalism, the art historian Stephanie Pratt (Crow Creek Dakota) has pointed out that White's 'imagining processes' were taking their cue from classical visual culture.[14] There was a whiff of Botticelli's three graces in the figures at the centre of the harvest ceremony depicted in 'A Festive Dance'. Some of the gestures look suspiciously similar to those in popular travel books published in Venice in the mid-sixteenth century. The conjurer in 'The Flyer' seems to have been modelled on a reproduction of Giambologna's bronze figure of the god Mercury from 1580, down to the parallels between the Algonquian's bird adornment and the wings on the god's helmet.[15]

White's drawings are representations of Indigenous lives filtered through a tradition of Continental art. His impressions of the inhabitants of Roanoke, as he himself wrote, were 'counterfeited according to the truth'. They were artificial creations, even as they gestured to something higher and greater; evidence and aesthetics combined.[16] They emphasised the humanity of Roanoke's inhabitants, yet served to encourage English colonial efforts. They were designed to be persuasive, signalling a proximity to the subject, but their knowledge of that subject remained opaque, like a pigment stiffened by lack of water.

In the months and years that followed, these images were copied and circulated to national and international audiences. Multiple versions of his watercolours survive, including an album of images 'after White', which may or may not have been painted by the artist, or another limner in Ralegh's circle. His Algonquian figures appeared as thumbnails on the edges of maps and in European costume books printed in Amsterdam and Venice. Two resurfaced in a miniature painted by a Mughal artist in India in 1620.

In 1590, the Flemish engraver Theodor de Bry produced a series of engravings based on White's images to accompany Thomas Hariot's *A Briefe and True Report of the New Found Land of Virginia*. John Smith included figures based on de Bry's engravings in *The Generall Historie of Virginia, New-England, and the Summer Isles* (1624). While the mass-market format of print made White's images widely recognisable, something was lost in translation. The watercolours were turned into graphic images that lost their finesse and subtlety, becoming a cog in de Bry's larger tale of European 'discovery' and conquest. Print Européanised White's originals, making the classical connections with Continental artwork even more apparent.

De Bry's engravings of White's drawings were successful enough that he followed these with images of French colonial projects in Florida the following year. These were based on the watercolours or 'Florida illustrations' that Ralegh had asked Le Moyne to paint in London. Unfortunately, only one of Le Moyne's original paintings of the Timucua survive, and even then, they are hardly reliable: Le Moyne was creating images based on societies he had witnessed some two decades before. All we have are de Bry's copies of these hazy memories, which he claims to have based on the originals he purchased from Le Moyne's widow in London. The result is another set of images of America by a European engraver, based on the drawings of an eyewitness who remained on the outside looking in.

In 'Floridians Crossing Over to an Island to Take Their Pleasure', a woman wades through the waters of her homelands with children on her back, her long tresses waving through the water like a nymph's. In 'The King and Queen Taking a Walk for Their Amusement', the 'queen and her handmaidens' wear moss adornments, interlaced with tresses 'so pretty that one would say they were filaments of silk', superimposing European royal ceremonies with hints of Timucua self-display. Even filtered through European notions of kings, queens, and attendants, however, de Bry alluded to aesthetics and story-telling practices that seemed unalterably different: these individuals pricked their skins, the caption informed readers, and filled them with 'a special herb whose sap gives an indelible stain'.[17]

For a short window of time, White and Le Moyne painted their North American watercolours in close proximity to one another in London, funded by Ralegh. Le Moyne died in 1588, as White desperately tried to find a way back to the colony and the family he had left behind. White's images show some evidence of interaction with the French painter. His drawing of a woman 'Of Florida' shows a Timucua woman covered in tattoos, holding a large earthenware bowl. One hand is outstretched, seeming to offer a handful of maize cobs. White's map of 'La Virginia Pars', stretching from the Chesapeake Bay to the Florida Keys, and decorated with English ships, sea monsters, and Ralegh's coat of arms, also included details of the French settlement of Fort Caroline.

As Ralegh's interest in a French Huguenot artist indicates, English views of the Americas and its peoples were framed by religious rivalries and alliances closer to home. In the years leading to the Armada, Protestant patrons like Ralegh cultivated writers and artists who might paint a picture of transatlantic geopolitics that marginalised

Catholic Spain. Together, White and de Bry's images signalled English involvement in the Atlantic, but also the character of English aspirations. In these artworks, there are no rosaries or extractive systems of tribute. There is grace, and abundant nature. The Spanish are nowhere to be found.

But Le Moyne's own life tells a different story. Le Moyne and de Bry's images of the Timucua, like White's of Algonquians, offered slight evidence of the profound changes that had come with European competition in their territories. Multiple Spanish campaigns in the early sixteenth century had brought conquistadors into Florida from Cuba or Central America. As many as 200,000 Timucuas may have lived in the region before Spanish colonisation. Reconstructing their ways of life on their own terms is immensely challenging. Commercial mining in Florida in later centuries destroyed many shell heaps and other archaeological sites of previous Timucua habitation that might have offered clues. Ancient mounds are still destroyed for building, interfering with landscapes where Native people buried their dead for thousands of years.[18] Surviving objects from Fort Caroline and other settlements testify to the multicultural reality of day-to-day life. There are brass buttons that once fastened the coats of Spanish soldiers; small amulets or *higas* carved of bone and shaped like closed fists, worn to protect against evil and death; a plaquette of hammered silver, perhaps made by Timucua artists using South American metals salvaged from Spanish shipwrecks.

In the 1530s, Hernando de Soto and his large retinue of soldiers, artisans, and war dogs settled on the banks of Little Manatee River, living in a village in the Uzita chiefdom and attempting to gain ascendancy over the region. Though they failed to establish long-term settlements at the time, the Spanish used these previous efforts to justify their conflict against the French thirty years later, when they sacked French Florida and redoubled efforts to establish outposts in the region. In the years following Mary I's death in 1558, as England turned back towards Protestantism, Spanish soldiers acting on Philip II's orders ransacked French settlements, creating alliances with Timucua groups to navigate the region's coasts and forests. As Le Moyne arrived with René de Laudonnière in Florida in 1564, whispers in the courts of Madrid and Paris suggested that the Spanish were preparing to renew their campaigns against the French.

Travelling through extreme winds, storms, and flooded lowland terrains, rain-sodden Spanish armies massacred French settlers, establishing their own presence in the region in their stead. Religion lay at the heart of this conflict. Reports circulated in France and England that the notorious captain Pedro Menéndez hanged prisoners with inscriptions that read, 'I doe not this as unto French men, but as unto Lutherans.'[19] Le Moyne barely survived one such attack, narrowly escaping death by retreating into the woods, and ignoring the searing pain in his leg, being 'not yet recovered from a wound I had received in the campaign against Outina' (Utina, the paramount Timucua leader).[20] At the time of White and Le Moyne's painting, the rumours of Menéndez's inscription were reprinted in English texts to foster anti-Spanish feeling, translated by the geographer and colonial enthusiast, Richard Hakluyt. Elizabethans were still hopeful that a Protestant league in the Americas, with French and Dutch allies, could offer a challenge to Spanish imperial ascendancy. John Hawkins had stopped at Fort Caroline in Florida in 1565, after all, helping to ensure the survival of the colonists by trading a ship and provisions for weapons. Le Moyne and White's watercolours wash over the shaky alliances, ambitions, and failures that undergirded European colonisation. The result is something far outside reality; an appealing, even hopeful depiction of Timucua life, but counterfeit.

In addition to humans, both White and Le Moyne were dedicated to recording the flora and fauna of southern North America. The watercolours in the British Museum's two White albums include silvery-blue flying fish, a brown bird snacking on a multicoloured maize cob, a leathery-skinned iguana awash in colours of emerald and sage, and a *nahyápuw*, or bald eagle. Physicians, apothecaries, and natural philosophers who lived in and around Lime Street, a hub for botanical experimentation in London, were already growing Atlantic specimens such as sunflowers, and they avidly requested copies of White's work.[21]

While White and Le Moyne were turning Algonquian men and Timucua women into classical gods and nymphs, a pair of unknown artists were painting their own vision of the Atlantic from on board one of Francis Drake's ships. These illustrations survive in an album known as the 'Drake manuscript', or the *Histoire Naturelle des Indes*. Several collaborators produced the manuscript, including at least two artists and two scribes. Through nearly 200 images, these artists catalogued a range of people, plants, and animals from various Atlantic places, including multiple Caribbean islands and Central American ports. The handwriting of the captions, and the religious language used in some of them, suggests these artists and authors were French. Many of the locations depicted in the album, meanwhile, were regular stops on Drake's voyages. The few exceptions to the West Indies as a location both relate to Drake: Gilolo, a Moluccan island that Drake visited on his circumnavigation of the globe, and Loranbec, a region between Florida and the Carolinas near where Drake stopped to collect the Roanoke colonists in 1586.[22] These artists, potentially among the Frenchmen who boarded Drake's ships in Cartagena, may have been on the very vessel that brought White and Hariot, with their plants and sketches, back to England.

The illustrators' drawings of plants, animals, and scenes of human labour and industry are not the drawings of expert limners. They have not exactly attained the 'perfection' of cataloguing a person's 'best graces and countenance' through classical training. But there's a vigour to these images, and they add something new to our understanding of the colonial, artistic gaze. These artists did not paint their subjects as specimens, but as denizens of entire ecosystems. There are mussel shells, but also enslaved African divers fishing for pearls. There are flying fish, but also Native women carrying silver from mountain tops. Indigenous messengers cross the Chagres River and its environs, carrying letters in gourds sealed with wax when wading through water, in an area of Panama that Drake navigated with English ships. Multiple images show the presence of Native and African people mining and paying tribute to the King of Spain, in dwellings where Spanish authorities stamped coins with Philip II's royal arms.

These images of labour are rare in watercolours. While court jewellers like Arnold Lulls drew cut and set emeralds in albums, removing the sparkling green gems from their Colombian origins, these artists drew men excavating emeralds in perilous conditions: 'The precious stone called emeralds grows on the very high mountains ... [The enslaved] usually end their days there because while digging in the rocks masses of stone fall on them which pin them underneath and they die miserably. There also is found a great quantity of beautiful rock crystal in large pieces richly adulterated with gold.' The caption described the coveted resource with attention to the lives and skills of those who lived there. 'The [Muzo and Muisca] Indians of this region are good workers with great skill and intelligence, working and making beautiful cloth of fine wool with which the Spaniards dress and fit themselves out.'[23]

In these watercolours, materials have connections to many different meanings and values. Despite the severe disruptions caused by the arrival of Europeans, the plants in the Drake manuscript remain rooted in the soil, allowed to grow without interruption. Potatoes and cashew nuts are stewed with meat for sustenance, the leaf of green peppers added to salads for zest and freshness in the intense heat. In Florida, the Timucua boil an orange tree with 'an excellent odor like a rose', making a paint to adorn their bodies. The variety of fish in Antigua, presented between paintings of oysters and conches, are caught by fishermen in a canoe. The ferocious glare of a manta ray does not float freely on the page, but chases an African man, in hopes that the pearl diver might drown.

Here, unlike John White's plantains and sassafras, the extracted resources that end up in Renaissance cabinets and portraits are not cut off from their origins. Transported Africans labour in emerald and silver mines, but the captions also relay Spanish fears of having 'the gold and silver transported by land from Panama . . . because of the many runaway [Africans] . . . who steal and plunder everything they find on the road belonging to the Spaniards', a reference to the autonomous *cimarróns* or maroons with whom Drake had allied in the early 1570s. Indigenous women and men live among Europeans, but they resist them, too: the Loranbec people in or near the Carolinas 'are extremely skillful in battle . . . as the English could tell fighting under Sir Francis Drake in 1586 when they attempted to conquer this land, but were forced to weigh anchor and retreat because of the resistance they encountered'.[24] Sometimes, the flora and fauna of the Americas came into London as a result of the *failures* of settlement, packed onto ships navigated by captains whose conquests had been unsuccessful.

Whoever viewed those humbler, at times whimsical illustrations in the Drake manuscript would see an industrial Atlantic that tugged at English interests just as much as the pristine naturalism of White's idyllic Roanoke scenes: gold and silver mining, multilingual villages situated at the edge of tropical mountain ranges, Native inhabitants spinning cotton and tending gardens brimming with papayas, maize, beans, and gourds. These were the environments that Elizabethans needed for their golden world. These were the soils, temperatures, rock formations, and waters that produced the emeralds, metals, and pearls so alluring to consumers in England.

Together, the watercolours of White, Le Moyne, and the Drake manuscript's artists present a particular visual archive of transatlantic encounters in the time of the Spanish Armada. They exhibit a clear gravitational pull towards southern North America and the West Indies. And they expand how we might think about Tudor tastes. The 1580s, after all, were a dazzling time for Elizabethan art. Alongside his portraits of the queen, Hilliard's magnificent 'Young Man among Roses' is one of the most iconic images of the Tudor court. A melancholic gentleman, adopting the pose of a mournful lover, leans against the trunk of a tree, his cheek pressing against the curls of his hair and the large ruff around it. His right hand rests against his heart. Nature invades the composition, covering the man in leaves, diluting the divide between artifice and nature. The prickly leaves and thorny branches of a rose bush cover the gentleman's legs, threatening to snag his costly white hose.

Hilliard painted this portrait in 1587, at the same time as White embossed the scales of a flying fish with real silver. A wealthy Elizabethan who commissioned a portrait of themselves or a beloved from Hilliard could also have acquired copies of White's illustrations, turning from the opulence and perils of the court to other lands, peoples, and ways of life. They could have gazed into the discerning eyes of an aged elder in fringed deerskin, or observed the 'mammee apple' (Santo Domingo apricot), a thick-rinded Caribbean berry that also grew in Florida, Nicaragua, and Peru. Avocados sprang to life as well as Tudor roses. At the same time, the Drake watercolours add a valuable discordance to these harmonious images. They offer a reminder that the visions presented by White and Le Moyne were part of a distinct tradition, following courtly conventions that offered very specific images of the Americas to their audiences. All the artists who travelled to Roanoke, Florida, and the Caribbean witnessed firsthand the brutal effects of settler-colonial projects. White's paintings were exquisite fictions.

Rakiock Canoes

Scratch the bark of the flowering sassafras tree and it releases a warm, sugary scent of cinnamon-like spice, its leaves smelling like sweet lemons. Longleaf pine, red maple, cypress, and grey elm dot the many ecological borderlands of eastern North America. Textures and colours bring infinite variety: prickly evergreen juniper, the apple red of maple leaves. Along the coast, marine waterscapes bring the sharp smell of seawater. Shifting tides reveal clusters of oyster reefs, and estuaries where otters forage.

Over time, the mystical enticements of apothecary shops in London would carry these scents from the Carolinas, passed through bark, berries, gums or saps. Many of these substances would have been transported from forest to coast, swamp to sea, by canoe before making their way onto English ships. The kinds of shells that White used to mix his paints were also the tools that Algonquian canoe-makers used to hollow out the charred interiors of trees.

The desire for flora and fauna from the Americas was partly why the accomplished mathematician, astronomer, and linguist Thomas Hariot came to publish *A Briefe and True Report of the New Found Land of Virginia*, about his journey to the Carolina Outer Banks. His book was published in 1588, and expanded in 1590 to include images by the famed engraver Theodor de Bry. These images were based on the watercolours by John White, a painter 'sent into the contrye by the queenes Majestye' to draw and 'describe the shapes of the Inhabitants their apparell, manners of Livinge, and fashions.'[1]

Hariot's text initially seems very different from White's fluid and elegant portraits. His account is all about things, outlining what resources might be turned into commodities, and how the landscape could be modified to benefit European trades, manufactures, and demand.[2] He related English colonial ventures to a host of ideologies about civility and European 'progress', whereby English exports, from language to technology, would benefit those who attained them. Yet despite Hariot's promise of luxury and profit, his book is also a document that wonderfully refuses, or fails, to fully incorporate Algonquian lands into English belief systems. Some resources lay beyond categorisation. It was hard to commodify something you didn't even have a name for.

It was 1585. Elizabeth's spymaster, Francis Walsingham, had been busy uncovering covert Catholic plots to put Mary, Queen of Scots on the throne. England and Spain were newly at war. Soon, Frobisher would accompany Francis Drake on his attack on Spanish settlements in the Atlantic, a voyage that would be key to Hariot's own return home. A recently knighted Ralegh busily advanced plans for colonial expansion, assembling a group of servants and advisors to gather intelligence about North America. It was in this moment of Anglo-Spanish competition that Ralegh sent Hariot to Ossomocomuck. The scholar had studied science and mathematics at Oxford, and Ralegh relied on Hariot to teach him and his sea captains navigation and cartography at his London mansion, Durham House. But Hariot was also a pupil. In his patron's house on the Strand, Hariot collaborated with two Algonquian men, Manteo (Croatan) and a more reluctant Wanchese (Roanoke), to produce the Ossomocomuck orthography, transcribing Roanoke and Croatan into an alphabet. Manteo and Wanchese had arrived in London in September 1584, following a brief, initial English expedition to Roanoke.[3]

Spanish spies who observed Ralegh's preparations sent covert letters home, reporting on the project's developments. Ralegh tried to keep information secret, but curiosity and speculation surrounded the affair. A cohort of gentlemen were conferring closely with 'two tall Indians whom they treated well, and who spoke English'. Manteo and Wanchese served as interpreters for Ralegh and his circle, but their attitudes to the English differed greatly. When they returned to Roanoke the following year, Manteo continued to establish friendly diplomatic relations between his Croatan people and the colonists. Wanchese, perhaps disturbed by what he had seen of England, and aware of how drastically his homelands might change if the English remained there, actively resisted their presence and encouraged the Roanoke to do the same.[4]

Hariot stayed in Ossomocomuck for a year. He arrived in June 1585 and returned home in June 1586, catching a ride back to England with Drake and Manteo, in a ship laden with spoils following Drake's raids on Spanish settlements from the Caribbean to Florida. Drake carried 300 Indigenous travellers, mostly women, from the Viceroyalty of Peru, along with 200 Africans and 'Turks and Moors'. The fate of these individuals is almost wholly unknown. A number of them may have been left in North America to make room for the colonists on the ship. Some made it to London. In October that year, a man known as 'Chinano the Turk', who had been with Drake in Cartagena, converted from Islam to Protestantism near the Tower of London.[5] An Algonquian man named Towaye living in London in 1587 may also have been part of this group of travellers, as well as several Caribbean men, Pedro and Juan, who had long served as interpreters in Drake's fleets.[6]

Hariot had returned home at a good time. English relations with neighbouring groups were ridden with conflict. Despite the clear hospitality that Hariot received from the Algonquians who welcomed him and other settlers into their villages, he admitted that 'some of our companie to wards the ende of the yeare, shewed themselves too fierce, in slaying some of the people'.[7] This was all Hariot wrote of the last few months of the colonists' stay in Roanoke, as the English alliance with Wingina (Pemisapan), a Secotan *werowance* or leader, began to break down. In early June 1586, under escalating tensions, colonists attacked a Secotan settlement, and an Irish soldier in Ralph Lane's company decapitated Wingina. The colonists left Roanoke in a hurry.

The Spanish Armada and ongoing conflict with Spain delayed further ventures in the months and years that followed. English ships were required closer to home, preventing Ralegh from sending more provisions. When Richard Grenville finally returned to Roanoke in 1590, the English had all vanished. Decades later, in his discourse promoting the colonisation of 'Virginia' (loosely taken to encompass the land 'from *Florida* to Cape Breton'), the geographer Samuel Purchas referred to the 'former Plantations of Sir *Walter Raleigh*' and what he took to be the inevitable deaths of the colonists. The 'carkasses, the dispersed bones' of the dead 'have taken a mortall immortall possession, and being dead, speake, proclaime and cry, *This our earth is truly English*'.[8] For Purchas, spilled English blood had changed the identity of the earth itself. No one wanted to imagine another possible scenario, which was that colonists had been incorporated into local groups as kin. For English Protestants, the project of assimilation only worked one way.

Apart from a few references to violence and disease, Hariot deliberately focused on things pleasant and useful. He told his readers about sassafras and copper, and how sugarcane, if grown alongside quinces and oranges, might be used to make jams or suckets, a popular sweet dish in England. He wrote of otters with lustrous fur that would yield easy profits. There were silkworms as big as walnuts, suggesting that, over time, an English silk industry might become as lucrative as it was for Italy or Persia. Through his eyes, the 'raw' goods of Ossomocomuck were there for the cultivating. The symbiotic relationship between beans, maize, and squash and other harvests were reconfigured as merchandise in an industrialised landscape.

To Hariot, civil refinement was not just gained by using resources from the Americas to create European objects – cedar for bedsteads, crushed berries for clothing dyes – but by bringing European-manufactured objects into the Americas. Mathematical instruments, sea compasses, books, clocks, and perspective glasses ignited curiosity among the 'naturall inhabitants'. 'In respect of troubling our inhabiting and planting, [they] are not to be feared,' Hariot wrote, 'but they shall have cause both to feare and love us, that shall inhabite with them.'[9] This 'inhabiting with them' also led Hariot to comment on Indigenous craft. He wrote of the fur mantles constructed with rabbit pelts, and the 'excellently wel dressed' Secotan women who decorated their bodies with pearls and copper beads.[10] He described woven mats and baskets, and the preparation of animal skins stitched into garments. The silver hanging from the ears of a '*Wiroans* [*werowance*] or *chiefe Lorde*' were small and round, reminding Hariot of a testoon – a Tudor coin.

As a result of these cross-cultural encounters and Hariot's interest in Native dialects, an influx of Algonquian words came to be stamped into the pages of this Elizabethan book. Colonial writers had long described the Americas as a *tabula rasa,* a blank slate on which Europeans might make their mark. But in the microcosm of Hariot's text, as Native words were pressed into paper, a product manufactured in London became a dwelling place for words intimately connected to Algonquian lands.

Hariot used Algonquian words for hard-to-translate, less-familiar tree or vegetable varieties, such as *metaquesúnnauk* for prickly pears, 'a kinde of pleasaunt fruite almost of the shape & bignes of English peares'. His text became a meeting place for English and Algonquian viewpoints. He noted that sassafras was 'called by the inhabitants *Winauk*'. *Ascopo* is 'a kinde of tree very like unto Lawrell', a sweet bay tree with a cinnamon-like bark. *Pagatowr*, or maize, appeared like clusters of multicoloured peas in hues of yellow-white, red, and blue. It is here that Hariot mentioned the golden flower, the *planta solis* or sunflower, extending its leaves towards the Upper World. Algonquian women planted sunflower seeds alongside beans and *macócqwer* ('pompions' or squash).[11]

Then there were the woodlands, full of trees, the Standing Ones reaching to the Sky World. Roanoke seemed to have infinite stretches of woodland, including ancient cypress and cedar, 'a very sweet wood'. Hariot imagined North American cedar furnishing Tudor interiors. The material could make chests, he proposed, or be fitted to make 'sweet and fine bedsteads, tables, desks, lutes, virginals, and many things else'.[12] Roanoke cedar, cut and carved into instruments, could entertain Elizabeth at a banquet. When the sea captain Arthur Barlowe travelled to Roanoke in 1584, he had been awed by the 'highest and reddest Cedars of the world'.[13] He believed the trees of the region surpassed the quality of spicy canelo tree bark that Captain John Wynter had obtained from the Strait of Magellan during Drake's circumnavigation four years before.

One bark evaded translation altogether. Barlowe had noted that Algonquians made their canoes from a 'wood not commenly knowen to our people, nor found growing in England'.[14] Hariot also commented on a sweet wood with which the inhabitants 'doe commonly make their boats or Canoes'. They called it *rakíock*. Hariot celebrated the way craftspeople made their *rakíock* canoes from a single tree, charring the trunk and hollowing it out with sharpened stones and shells. De Bry's 1590 engravings depicted Algonquians pushing their canoes through clear waters, filling their boats with shimmering fish. It was 'a pleasant sighte to see the people . . . sailinge in those Rivers', he reflected in the caption, 'free from all care of heapinge [u]pp Riches for their posterit[i]e, content with their state, and livinge frendlye together'.[15]

As settlers quickly recognised, this tree was central to Algonquian life. The inhabitants of Ossomocomuck, after all, had been using these techniques to make canoes for millennia. The region was a network of waterways intimately related to the identities of those who dwelled there. In 1984, four centuries after the English first arrived in Roanoke, thirty dugout canoes dating from 2430 BC to AD 1400 were found in the region, after the shallow waters of a North Carolina lake were used to quench a series of wildfires. As the water levels dropped, the charred and splintered bow of a canoe appeared under the dappled waters.

Rakíock was a soft and durable wood, possibly white cypress or white cedar. It might find fit use, Hariot suggested, as masts for English ships, eventually brought to serve imperial expansion. But first and foremost, it remained central to Algonquian communication, sociability, and survival, as subsequent colonists knew. Summarising Hariot's observations in his history of Virginia and New England, John Smith wrote that 'their woods are such as ours in England for the most part, except Rakeock a great sweet tree, whereof they make their Canowes'.[16] In the Chesapeake in the early seventeenth century, the Jamestown secretary John Pory wrote of an elder who invited him to his house, presenting him with 'twelve Bever skinnes and a Canow' as gifts.[17] The English travelled to the settlements of Indigenous allies in canoes. Roving up the coastline to Massachusetts, Smith also recorded English tactics of stealing or ransoming boats. In a 'quarrel', 'we tooke six or seven of their Canowes, which towards the evening they ransomed for Bever skinnes'.[18]

Hariot, who had chatted in broken Algonquian to Manteo while dining on silver platters at Ralegh's London mansion, disapproved of the 'too fierce' activities of the military men. From their side, soldiers like Lane, and later Smith, criticised the courtly manners of wealthy gentlemen, those Oxford boys with their 'tender educations, and small experience in Martiall accidents'. They expected feather beds, pillows, and taverns, Smith scoffed, even in swamps and forests, whining incessantly about the lack of 'gold and silver and dissolute liberty'.[19]

It was clear that Hariot put a premium on the materials of European civility, and believed in the value of the colonial project. But even in his account of settlement, acts of unsettlement were taking place. To unsettle something, the translator John Florio wrote in 1598, was like dismounting artillery. You removed, piece by piece, the iron mechanisms that had appeared so immovably fixed. Faced with the task of translating the untranslatable, Hariot was learning through unlearning.

In bringing Algonquian words and associated knowledge into his text, Hariot, whether consciously or not, tempered the language of commodification that at first seems to dominate his book. Luscious grape varieties, laurel trees, and sweet barks would have appealed to investors back home. Grapes and bay trees might have conjured associations with Greco-Roman villa life, where the tendrils of vineyards and laurel wreaths crowned the heads of gods and poets. But Hariot's descriptions also located these travelling objects within specific ecosystems. To know about gum sap and cedar, he seemed to be telling London investors, you'll also have to find out about *metaquesúnnauk* and *rakíock*. These confluences point to very different worldviews that inhabited the contact zones of colonial settlement, but it also expresses a plurality. In Hariot's text, Native knowledge seeps through and cracks the confidence of the colonial project. 'There are many other strange trees,' he wrote, 'whose names I knowe not but in the *Virginian* language.'[20]

Hariot's sense of strangeness is important. It plays a role in his understanding of the limits of translation. The word 'strange' appears frequently in the book, as it does in many travel stories. Hariot describes 'strange' customs, gestures, words, and beasts. But what, or who, is strange, is not so clear-cut. At times, the perspective shifts. The English bring 'strange diseases'. They carry 'strange weapons'. In another instance, Hariot recognises that value judgement depends on perspective. As part of their travels, the colonists were forced to eat food 'of which some sorts were very straunge *unto us*'.[21] Hariot imagines lutes and furniture, but *rakíock* lives in the shape of a canoe.

Over time, Londoners came to see North American cedars and Indigenous craft in their own rivers and wood-panelled interiors. In 1599, a Swiss traveller marvelled at Walter Cope's collection of global wonders, including fireflies from North America, and 'a long narrow Indian canoe with the oars' that hung from the ceiling. In 1603, several Algonquians delighted passers-by when they navigated their canoe on the Thames. Though they were reputedly paid for their activities, they may have been the men captured by English colonists along the Chesapeake Bay's Rappahannock River some months before.[22]

There are many constraints on how well we can understand or access the Indigenous Roanoke that Hariot and other colonists entered. Acknowledging this stands as a corrective to the mentality of the time, in which mapping other lands, and altering other ways of life under the banner of civility, were mechanisms of colonial control. 'The Country is now also Described & drawne into Mapps & Cardes,' the lawyer John Davies wrote from Ireland in 1609. In Davies' view, Virginia would come to be known in the same way. To 'know all the passages, [and to] have penetrated every thickett & fast place, and have taken notice of every notorious Tree or Bush' would 'not only remayne in our knowledge & memory during this Age; but . . . [be] layd open to all posterity'.[23] For Davies, unknowable environments were alien and dangerous. Unfamiliar trees were 'notorious'. Processes of gaining knowledge were described in invasive terms, requiring exposure and surveillance. Hariot does not depict a land that the English have brought meaning to. For him, Roanoke is a place whose environment can only make sense with the knowledge of its people.

An Aztec Codex in Oxford

In the 1580s, the English geographer Richard Hakluyt, then resident in France, purchased a 'painted book' of Mesoamerican pictorial writing. As English captains travelled to Roanoke and circumnavigated the globe, images drawn on European paper by Nahua painter-scribes brought Mexica (or Aztec) history, tributary practices, and the life cycles of Nahuatl-speaking women and men into the Elizabethan realm.

Now known as the Codex Mendoza, the manuscript Hakluyt acquired had been created in the early 1540s, some two decades after the Spanish invasion of Mexico under Hernán Cortés. The codex may first have arrived in Paris through French privateers, ransacked from a captured Spanish ship. The figures populating the codex provided the basis for an oral account of Aztec/Mexica history, beliefs, and practices. One or several multilingual interpreters explained these pictographs to a Spanish scribe, who then 'translated' the images and their meanings into Spanish. The result is a collage of Mexica lifeways and Spanish glosses on Mesoamerican history, rushed, the scribe noted on one page, so that it could board the ship on time.[1] The codex isn't a case of Europeans subjugating or assimilating Nahua voices, but of working around and in response to them.

Though he would never travel to the Americas – nor even beyond France – Richard Hakluyt spent his life collecting stories from sea captains and merchants who travelled across oceans in the pursuit of trade or land. Hakluyt was convinced that he lived in a critical moment in English history. It was God's plan that the English would subvert Spanish imperial expansion, leading to a different world order. His writings conjure secret conversations and firsthand knowledge, hearsay and rumour. For a moment, we are in the room with weather-beaten travellers eager to impart tales of merchant ships and secret kingdoms.

Hakluyt is best known for *The Principal Navigations, Voyages, Traffiques and Discoveries of the English Nation,* an immense compendium of travel writing that appeared in print in 1589. The second, expanded edition, published ten years later, consisted of some million and a half words. It contained everything from a list of the porcelain and spices captured in 1592 from the fabulously rich cargo of Portuguese carrack the *Madre de Deus,* to the activities of merchants in Russia and the Ottoman Empire. But in 1583, years before *The Principal Navigations* brought global travels together, Hakluyt, then a fellow at Christ Church in Oxford, was especially interested in western plantation. He had recently published *Divers Voyages Touching the Discoverie of America,* dedicating his volume to the courtier Philip Sidney and catching the attention of prominent statesmen at Queen Elizabeth's court. Sensing his enthusiasm, Elizabeth's Secretary of State, Francis Walsingham, sent him to France to serve as a chaplain and secretary to the English Ambassador in Paris.

Hakluyt arrived in a bustling commercial city, its winding medieval streets leading to Catholic churches and elegant *hôtels particuliers,* or private mansions. The spectre of the 1572 St Bartholomew's Day massacre, a targeted attack against Huguenots that led to the death of thousands of Protestants, lingered, and religious tensions ran high. Still, as any good humanist knew, travel was a means of serving one's country; gathering evidence of life elsewhere could be useful for national diplomacy and politics. French forts and settlements in the

Atlantic spanned from Tupi Brazil to Iroquois Canada, and Hakluyt busied himself meeting merchants and collecting and translating travel accounts. He tracked down the testimonies of sailors returning from Mexico or the Caribbean, met with fur merchants trafficking otter and beaver skins, and learned of the uses of Atlantic plants from physicians who had studied botany.

A sadness may have hung over him at this time. Hakluyt had recently encouraged his Oxford friend, the Hungarian poet Stephen Parmenius, to travel to Newfoundland with the soldier and adventurer Humphrey Gilbert. In August 1583, Parmenius drowned on the voyage home. Before his death, the poet had written a Latin poem expressing his fervent belief that North America was key to England's search for the Golden Age. 'They say that the passing of time, running through the ages of silver and bronze, once it deteriorates and cheapens into hard iron, returns again, in time's turning, to the ancient gold. Am I wrong, or is that time?'[2]

In Paris, Hakluyt met André Thevet, the royal cosmographer and chaplain to Catherine de Medici. Thevet was a Catholic priest who had been to Brazil in the mid-1550s, spending several months in the short-lived colony of France Antarctique. Although a Catholic with a reputation as an unreliable storyteller, Thevet had witnessed South America with his own eyes, and Hakluyt could now freely ask Thevet about anything that piqued his interest. Having read Thevet's travel books, Hakluyt might have asked about the Tupinambá creation myth of how a young girl first learned to plant and cultivate sweet potato, for example, or about how animals moved through Brazilian forests, or what the plants and trees smelled like when you stood underneath their thick and fragrant canopies. We know he borrowed a copy of Thevet's manuscript charting René de Laudonnière's journey to Florida, since he eventually helped see it into print. Hakluyt could also have viewed items brought back from Brazil.

Thevet was keeper of the king's cabinet of curiosities, which contained toucan beaks and a Tupinambá club, decorated with feathers and cotton fibres.

Hakluyt acquired the Codex Mendoza from Thevet. In his 1625 account of this 'Mexican Chronicle', Samuel Purchas – also a chaplain, and Hakluyt's successor in compiling the voyages of the English after Hakluyt died in 1616 – noted that 'Master Hakluyt (then Chaplaine to the English Embassadour in France) bought the same for 20. French crowns.'[3] The first image in the codex is a map that depicts the founding of the Mexica capital of Tenochtitlan at its centre. An eagle astride a cactus dominates the centre. Rich turquoise represents the city in relation to its waterways; numerous Europeans compared it to Venice. Military strength was conveyed through the inclusion of Mexica warriors on the lower third of the page, claiming victory over other cities and communities.[4] Among the temples, houses, animals, and human figures painted by Nahua artists, we see another hand at the top: A. *Thevet, cosmographe du Roy.*

Leafing through the codex, Hakluyt would have encountered the names of hundreds of towns and cities conquered by the Mexica, and the types and amount of tribute they delivered to Tenochtitlan. Regional crafts and economies emerge in the lists of particular tributes expected of different provinces, giving a sense of the range of resources and luxuriously crafted items that the Mexica could access in their dominions, from cacao to conch shells, turquoise sandals to blue cotinga feathers. The codex records that the capital of Techtepec, to take one example, sent thousands of mantles and tunics biannually, along with a warrior's quetzal costume, gold diadems and beads, bundles of green feathers trimmed with yellow feathers, 100 pots of liquidambar (gum tree sap), 8,000 handfuls each of blue, red, and green feathers, and 200 loads of cacao.[5] A later codex, created in the 1570s and sent to the Medici family in Florence, contained a description of how wealthy Mexicas might have enjoyed such varieties of cacao: 'green, made of tender cacao; honeyed chocolate made with ground-up dried flowers – with green vanilla pods; bright-red chocolate; orange-coloured chocolate; rose-coloured chocolate; black chocolate; white chocolate.'[6]

In addition to details about Mexica wealth and power, Hakluyt could learn about the life cycles of girls and boys from birth to death. In the third part of the codex, a woman gives birth. Four roses over the cradle signal the days that pass before the child is washed, named, and brought signs of their future. For a boy, these consisted of martial objects or the instruments of a trade; for a girl, implements for food preparation and domestic work. At five, children exercised bodily labour, carrying small burdens of wood to the marketplace, or learning to spin. At thirteen, the boy would collect wood from the mountains, or travel by canoe to find herbs and plants. Girls would grind cakes and weave yarn. We lose sight of the girl, after marriage, though women and children appear later as prisoners of war. The boy might become a merchant, or a high-ranking servant to those in the highest political offices, or a feather-worker. If he is especially favoured, he might become a warrior and come to wear the rich mantle of a champion, tasselled with iridescent feathers.

In the fierce, exquisite language of Aztec/Mexica poetry, songs are flowers, flowers are warriors, warriors are songs: 'Ah, let me pass away and be arrayed, singer that I am ... / Only thus would I pass away, my hearts as flowers twirling, scattered as jades.' Interspecies dialogue illuminates a world where butterflies' wings are sharp but brittle like obsidian, where 'plumelike popcorn flowers come spinning. Jaguar cacao flowers are massed at the place of sprinkling down ... / Their diffusing fragrance in our midst.' Words and music intoxicate, create artworks, vivify and commemorate: 'Here, through art, I'll live,' proclaims one poem or 'canto' in a surviving Nahuatl-Spanish manuscript, transcribed by Nahua peoples around the time of the creation of the Codex Mendoza. 'In song I cut great stones, paint massive beams, and this, in future time when I'm gone, shall be uttered ... / My hearts will be alive here: they'll have come, a remembrance of me.'[7]

What did Hakluyt think of his newly acquired codex? Did those graphic impressions – baskets of chillis, warriors wearing pelts – linger in his mind as he walked through the streets of Paris? Jaguars, hovering over the Seine. It is impossible to know, but we do have other European impressions of Mexica life from around this time. Hakluyt was in France not long after the philosopher and diplomat Michel de Montaigne published his famous essays, which ruminated on everything from eating melons to 'How the Soul Releases its Emotions on False Objects When Real Ones are Missing'. The Englishman could have picked up a copy from a bookseller's stall, rifling through its pages to find Montaigne's essay 'Of Cannibals'. Montaigne had met several Tupinambás in Rouen in 1562, and he drew on his encounter, as well as rumours and stories about Indigenous Americans, to engage in a bit of cultural relativism. He concluded that the French had proven themselves to be far more barbarous in their violences than even the fiercest warriors who were rumoured to eat their enemies. 'Prying so narrowly into their faults,' Montaigne wrote, 'we are so blinded in ours.'

Montaigne expanded his essays in 1588. Hakluyt might have read these in the original French; by 1603, he could read them in English, thanks to John Florio's popular translation. In this second edition, Montaigne turned to the Mexica. Whereas he saw the Tupinambá of Brazil as representing, in an idealised way, inhabitants of the classical Golden Age – close to nature, uncorrupted by luxury – he admired the 'amazement-breeding magnificence of the never-like seene Cities of *Cusco* and *Mexico*', in all the artifice of their gold-wrought gardens, cabinets, and striking textiles. In 'the exquisite beautie of their workes, in precious Stones, in Feathers, in Cotton and in Painting; [they] shew they yeelded as little unto us in cunning and industrie'. Montaigne mourned the lost potential that came with toppling an empire, imagining what European and Mexica diplomatic alliances might have looked like.

> Who ever raised the service of marchandize and benefit of trafficke to so high a rate? So many goodlie cities ransacked and razed; so many nations destroyed and made desolate; so infinite millions of harmlesse people of all sexes, states and ages, massacred, ravaged, and put to the sworde; and the richest, the fayrest and the best part of the world topsyturvied, ruined and defaced to the trafficke of Pearles and Pepper.[8]

People and their material culture – edifices, exquisite works of artistry and skill – all destroyed by Europeans for mere commodities.

For a while, the codex slips from view. But, like Montaigne and Hakluyt, Samuel Purchas viewed Mexica history as a civilisation whose history mattered. He made the extraordinary decision to print the Codex Mendoza in his *Hakluyts Posthumus, or, Purchas his Pilgrimes* (1625), published nine years after Hakluyt's death. Creating new woodcuts of Mexica pictographs was a fabulously expensive undertaking. It was clear to Purchas that the Inca and Mexica had been prodigious civilisations. Elsewhere in his book, he compared Peru and Mexico to ancient Greece and Rome, empires 'growne great, civil, rich, and potent, after their manner, as our *Mexican* and *Inca* stories will shew in due place. This their greatnesse produced stories of their Acts by *Quippos,* Pictures and other Monuments, which derived to posterity the knowledge of former times and acts.'[9] Like monuments and *quipus* (the Incan system of knotting cords to record information), 'pictures' were ways of relaying histories that conveyed the wonderful diversity of God's earth, while imparting the urgency of Protestant conversion projects in the yet-unconquered regions of the Americas.

Purchas called the codex a 'Mexican picture historie' and a 'Mexican historie in pictures'. Significantly, he removed the Spanish glosses on the text, bringing the focus onto Mexica culture and downplaying the Spanish presence in the document, muting the colonial conditions that originally produced it. Purchas's influential book was a staple in the merchant and elite libraries of those who could afford it. Jacobean and Caroline readers who flipped towards the end of his thousand-page tome would have seen eagles and strings of beads, bundles of quetzal feathers, and flat cakes made of maize.

Hakluyt and Purchas were not alone in their fascination with Mesoamerica. In the Tudor era, translators 'English'd' Spanish books about the conquest of Mexico. By then, some writers professed a kind of antiquarian interest in the powerful polities of Central and South America, while showing little awareness of the travels and presence of Nahua, Inca, or Maya peoples and their descendants in Europe over the course of the sixteenth century.[10] Records of lost plays with titles such as *The New World's Tragedy* (1595) or *The Conquest of the West Indies* (1601), though their contents have not survived, suggest an appetite for transatlantic tales of conquest and plunder, performed around the time that Shakespeare wrote *The Merry Wives of Windsor* (which includes references to potatoes, pumpkins, and South American gold). The Black Legend of Spanish atrocities fuelled Protestant propaganda about England's ostensibly gentler colonial designs, an opposition which flattened the complex societies that had formed across the Americas as European, Indigenous, and African peoples built their lives together.

An artefact like the codex brought Mexica life to Tudors and Stuarts through the mediation of the *tlacuilo,* or scribes. For a moment, they encountered the world through animals, flowers, the translucent green of jade, and the dappled waters of Tenochtitlan. Before illustrations of cactuses appeared in English plant books, they sat at the heart of the Codex Mendoza, conjuring Mexica foundation stories on the same page that Thevet inscribed with his name. 'Live and blossom here on earth,' went one Nahuatl song,

> As you move, shaking, flowers fall. Eternal are the flowers, eternal the songs that I, the singer, lift . . .
> Not forever on earth, but briefly here. Even jades are shattered. Gold, broken. Ah! plumes, splintered. Not forever on earth, but briefly here.[11]

Purloined in an act of Atlantic piracy and then carried across the Channel among Hakluyt's belongings, the codex had moved, like many Native travellers and their belongings, through an Indigenous Atlantic.[12] In their language, the Mexica had always dwelled on the sea: the earth was known as *cemanahuac*, a place surrounded by water. Across the Sky Water, an English geographer carried the codex into Elizabethan England, where it was prized by geographers and antiquarians who were using texts and chronicles to reformulate their ideas about the world.

Not forever on earth, but briefly here. This fragment of Mexica life now rests in a university library. In the 1650s, the codex passed from the jurist and scholar John Selden's possession to the Bodleian Library at the University of Oxford – the same library that now houses Ketel's portrait of Frobisher in his yellow jerkin, and a chair constructed from the timber of Drake's ship, the *Golden Hind*. It sits, stored away, in Special Collections, in the company of several other codices. Selden also left a Mixtec codex (the Selden Codex); a document that preserves the genealogy of the Jaltepec dynasty; and a sixteenth-century manuscript depicting the founding of a city-state in the region that is now Oaxaca. In 1636, William Laud, the Archbishop of Canterbury, had donated a codex from Central Mexico, known as the Codex Laud, or Book of Death, full of divination rituals and offerings. And a Bodleian catalogue drawn up around the time of Elizabeth I's death lists a manuscript known as the Codex Bodley, containing a history of the dynastic networks of Mixtec families.

As Elizabeth I approved the foundation of Jesus College and elaborate portraits of the queen were hung up to commemorate its royal foundress, some of her more eccentric subjects were consulting glyphs of death deities, turkeys, and rain predictions, rendered in indigo and cochineal. They collected pendants made of the teeth and claws of predatory jungle cats, woven with vegetable fibres. Elizabeth's astrologer, John Dee, owned an obsidian mirror from Mexico. One of these codices may have been in his possession before it ended up in the hands of later Stuart collectors. Now, in the midst of Oxford's golden spires, among its medieval chapels and Jacobean dining halls, a jaguar skin carries Mixtec stories; between the city's own waterways lies a codex that depicts the waters running through Tenochtitlan.

Silver Vessels and
Pieces of Eight

'Parnassus is out of silver.' Past hills and olive groves, two young travellers push forward through the warm terrain, determined to reach the site where wit and poetry flourish. They are making a pilgrimage to Parnassus, home of Apollo and the muses. A host of unruly characters attempt to distract them from their virtuous quest for knowledge with intoxicants and hedonistic poetry. Parnassus, a former student warns, is full of golden phrases, but it is clean out of silver – there is nothing but poverty there.[1]

In this allegorical play from the late 1590s, the upstanding protagonists of *The Pilgrimage to Parnassus* understand that intellectual achievement outshines material wealth. But the play also reminds us that the literature of the Renaissance often depended on metals for the force of its imagery. Ideas about cultural refinement and linguistic purity found apt metaphors and allusions in the metallurgic language of separating true essence from what was inferior or base. The way metals could be transformed through processes of refinement brought together purity and impurity, beauty and corruption, pleasure and utility. 'I, when I value gold, may thinke upon / The ductilleness, the application, / The wholesomeness, the ingenuity, / From rust, from soyle, from fyre ever free', wrote the poet John Donne.[2] For Donne, the pliability of precious metals, the way they could be melted, spun, and twisted, the way they resisted obliteration, made the metalworker something of a poet, and the other way around. But Donne's writings, like those of many poets of the time, were also rife with references to the Americas as the source of the most covetable gold and silver that the world had to offer.

The most abundant source of silver in the time of Donne's writing was not found in Parnassus but on another sacred mountain, located in what is now Bolivia. As Elizabethan courtiers developed schemes for settlements in North America, the Tudors had already long benefited from a colonially sourced commodity found in the mines of Central and South America. In 1545 – Henry VIII was on the throne, busy waging war with France and Scotland – a Quechuan herder came across a vein of silver on a mountain within the jurisdiction of the Viceroyalty of Peru, or so the story went. In some versions, Diego Huallpa came across the vein while herding his llamas through the highlands. He relayed his finding to an Indigenous metallurgist, who was likely in the service of Spanish prospectors already overseeing silver extraction on a small scale in parts of Bolivia and Mexico.

Potosí was silver-rich beyond what could be imagined. Sumaj Urku (meaning 'pleasant or good mountain' in Quechua) or Cerro Rico ('rich mountain' in Spanish) dominated the view from the bustling, multicultural city that soon formed around it. By 1600, this city housed some 100,000 residents. Tens of thousands of Andean men worked in its hundreds of cramped and dangerous mines. Native women cultivated and sold food and cloth in the city's markets. Enslaved West Africans worked in wealthy households and the Royal Mint. Children ran between marketplaces, mills, and municipal buildings as pages and messengers. The large quantities of food and wood needed to keep people alive and operations functioning had to be brought in from outside towns and villages. The work was so dangerous, one Spanish priest observed, that pious converts took the sacrament of communion each time they entered the mines.[3] Death waited in the wings.

In the early 1560s, mercury was found near Huancavelica in the region of Wankawillka ('sacred stone'). Used to extract and refine silver particles from silver ore, this chemical process of amalgamation was more cost efficient than the heating method used before. But it introduced new risks: the deadly emissions that arose from cinnabar-smelting. Spanish Jesuits in the region witnessed the clear effects of mercury poisoning when they administered last rites. Mining involved complex technologies and systems of labour – extracting the metal from the mountain, but also crushing and sorting minerals, mixing reagents such as salt or iron into silver mounds, adding mercury, washing metals, removing amalgams of silver from mercury, and melting the silver into bars or ingots to further process and stamp. Women were involved at various stages, putting themselves at risk of severe illness; and, if they were pregnant, exposure *in utero* risked harming the baby.[4]

Under these hazardous conditions, the boomtown at Potosí went on to produce an estimated 60 to 80 per cent of the world's silver supply. The wealthier poets who wrote their odes to Parnassus may well have dipped their pens in inkwells made from this silver, extracted from an extinct volcano thousands of miles away. How did this silver from Potosí and Mexico make its way into Tudor and Stuart England?

When Mary I married the soon-to-be Philip II of Spain, heir to his father Charles V's vast Atlantic empire, she received South American treasure as a betrothal gift. As part of the public marriage celebrations in October 1554, a procession of carts laden with wedges of silver and gold made their way to the royal treasury, part of Philip's commitment to replenishing England's money supply and furnishing his new royal household in England. At the Tower of London, the load was valued at £40,507, a sum so large that it caused a 7 per cent increase in England's real wealth. In the following decades, a steady stream of 'pieces of eight' – often known as 'Spanish money' – entered into the realm.[5] In 1577, one chronicler noted that, from the time of Queen Mary, 'Spanish money was very common in England, by reason of hir mariage with Philyp King of Spayne.'[6]

These hammered discs of silver, also known as a Spanish *real* or 'cob', were minted across the Americas. Though irregularly shaped – their designs varying depending on which mints they were stamped in – pieces of eight were carefully weighed for accuracy, making them a standard monetary unit used across the globe. Silver *reales* have been found in the wrecks of English ships. In the 1560s and 1570s, Elizabeth's financial agent in Antwerp, Thomas Gresham, coined silver out of *reales*. In 1572, he sent 120 chests of *reales* to the Tower of London.[7] Less directly, silver became responsible for the presence of other covetable goods in England, such as Asian textiles. When the East India Company was established in 1600, many English merchants and agents used silver, which could be sold at a high premium in Asia, to buy the calicoes and porcelain that wealthy Tudors coveted. Behind many luxurious 'Indian' goods in England, therefore, lay the Andean silver that had been re-exported to China and Japan, or shipped across the Pacific to the Spanish port at Manila.

In the sixteenth century, and especially in the second half of Elizabeth's reign, pirates and privateers became crucial economic agents who redirected bullion to the Crown and aristocracy. With England and Spain at war for much of the late Elizabethan period, naval commanders including John Hawkins and Francis Drake became celebrated heroes for their attacks on Spanish forts and ships in the Atlantic. Ambushed storehouses in the jurisdiction of the viceroyalties of Peru and New Spain yielded large amounts of silver from mines in Potosí and Zacatecas. This spike in English piracy coincided with a boom in silver production at Potosí from the 1570s, caused by new refining processes and the development of the *mita* labour system, an Incan practice deployed and repurposed by the Spanish to ensure a steady supply of Indigenous labourers to extract and refine ore. As late as the 1590s, Elizabeth's Secretary of State solicited reports that explained 'the change of the value of money in England and Europe, caused by the discovery of the Indies, and opening of the mines there'.[8]

In the spring of 1573, seven years before he completed his circumnavigation of the globe, Drake made his name by intercepting a Spanish gold and silver train in Panama. In historical retellings, Drake often seems to stumble haphazardly on the rich metals in transit from Potosí to the port of Nombre de Dios. But the operation had involved months of preparation and collaboration with a 'troupe of *Simerons*'. These *cimarróns*, or maroons, were a community of previously enslaved African men and women who resisted Spanish oppression and lived in settlements removed from Iberian oversight, merging with Indigenous communities. The *cimarróns* were integral to Drake's success, helping the English navigate forests and waterways, find sustenance, and avoid enemy settlements.[9] During this time, the English set up their own coastal camps while visiting maroon towns and gathering information along the coast.

Secret Spanish intelligence revealed the centrality of the *cimarróns* in Drake's operations. One eyewitness reported that at least 'twenty of the English, along with forty . . . *cimarrones* with whom they are allied, assaulted the road that passes between this city and that of Nombre Dios'. The English had 'shamelessly opened a door and a path by which they can attack, whenever it suits them, the pack trains that frequent this overland route, which . . . carries to gold and silver of Your Majesty'. These accounts are clear: the *cimarróns*, who often outnumbered the English and were 'very skilled in the things of this land', were far more adept at navigating the terrain.[10] With the assistance of the *cimarróns*, and by joining forces with French privateers,

Drake's famous raids in the 1570s brought several dozen tonnes of silver and gold into England. The exact amount is impossible to verify because state authorities were intent on keeping it secret.

Andrés Sánchez Gallque, an Indigenous artist in Quito, conveyed the power and status of some members of these mixed Central American communities in his 1599 *Portrait of Don Francisco de Arobe and Sons Pedro and Domingo* (also known as *The Mulattos of Esmeraldas*). Francisco de Arobe, born to an enslaved Madagascan man and a Nicaraguan woman, is depicted with his sons, all wearing Spanish fashions, including doublets and ruff collars, as well as gold ornamentation in the Andean style. Arobe had converted to Catholicism and pursued alliances with the Spanish, but this spectacular portrait gives a unique sense of the hybrid environment Drake stepped into when he conducted negotiations with Indigenous and African communities in the region. Twenty years before Sánchez Gallque painted the image, Drake had steered the *Golden Hind* in the vicinity of the Esmeraldas, where Arobe was already an established community leader.

For the next twenty years, English attacks on Spanish settlements brought silver into England along with gold, pearls, and other precious cargo. In Spain, at the Casa de Contratación (the House of Trade of the Indies), state officials read the complaints of governors in the West Indies who had suffered at the hands of 'los corsarios ingleses', English pirates.[11] While Catholic plots brewed and new grammar schools were established to advance classical learning, transatlantic tales recounted sparkling silver wedges stacked high on pack animals; soldiers burying stolen cargo, returning in the veil of night to recover it; and merchant storehouses in Nicaragua, raided for silver, spices, and silks. Arica, a province in Chile, became a repeated target for Drake, Hawkins, and Thomas Cavendish, since the port served as a key entrepot for Potosí silver on its route to

Seville. In 1586, one alderman reported that English privateers had returned with six tonnes of silver; the spoils of two ships from Brazil; and a prominent Spanish admiral as prisoner.[12] After the defeat of the Spanish Armada in 1588, English access to silver became more closely tied to nationalist triumph than ever before. Treasure came into the realm from captured ships on English and Irish shores, while privateers continued to target Spanish galleons further west. The memory of these exploits loomed large in the minds of Jacobeans. Drake's *Golden Hind* had 'traversed the world round, and returned a golden Hinde indeed, with her belly full of Gold and Silver', Samuel Purchas wrote in 1613.[13]

It's impossible to know how much of the silver in England was created from metals extracted in the Americas, but part of that was deliberate obfuscation. In 1602, Elizabeth complained to her officers of the Exchequer that a significant quantity of silver and gold 'embezzled from ships of the Spain navy . . . still remains concealed'.[14] Surviving letters, diaries, reports, and interrogations in the State Papers archives provide ample evidence that hopes for finding and controlling flows of silver remained a matter of government concern. In 1591, an anonymous report offered details about identifying stamped metals that were marked in South America, noting the passage of silver through territories across New Spain and the importance of Lima for minting gold and silver from Peru. Silver and gold flowed to Cartagena in vast quantities, while 'Havana is the key of the Indies, insomuch that he who is Lord of that obtaineth the rest.' 'Great secrecy is needed,' one intelligencer urged, 'for the Spaniards have often prevented the intentions of the English . . . Good ships should be prepared, not many in one place, but scattered in the divers ports with order to meet at the secret appointment.'[15] Details and misinformation circulated about private meetings and covert operations. The activities of those many agents who moved across the seas and through Indigenous lands at the behest of Tudor government officials have been lost to us forever.

As privateers brought sensational cargoes of metals into the realm, other Elizabethans found themselves experiencing life in the mines in Mexico and Peru. In 1567, when he was around thirteen, a boy named Miles Philips sailed on John Hawkins's voyage across the Atlantic. For some fourteen years, Philips travelled through Central America, working in silver mines and Catholic monasteries.

Philips made clear that Hawkins's aim for the voyage was to buy enslaved people on the West Coast of Africa and sell them to the Spanish in the Caribbean. The opening pages of his account describe how the English met Africans near Cape Verde, only to be beaten back in retreat: they 'hurt a great number of our men, so that they were inforced to retire to the ships'. Hawkins later forced 150 people onto his ship, and hundreds more near Sierra Leone. After selling them to the Spanish in the West Indies, Hawkins left Philips and other crew members behind 'northward of *Panuco*'. Philips went on to spend his formative years in the company of 'Indians, or *Mexicans*' and Africans. In the late 1560s and early 1570s, he and his English companions served members of the Spanish elite in Mexico City, as household servants and then as overseers in their mines. In the mines, Philips admitted, 'many of us did profit & gaine greatly'. Sometimes, on Saturdays, enslaved African and Indigenous workers would 'labour for us [blowing silver] ... Sundry weekes we did gaine so much by this meanes besides our wages, that many of us became very rich' by acquiring thousands of pieces of eight.[16]

Philips did not offer a moralising gloss on the silver industry or the brutality of mining life. Drawing on experience and observations, he presented a world populated with Indigenous metalworkers, carpenters, servants, entrepreneurs, and farmers with political systems, alliances, and agendas of their own. He recorded Nahuatl words and took pleasure in eating Native sweet breads made from corn. When the opportunity presented itself, he left his job as an overseer and apprenticed himself to a silk-weaver. Forsaking mines for ribbons, he learned the science and art of weaving taffeta.

In his years in Mexico, Philips lived in the reach of the Inquisition, continually threatened with being 'stript of all, with losse of life also'. He witnessed the ardour of Catholic priests seeking to uproot heresy and stamp out unorthodox beliefs and practices. He may have come across those on public trial for witchcraft, for example; African-descended women who worked as healers faced severe punishments. In 1573, his goods were confiscated and he was imprisoned by the Spanish Inquisition alongside other Englishmen. He escaped death by dint of his age, sentenced to work in a monastery where he might be indoctrinated in the Catholic faith.

Philips and his companion, William, helped oversee the building of a new church. There, 'among [these] Indians I learned their language or Mexican tongue very perfectly, and had great familiaritie with many of them, whom I found to be a courteous and loving kind of people, ingenious, and of great understanding'. In the years that followed, Philips travelled through Mexico and Guatemala, moving between languages as he navigated his surroundings and tried to find a way back home. Occasionally, he was brought before Spanish authorities to be examined about the activities of a certain pesky Englishman named Francis Drake.[17]

Philips tells us he pretended to abandon Protestantism as a strategy for survival, but resisted the Spanish authorities' attempts to see him settle down. He is frank about his companions' marriages to African and Indigenous women. Three men, David Alexander, Robert Cooke, and John Storie, married African women; Paul Horsewell married 'a *Mestisa,* as they name those whose fathers were

Spaniards, and their mothers Indians'. Horsewell's wife was rumoured to be 'the daughter of one that came in with *Hernando Cortes* the Conqueror'. But, as Philips claimed after finding his way back to England, he had always had a longing to return home. Using 'the *Mexican* tongue' and buying a horse with the gold he quilted into his doublet, 'Miguel Perez' eventually found passage to Seville, riding on a fleet laden with silver, cochineal, sugar, and drugs. In Spain, he pretended to be a student who had gone to improve his language skills. He finally found passage to English soil with the help of some pieces of eight.[18]

In 1604, the year after Elizabeth I's death, England and Spain signed a peace treaty, and attacks on Spanish ships were no longer sanctioned by the Crown, even unofficially. The use of 'Spanish silver moneys' persisted, though these were often minted into new coins at the Tower, or exported across the Pacific in the hands of East India Company merchants. In 1613, James issued a proclamation against the use of Spanish silver coins, declaring that 'there is daily brought from forraine Countreis into divers parts of this Kingdome, an exceeding great quantitie of . . . Spanish Moneyes'. These stamped pieces were 'so clipped and impaired' that they caused a 'disturbance betwixt the Buyer and Seller, and the Creditour and Debtour'. Spanish silver should be brought to the Royal Mint in the Tower of London 'to be coyned of new into currant Moneys of this Realme'.[19]

In the Tower, silver from Mexico and Potosí underwent further transformations, stamped with the faces of Stuart rulers and melted into new forms. Large quantities of wedges and bars, acquired directly from the Americas or via Seville, Paris, or Antwerp, were reworked into spoons, devotional objects, cases and boxes, goblets, and table decorations. Large porcelain bowls from China were fixed with bright silver handles. Drinking vessels made from carved coconut shells or ostrich eggs were mounted with silver decorations, embossed with Tudor roses and heraldic lions. Venetian ambassadors attending court dinner parties were awed by 'the great number of silver-gilt vases upon the side-board, piled up to the ceiling'. In giving Drake a gilt cup topped with a tiny replica of the *Golden Hind* sailing the globe, Elizabeth I linked her privateer's exploits to the precious metals that his travels made available. It was rumoured that Drake had furnished his own ship cabin with pure silver, from dining vessels to 'divers shewes of all sorts of curious workmanship', to proclaim 'the civilitie and magnificence of his native countrie' and to celebrate its overseas exploits.[20] The explosion of silver objects in English interiors around the time of Drake's voyages, and the half-century that followed, was unprecedented. Until the English began turning to African gold later in the seventeenth century, after the Restoration, the Americas were fixed in merchant writings as the place 'abounding in Mines of silver and gold'.[21]

Many of the artisans who worked with silver in England were Protestant migrants from the Spanish-ruled Netherlands. They brought a taste for mannerism to English silverworking – an eccentric style of ornamentation that developed in Italy in the 1530s, characterised by foliage and scrolls, marine imagery and grotesque figures. Fantastical iterations of gods straddling dolphins, or twisting flowers with exuberant stems, encircled goblets and silver-gilt ceramics.[22] Glittering or rusted, perfectly curved or clipped and uneven, silver was passed through generations as family heirlooms, left in wills and documented in inventories. Births were commemorated with sugared confections served on silver plates. Servants polished silver cups, and thieves purloined them: goblets and boxes appear as evidence in trials against pickpockets.

It is notoriously difficult to work out the origins of all this silver. In the 1530s, Catholic ceremonial silver had been melted or redistributed after the dissolution of the monasteries, bringing an influx of

Northern European silver into the households of the ruling elite. A hundred years later, silver would be melted down to fund armies and create new coinage during the civil wars, meaning that much Tudor and Stuart silverwork no longer survives – we can't test it even if we wanted to. Elizabeth, in 1574, possessed at least forty sets of silver or silver-gilt ewers and basins, often used to wash hands with scented water after a banqueting course; but less than a dozen sets made in London before 1600 are known to survive.[23] We don't know whether the silver artefacts in princely collections, such as the ewer and basin made for James's son, Henry, by the goldsmith Symon Owen in 1610/1611, are composed of transatlantic metals, though it is tempting to imagine that Henry connected such gifts to his enthusiasm for colonial expansion. Henry had, after all, sent Thomas Roe to the Amazon in February 1610, tasking him with searching for Manoa and other sources of precious metals. Tests on Tudor coins, meanwhile, do contain high amounts of silver from Mexico as well as Europe.[24]

When William Heath, a clerk in the king's navy, compiled a treatise about currency and wealth called *The Goulden Arte* in the early years of the Stuart accession, he knew he couldn't write about metals without discussing the silver mines 'furnished' by God in the mountain at Potosí. Relying in large part on an influential account by the Spanish Jesuit José de Acosta, who had visited Potosí in the 1580s, he explained how the 'force of Silver' had drawn people to the mountain, until it now had 'the greatest trafficke and commerces of all [P]eru'. The Spanish 'had no knowledge of Potozi nor of the wealth therof [until] . . . An Indian Called Gualpa, of the natione of Chumbiblca which is a province of Cusco' had gone hunting in the region. According to this version of events, Gualpa had metalworking experience from the mine at Porco. He took some metal to be tested, keeping his information secret until 'an Indian called Guanca of the Valley of Caura' came to Porco and noticed Gualpa's experimentations, eventually passing this inform-ation to the Spanish.[25]

Heath credited the metalworking knowledge of Indigenous Andeans, and lamented the horrors of the large-scale mining oper-ations that quickly followed. He was Protestant, after all, and the Black Legend was built on tales of Spanish atrocities during and after their conquests. In his section on 'How they Labour in the mines of Potozi', Heath wrote of the hundreds of mines within the mountain, divided between various prospectors. The mines were dark, he wrote, with nothing but candles for light. It was 'a fearefull thing', but the lust for silver had reached such heights that 'men indure any paines . . . and goe huntinge after riches even to the place of the damned'.[26] 'I thinke that more properly this age should be called the golden worlde,' he continued, because 'gold beareth so much swaye'. Humans had once deemed it immoral to break into the realm of Pluto, god of the underworld, 'to get gold and silver[,] the seeds of all mischeefe'.[27] In the decades that followed, Samuel Purchas would articulate the same idea. Precious metals never emerged to light 'but by violence . . . upon records written in bloud'.[28]

Heath was a civil servant, and his condemnation of excessive wealth did not prevent him from supplying information about colo-nial mining that might be useful to projectors. He was writing at a time when the silver and gold fever of the Elizabethan era had begun to develop into new ways of thinking about precious metals. The idea of mercantilism, emerging among some economic and political thinkers in England, was concerned with how best to accumulate and retain wealth within the realm. Most agreed that a balance of trade was the priority, so that England's exports always outweighed its imports.[29] In warning his readers that a golden world was an idol-atrous one, Heath was partly concerned with the circulation of finite resources, and their insufficiency for long-term national prosperity.

When Miles Philips abandoned life in the mines of Mexico to weave fabrics, he was, however accidentally, mirroring a broader pivot in English economic thinking. Even in the midst of silver fever, a staunch counternarrative persisted about national strength and bounty, whereby cloth manufacture won out over the 'cursed riches' of the earth's forged and hammered metals.[30] English merchants, pushing for the expansion of their cloth industry to other parts of the world, expressed the belief that 'honest', homespun cloth would provide the basis for a greater empire than one built on extraction: 'our *Wooll* [is] so rich a Jewell . . . that it exceeds in worth the *Spanish Silver Mines* in *Western India*'.[31] Who needed gold, the Welsh colonial promoter William Vaughan asked in 1626, when the English had their 'Golden Fleece'? Vaughan cited the classical myth of Jason's quest for the fleece of a magical ram or sheep, one that had long served as the emblem of English drapers and cloth merchants. Grazing sheep on estates and farms on both sides of the Atlantic, not extracting minerals, would be '*Great Britaines Indies,* never to be exhausted dry'.[32]

Emphasising manufacture over metals enabled English colonial administrators to endorse their own emerging colonies as microcosms of agricultural England, ripe for husbandry, rather than as sites of mass industrial exploitation. Potosí served as shorthand for avarice and corruption, representing an economic model that prioritised short-term gain. Ben Jonson satirised the culture of global projecting in *The Staple of Newes* (1631), in which Lady Pecunia, personifying money, breathes a sigh of relief when she discovers that her pedigree partially locates her in the 'rich *mynes* of *Potosi*'. By the time of the Restoration, one author condemned the 'slimy path' to 'steep *Potosí*': 'Better the latter World had ne're been known, / Than thus to swallow up the former one' through greed.[33]

The lives of Indigenous and African miners and farmers are rarely considered in histories of English silver, but they are there when we look for them, nestled in secret intelligence reports, manuscripts about metallurgy, and unlikely travel accounts by English teenagers. Andean mountain ranges and conquistadors may seem far removed from English banqueting tables, but the division that Protestant writers created between the cruel Spanish and the liberating English collapses when silver comes into the picture. When we follow the money, Mexico and the Bolivian highlands are part of English history, too.

The connections have partly been lost because malleable, shifty silver has evaded our grasp, transmuting from raw ore to wedge, coin to cup, making it difficult to trace its origins and its many possible forms. But English connections to Indigenous lives and labour have also been lost because Elizabethans and Jacobeans preferred it that way. It was morally convenient to view Native labour as the product of the cruel systems of other nations. As the moon-white gleam of silver drew captains and their ships across the Atlantic, English merchants, politicians, and economic thinkers justified their access to silver by emphasising the brutality of Spain's large-scale mining operations. Potosí became a kind of anti-Parnassus, a place where creativity and the nobility of human endeavours went to die. But English involvement in trafficking and acquiring silver also became the means through which travellers and wealthy consumers developed their own sophisticated tastes. Coins and mannerist drinking vessels, but also calicoes and porcelain purchased in Asia with American silver, are testaments to what these shifting flows of metals enabled, and took away.

When writers began to make explicit connections between Parnassus and the landscapes of the Americas in the early seventeenth century, they kept Potosí out of the picture. In poems prefacing a 1602 mock epic about tobacco, it is not silver but the divine leaf that sprouts on the hills of Parnassus, before the muses find it in greater abundance in North America. The colonial investor William Vaughan set his discussion of the benefits of Newfoundland's colonisation in Parnassus' amphitheatre. Verses dedicated to the courtier Susan Herbert, Countess of Montgomery, described the goddess Flora decorating the arid lands around Parnassus with flowers and 'Cuchenella' – cochineal from Mexico.[34]

To describe the stark divide between flourishing ecosystems and extractive wastelands on the border between Mexico and Guatemala, the traveller Thomas Gage also evoked that mythical mountain. Gazing over one of the region's active volcanoes, one might 'fancy a new *Parnassus,* find out new steps of flying *Pegasus,* and greet the Nymphes', he wrote. But the other side of the mountain was a horror to behold, full of ash and shadow. In the place of whispering waters and murmuring fountains, one heard the 'thunders and roaring of consuming metals . . . a Paradise on the one side and a hell on the other'.[35] While Renaissance writers pursued the silver words and golden phrases sparked and polished in Parnassus, the volcanoes and mines in the Americas rumbled and churned. If you stood in the right place, it all came into view.

'A Guiana Idoll of gold & copper'

In the summer of 1618, a fallen favourite facing death clambered into a rowboat and tried to flee to France. On his finger, he wore a diamond ring, a cherished gift from a long-dead queen, harking back to the days when he had been adored by Elizabeth herself. He also carried a less expected object, one that had been crafted far from the artisans' workshops of London: a copper-and-gold figure made by Indigenous metallurgists, acquired somewhere in the tropical forests of the Amazon.

This was Walter Ralegh's second recent attempt at evading his captors, but it was a half-hearted one, and he was soon wrested back into custody. Several months later, he was dead, executed on the orders of Elizabeth's successor, James I, who had always harboured contempt for him. When authorities drew up an inventory of everything Ralegh had been carrying with him at his arrest, the Indigenous artefact appeared first on the list. All we know of this figure is contained in these few words: 'A Guiana Idoll of gold & copper'. Likely a sacred entity, perhaps intended to be buried next to the body of a deceased ruler, it had travelled into a land whose beholders viewed it as an alien thing, used as evidence of the marvellous possibilities for precious metals in Arawak and Warao lands along the Orinoco Delta of what is now Venezuela.

For centuries, Indigenous metallurgists had used a process known as depletion gilding to give copper-and-gold alloys an appearance of pure gold, removing the base metals from the surface with plant extracts or mineral salts. To the Kalinago in the Caribbean who traded for gold in South America, these alloys were fashioned into bodily adornments known as *guanín* to the Taíno. The power of the metals lay in their colour, shape, and symbolic associations; in one Taíno myth, *guanín,* formed into crescents, related to the rainbow bridge that connected sky and underworld.[1] On the mainland, these figures, fashioned into frogs, bats, and jaguars, are known as *tumbaga,* a Southeast Asian term (possibly carried to Mexico via the Philippines) which came to refer to the copper-gold alloys from Central and South America.[2]

The English had already encountered *tumbaga* in travel books by the time Ralegh carried his. Some might have seen them in the cabinets of wealthy European patrons in the aftermath of Columbus' voyages. In 1583, an English translation of an earlier account of the Spanish invasion of the Americas described the 'copper and gylt' furnishings found in Guatemala, 'resembling golde' and taken by conquistadors.[3] Other accounts reported similar processes of mixing gold or silver with copper in jewellery among the Timucua in Florida, who created copper necklaces mixed with silver.[4]

The 'Guiana idoll' was one of many objects found on Ralegh at his capture that pertained to his singular obsession with South America. Authorities confiscated a seal set in gold with 'Guinana oare [ore] tyed to it'; wedges of fine and coarse gold; sixty-three gold buttons sparkling with diamonds; maps of Panama, Guiana, and the Orinoco River; reports on silver mining trials; and a description of chemical trials on Guiana ore.[5] Clinquant with minerals, the old courtier had made his escape as a sort of pedlar of American ecosystems, a walking advertisement for his decades-long infatuation with El Dorado, known to the Arawaks of the region as Manoa. 'Golde is our fate,' the poet George Chapman had written, weaving Guiana into the heroic future of the nation through its most enticing material.

To understand the significance of this object in Ralegh's possession, we need to go back further in time. In the 1580s, with Hakluyt in Paris acquiring codices and intelligence about Florida and Brazil, a tall, curly-haired Ralegh rose through the ranks at court, capturing the queen's fancy and acquiring land through colonial warfare in Ireland. As he built his fortunes, he retained close connections to his native Devon and his family's seafaring heritage. The adventurer Humphrey Gilbert was his half-brother, likely encouraging Ralegh's initial interests in North America. In 1592, however, following the collapse of the Roanoke colony, Ralegh fell into catastrophic disfavour after secretly marrying the courtier Elizabeth Throckmorton. *The Discoverie of Guiana* (1596), Ralegh's strange, entirely unreliable narrative about his first voyage to Guiana in 1595, is as much about finding a way back into court life as it is about encouraging trade and settlement in Greater Amazonia. It's as if Ralegh had become convinced that only the rivers of the Orinoco Basin would bring him safely through the labyrinth of the London court.

For many Tudors and Stuarts, Guiana embodied all the untold riches that the Americas still might contain, nearly a century after the Spanish first arrived there. In 1584, in an unpublished treatise written to endorse English colonisation, Hakluyt noted that vast regions in the Americas were occupied 'onely [by] the Caribes, Indians, and salvages [*sic*]', just waiting for English intervention.[6] In addition to Ralegh's voyages in 1595 and 1617, journeys were carried out by seafarers including Lawrence Kemys, Leonard Berry, Robert Harcourt, John Ley, Thomas Roe, Philip Purcell, William White, and Matthew Morton.[7]

Councillors kept themselves informed on English navigators employed by European rulers, too. In 1608, the captain Robert Thornton carried out a voyage to what is now French Guyana on behalf of Ferdinando I, Grand Duke of Tuscany. The English

Ambassador in Venice conceded that Italian voyages to Guiana were mostly possible due to the English mariners, shipwrights, and pirates under the duke's protection, who were experienced in travelling to the region.[8] Thornton promised his Florentine patron rosewood, wild sugarcane, marmosets, and cotton, but he also brought 'five or six Indians . . . which were of those Caribs, who eat human flesh'. These travellers reportedly spoke of Guiana's fertile lands, including 'a very rich mine of silver, which they called Perota'. This resuscitated hopes for Manoan splendours among a number of Englishmen, even as 'the Countries did affoord no such thing', as one surgeon on Thornton's journey flatly wrote.[9]

Since the Spanish invasion of Peru, the English had ravenously collected hearsay about extravagant riches hidden away in South America. Then, one day, Elizabeth's eccentric darling decided to find them for himself. Much of Ralegh's information about Manoa derived from conversations with a Spanish captive of his, Antonio de Berrío, who had conducted multiple expeditions in the 1580s in search of a kingdom of gold in the Orinoco Delta. It was through Berrío that Ralegh apparently got his hands on a testimony by the soldier Juan Martín de Albújar, who claimed to have been taken, blindfolded, to Manoa in 1569. For seven months, the Spanish soldier lived among the splendours of the palace, gaining enough favour with the city's emperor to be given a great store of gold at his departure. But soon after embarking home, the Orenoqueponi robbed Martín of his treasure, leaving him with only two gourds, filled with gold beads, that they tossed aside, assuming them to be food vessels. At his death, Martín delivered his testimony to a priest, offering up a *calabaza,* or gourd, full of gold beads as proof of his story.[10]

Equipped with a Catholic soldier's deathbed testimony and the intelligence of his Spanish captive, Ralegh gathered every rumour, every story of treasure or the briefest sighting of gold. For Ralegh,

'Indian gold' lay at the heart of Renaissance politics, for those 'princes which a bound in treasure have great advantages over the rest'.[11] South American gold mines, and the 'curiously wrought' *tumbagas* created by Indigenous metalworkers, showed 'riches and rarenes most marveilous & exceding al[l] in *Europe,* and I think of the world'. Even as he sought mass stores of gold, Ralegh acknowledged Indigenous goldworking and flourishing trade networks. Male and female lapidaries and metalsmiths traded gold for animals or dyewoods in market hubs along the Orinoco River. He seemed aware of the importance of the legendary region of Lake Parime/Manoa as a site of spiritual and political power.[12] For Ralegh, however, this wealth was conveniently destined for the English, according to an ancient Peruvian prophecy that had foretold that 'from *Inglatierra* those *Ingas* shoulde be again in time to come restored, and delivered from the servitude of the said Conquerors'.[13] There was a natural connection, a linguistic slipperiness, between 'Inga' and 'Inglatierra'. A common enemy might create a new world order, an alliance between England and South America – an idea he would revisit in that court entertainment staged for Elizabeth shortly after his return home.

Although Ralegh seemed intent on finding 'the greate and golden citie of Manoa', to the point of obsession – a palpable hunger and desperation pulses through his account of the journey – he navigated the waterways of the Orinoco Basin with the assistance of countless local inhabitants, 'those nations which are called *Arwacas* which dwell on the south of *Orenoque,* (of which place and nation our Indian Pilot was)'.[14] To get anywhere, Ralegh relied on 'my Indian interpreter, which I carried out of England', an almost haphazard acknowledgement of the presence of Arawakan and possibly Carib/Kalina or Warao individuals in London, depending on where these Indigenous guides initially came from. His 'Indian Pilot called *Ferdinando*', 'old Pilot of the *Ciawani* [Warao]', and 'my new hired

Pilot *Martin* the *Arawacan*' played key roles in negotiating between the English, Spanish, and local groups, probably communicating in Spanish. There was also the African man in Ralegh's retinue who met his violent end when a caiman attacked him in the water.[15]

As he navigated and charted the rivers, Ralegh established an alliance with Topiawari, the *casique* or ruler of the Orenoqueponi.[16] Topiawari's son, Cayowaroco, went on to accompany Ralegh to London, along with several others. Worried about the safety of his son in the midst of escalating conflict with the Spanish and their Indigenous allies, Ralegh claimed that the elderly Topiawari 'freely gave me his onely sonne to take with me into England', hoping that 'by our meanes his sonne shoulde be established after his death'.[17] Ralegh also brought an Indigenous boy to London who was baptised in Chelsea in 1597 and christened Charles. In return, Ralegh left two young servants, Francis Sparrow and Hugh Goodwin, in Topiawari's settlement.

By conversing with Topiawari, Ralegh learned more about the Epuremei, a local group rumoured to possess many golden objects. Like their Manoan counterparts, the Epuremei gathered pure gold nuggets from the rivers and 'put it to a part of copper … [mingling] gold & copper together' to make 'plates and Images'.[18] This description of creating *tumbagas* was not unlike the translator Richard Eden's description in *The Decades of the Newe Worlde* (1555), an influential compendium of transatlantic intelligence published during the reign of Mary I. Most of the gold in the Americas, Eden wrote, contained copper, but 'the Indians can very excellently gylte such vesselles of copper and base gold … [so] that all the masse whiche they gylte, appeareth as though it were of golde'. This 'secreate maner of gyldynge' made the artefacts appear as though made by the finest goldsmiths of Italy or Spain.[19] 'I have sent your Honours, of two sorts [of *tumbagas*] as such I could by chance recover,' Ralegh reminded Charles Howard, Earl of Nottingham, and the State Secretary Robert Cecil.[20] The fate of these figures is unknown, but perhaps they ended up in a curiosity cabinet or on a desk at Cecil's stately home in Hertfordshire.

Ralegh sought to make clear that he had not sent the figures as valuable gifts, but to give a sense of how they had been made. He knew they contained copper. Anxieties over the value of Indigenous goldwork went back to the writings of conquistadors, who complained that they had been deceived into believing the objects contained pure gold. In reality, the shimmering gold surfaces were the expert effects of deliberate chemical transformation. The Indigenous cultures that produced them did not intrinsically value gold in and of itself. What they valued was its brilliance, the way it connected humans to other forces through its light, signalling a connection to divinity. Gold is just stuff, the Sápara activist Manari Ushigua maintains, signalling little without the ceremonies and songs that allow the bearer to connect to the 'vital cycles' of nature – to the sound, texture, and movement of the rainforest.[21] There is nothing false about a play on light, or the alchemical artistry of an Arawakan or Muisca metalworker.

Even as he collected examples of Indigenous metalworking, Ralegh kept his sights on his patroness, Elizabeth. He distributed coins with the queen's image to those he met. As with painted miniatures, coins could be worked into jewellery and worn against the body. 'I gave among them . . . the new money of 20. shillings with her Majesties picture to weare,' Ralegh wrote, 'which they so admired and honoured.'[22] Everywhere he went, Ralegh seemed intent on reminding Elizabeth that she had been there with him, worshipped to an extent that bordered on idolatry. He assured her that he had conveyed her majesty with the help of interpreters by introducing himself as the servant of a queen who was 'the great *Casique* of the north, and a virgin, and had more *Casique* under her [than] there were trees in that land'. In the Orinoco Delta, Ralegh claimed, Elizabeth was known as '*Ezrabeta Cassipuna Aquerewana*', reconfiguring the Virgin Queen as an Arawakan *cacique*.[23] Somewhere in the soil, perhaps swept through the extreme floods of the earth's largest hydrological system, there might still be a profile portrait of Elizabeth I on a coin, her face eroded by a life submerged.

In another attempt to amuse Elizabeth, Ralegh reported rumours of a sensational all-female society who lived just beyond Guiana's bounds. The existence of Amazons harked back to classical mythology, which located them in places ranging from Greece to Africa. Tales of skilled women warriors who fought in battles and used men for pleasure appealed to elite Tudor ladies, who lived in an exhilarating and unprecedented moment for women in English politics. Every time they picked up their copy of the English edition of the Bible, produced by the Church of England in 1568, they could see a portrait of their queen, holding symbols of earthly and spiritual authority, flanked by virtues personified as women. In the aftermath of the 1588 defeat of the Spanish Armada, verses likened Elizabeth to an Amazon, 'a virago against men'.[24]

Once a year, for the space of a month – Ralegh gathered this was in April, an optimal time for a frolic – the 'queens' of the Amazons brought the kings of the area together, and 'cast lots for their *Valentines*', feasting, dancing, and drinking for a month. If they conceived and gave birth to a son, they returned the child to the father. If 'a daughter [is born] they nourish it, and retaine it, and as many as have daughters send unto the begetters a Present, all being desirous to increase their owne sex and kind'.[25] This Amazonian interlude brings a moment of levity to Ralegh's narrative. One imagines a lady at court, or a merchant's wife taking a break in her accounting, pausing to appreciate the lives and freedom of these women and their valentines. In a matrilineal society, having a daughter is not a disappointment, but a blessing. Somewhere in the world, women can live beyond the control of men. Somewhere, girls inherit everything.

Ralegh's hopes of finding a mythical city of gold never materialised. The Amazon and Orinoco's waterways, flowing across millions of square miles, swelled in floods and ebbs, interfering with plans for settlement. The rivers' seasonal flows washed over the land that Ralegh so desperately wanted to claim, sometimes submerging the lowlands entirely, threatening to carry travellers far from their ships.

After his return, Ralegh gained some glory in the capture of Cádiz in 1596, though there, too, hopes of acquiring Atlantic silver from Spanish vessels failed. In 1603, after Elizabeth's death, he was imprisoned in the Tower under suspicion of treason for his involvement in a plot to put James I's cousin, Arabella Stuart, on the throne. In his Tower chambers, Ralegh busied himself conducting botanical and alchemical experiments and writing a magisterial history of the world. Occasionally, he wrote letters to James's queen, Anna of Denmark, asking her to convince King James to pursue projects in Virginia and Guiana. The Arawakan interpreters who accompanied him to England continued to visit him in the Tower, perhaps advising him on his plant studies, or partaking in the tobacco that Ralegh kept rolled up with some clay pipes, in a leather pouch. Among them were Leonard Ragapo, 'the Indien who [had] bine with me in Ingland 3 or 4 years', and Harry, who 'had lived with mee in the tower 2 yeers'. Both would find their way to Guiana again. In 1609, Robert Harcourt encountered Leonard in the region and remembered that he had been 'heretofore in England with S[i]r *Walter Raleigh*, to whom hee beareth great affection'.[26]

In 1617, twenty-two years after he first navigated the Amazon, Ralegh went back. James I hated his predecessor's old favourite, but the prospect of bullion was too enticing. The king had inherited many of Elizabeth's debts, and spent extravagant amounts of money on drinking dens and hunting lodges of his own. No matter how lofty the justifications for colonial projects could be, the Crown supported such schemes in large part because they were a relatively low-risk way to make potentially high gains. Looking back on the ill-fated second venture, one book about Ralegh's trial commented that, although the king – showing all the good taste and discernment that a monarch should display – was sceptical of those promises of untold riches, 'neverthelesse Sir *W. Raleigh* had so enchanted the world . . . as his Majesties honour was in a manner engaged'. Moreover, the project aligned with the king's desire to 'nourish and incourage Noble and Generous enterprises, for Plantations, Discoveries, and opening of new Trades'.[27]

The journey was a catastrophe. Ralegh had promised the peace-loving James that he would avoid conflict with Spain. Recovering from a severe illness on board ship, he was not present when his longtime associate Lawrence Kemys attacked the Spanish settlement of San Tomé, causing a diplomatic furore in Europe. Ralegh lost his own beloved son Walter in the fight, and Kemys felt so racked with guilt about the outcome of the raid that he soon took his own life. The Spanish Ambassador in London, Diego Sarmiento de Acuña, Count Gondomar, used the whole debacle to press for Ralegh's execution and to try to quell English encroachments on Spanish-claimed lands.

Were Indigenous people in the crowd to witness Ralegh's demise on that late October day in 1618? A man named Guayacunda, known as Christopher to the English, may have been among those who saw him alive in his final moments. Guayacunda, from Sogamoso in present-day Colombia, had been serving the Spanish Governor of San Tomé when the English attacked it. He had come to London, Ralegh's gaoler reported, because of his purported knowledge of some '7 or 8 mynes of Gold'. The man 'who is now with me', Ralegh insisted, 'could have led [the English] to two gold mines . . . as well as to a silver mine' just a short way from the Spanish fort, had Ralegh only had more time.[28]

Even in the moments of Ralegh's death, Guiana, and perhaps his old interests in Algonquian Roanoke and Timucua Florida, lingered. Ralegh reportedly smoked tobacco in his cell before his journey to the scaffold. His dying speech included mention of that 'enterprise for a gold mine'. Some of his final words were directed to his friend Thomas Howard, Earl of Arundel. Ralegh recalled how Arundel had boarded the ship before that last journey, urging him to return regardless of what might happen in faraway lands. Arundel's concern seems to suggest that even those close to Ralegh viewed his voyage as foolhardy. But Arundel would also carry on Ralegh's legacy, attempting to establish new trading companies in South America in the years that followed.

Plans were quickly afoot to establish the Amazon Company, which might, like the Virginia or East India companies, help pour riches and marvellous objects into the realm while furthering English imperial aims. As English captains, metalworkers, and apothecaries scoured the banks of the Amazon with the help of their Indigenous guides, navigating its waters with galleys and canoes, Londoners met in the houses of merchants and aristocrats, planning ventures to Venezuela and Peru. In 1620, on Thursdays at two o'clock, leading courtiers met in Arundel's house on the Strand to confer about Amazonian affairs, discussing their hopes for cacao and cinnamon, yams and cashews, sugar and 'sheep of Peru'.[29] Sometimes, when the Duke of Buckingham sat drinking with James and Prince Charles, the topic would turn to the Indies, and the Spanish Ambassador, Gondomar, would get notoriously prickly about the subject. Letter-writers gossiped about how a disagreement over South American affairs had ruptured at a table at court, disgracing those involved and amusing all those who witnessed it.

By his death, Ralegh's chivalric brand of colonial fantasy seemed quaint and impractical. For the Trinidadian-British writer, V. S. Naipaul, Ralegh's strange romance was an elegy for a changing world, cataloguing an improbable knightly quest at a time of escalating plantation, industry, and enslavement in the region.[30] How assured Ralegh had been, the colonial adventurer Robert Harcourt wrote in 1613, of 'gaining to our Countrey inestimable riches, and subduing to the Crowne of *England* a potent Empire.'[31] Despite his admiration for Ralegh, Harcourt's own 1609 voyage in search of minerals, 'golden Mountaines', and suitable places for plantation left him frustrated. Those 'intelligences (of Mines already found) I had from other men in England', he admitted, 'I found them by experience false, and nothing true concerning Mines, that was in England reported unto me.'[32] Ralegh's text belonged in libraries and studies, Harcourt implied, but more for its myth-making than its geographical precision.

In the aftermath of his execution, criticisms of Ralegh's adventures included accusations that he had not gone to America prepared to conduct the hard work of actually extracting resources. He had brought pickaxes and shovels only for show. He had followed the stories of local inhabitants and interpreters, desperate for gold to fall into his lap like a fable in Ovid's *Metamorphoses*. He had enchanted the world, but he had been enchanted by it, too.

Of course, Ralegh hadn't actually returned from his voyages empty-handed. An 'image of Copper made in Guiana, which held a third part gold', had been among the transatlantic objects tested by refiners in 1590s London, along with those Ralegh gave to Howard and Cecil.[33] These gold-and-copper alloys introduced Londoners to longstanding Indigenous metalworking traditions. Harcourt, perhaps with the help of his Native interpreter, Anthony Canabre, had been given 'a halfe

Moone of mettall, which held somwhat more then a third part Gold, the rest Copper', 'a little Image of the same mettall', and 'a plate of the same (which hee called a spread Eagle)', images 'by them called *Carrecoory* [*caracoli* in Kalinago]'.[34]

As for the 'Guiana Idoll of gold & copper' found on Ralegh at his arrest? It may have been the same figure he had brought out of Guiana decades before, or one of the number of others that found their way to London from the many South American voyages that followed. The papers and sparkling items Ralegh carried in his desperate escape – diamond ring, copper-and-gold alloy – were an unusual assemblage, testaments to his interest in Atlantic projecting and to that Renaissance fascination with alchemical knowledge and the mystical power of metals. Ralegh struck his captors as somewhat madcap; a charlatan clinging to trinkets while his hour of death loomed, hatching a plan to flee to France to beguile other monarchs with tales of gold. We cannot know, but among the charts and reports, perhaps the *tumbaga* held a more personal significance for Ralegh. For decades, he had conferred with and learned from Indigenous nations, in South America and in London. Harry and Leonard had lived with him in the Tower. Manteo and Wanchese had lodged with him at Durham House. Native peoples had supplied the cassava that nourished him back to health months before, as he lay ailing in his ship. We can only imagine what the councillors thought of the figure when they confiscated it, laying it on the table for cataloguing alongside the maps of the Amazon's branching rivers. Perhaps its burnished surface flashed in the light, reminding Ralegh of the sun hitting the Orinoco Delta. Glimmering, diamond-bright, like some truth that lay ever behind human understanding.

Boy with a
Pearl Earring

The divers left the camps at daybreak. Past the thatched dwellings and hammocks, past the armed guards and the locked chests that store the supply of pearls, they carried their baskets, knives, and ropes to water's edge. Over the spray of the waves, they boarded canoes carved from local trees and paddled out to the place of harvest. As dawn seeped over scrublands and Caribbean waters, fleets of several dozen canoes rocked in the breeze. The boats were occupied by men who had been brought to Venezuela's shores from Sierra Leone, Senegambia, and Brazil.

By weighing themselves down with a rock, the divers could make their descent more quickly. Underwater, the temperatures grew colder. Holding their breaths for extraordinary periods of time, they swam deeper, fending off sharp-toothed creatures in search of pearl-bearing molluscs. All day, they dived into the sea and back to the surface, plucking oysters from their rocky beds. As they filled their bags, agents of the Spanish Crown looked on, ensuring their moments of rest were only long enough to enable them to carry out the work.

Across the Atlantic, an Elizabethan poet playfully chided the sun for interrupting his sleep. He was entwined in the arms of his mistress. Go chide school boys and apprentices, the dishevelled speaker commands, blinking in the light. Go see whether the riches of the Indies are really in America, or whether they lie here with me.[1]

The pearls that writers imagined spilling from the earth in such abundance were the result of large-scale colonial operations that had been in place for about a century. In the early 1500s, Lucayan conch divers from the Bahamas were trafficked to Cumaná and Cubagua Island to fish for pearls. As with sugar-plantation labour in Brazil, the Spanish and Portuguese soon began replacing Indigenous with African workers in far greater numbers. As ramshackle settlements developed along what became known as the Pearl Coast in eastern Venezuela and its nearby islands, pearls entered Tudor England on an unprecedented scale.

For centuries, pearls had been sourced in the Indian Ocean, especially the Persian Gulf, and in freshwater streams in Scotland and Sweden. But Columbus' third Atlantic voyage drastically altered supply and demand. In the decades after 1498, millions of Atlantic pearls flooded into Europe. These sea gems came to adorn jewellery, purses, clothing, fans, book coverings, garden grottoes, devotional objects, even toothpicks. Smaller, cheaper seed pearls decorated buttons and purses, and were sold in apothecary shops alongside coral and bezoar stones. Merchants and goldsmiths sent their agents to inspect ships arriving from the West Indies, their cargoes rumoured to be laden with these gems. The large irregular pearls that Portuguese merchants called *barroco*, from which we get 'baroque', brought a dash of irreverence. Boys with pearl earrings skulked and pranced around the English court. Satirists scoffed at the nation's prodigal sons, who spent too much time preening themselves with 'haires curl'd, eares pearl'd'.[2]

How did the secretions of molluscs, triggered by unwelcome substances lodged in a bivalve's mantle, become such a sought-after commodity in England? How important were pearls' distinct associations with the sea? And what did empire have to do with it? For the Roman Pliny, whose first-century writings on pearls were endlessly cited in the Renaissance, pearls were emblematic of the folly behind people's desire for things. Humans were infinitely strange creatures, he wrote, and pearls were a prime example of their inexplicable obsessions. Women bedecked their hair and clothes with them, even their shoes. It did not suffice to accessorise oneself in them, 'but they must tread upon pearles, goe among pearles, and walke as it were on a pavement of pearles', as the Stuart translator Philemon Holland wrote in his edition of Pliny's *Natural History*. Pliny cited the famous story of the fairest pair of pearls ever known, 'the singular and only jewels of the world, and even Natures wonder', possessed by Cleopatra. When the enamoured Mark Antony failed to impress the Egyptian queen with his opulent banquets, he defied her to surpass his lavish spending. Cleopatra invited Antony to a supper of her own. When Antony smugly commented that the meal had hardly been more luxurious than those he regularly offered her, Cleopatra took a priceless pearl from one ear, steeped it in vinegar until it dissolved, and drank it, winning the wager.[3] Where pearls went, wasteful extravagance followed.

In their luminescence, pearls symbolised purity, even divinity. Through their inception in oysters deep within mysterious seas, they evoked sex and carnal desire, formed as 'a certain moist dew as a seed, wherewith they swell and grow big'. Fair, white pearls had been forged with pure and clear matter, Pliny wrote, while dim or dusky pearls, 'grosse and troubled', were conceived under dark and foreboding storms. Pearls only made it into human society through the violence of greed. Pliny had seen Lollia Paulina, third wife of the Emperor Caligula, clad in rows of pearls, glittering like the sun. But her pearls were gifts from her profligate husband and inheritances from martial relatives, acquired 'by the robbing and spoiling of whole provinces'. Pliny lamented the folly of humankind, where 'there is nothing that goeth to the pampering and trimming of this our carcasse . . . that is not bought with the utmost hasard, and costeth not the venture of mans life! . . . The richest merchandise of all, and the most soveraigne commodity throughout the whole world are these Pearles.'[4]

Pliny's writings about pearls were widely quoted by sixteenth-century chroniclers and travellers, and by merchants who puzzled over how to value the new West Indies varieties. Spanish and English writers combined Pliny's critiques of imperial extraction with details about the particular conditions of the enslaved people who now cultivated the gems under perilous conditions. The story of Cleopatra dissolving her pearl became a means for writers to reflect that 'these were the follies of those ages, and those at this day are nothing lesse, for that we see, not onely hattes and bandes, but also buskins, and womens pantofles [slippers] . . . imbrodred all over with pearle'. The Jesuit chronicler José de Acosta reported on pearl fishing, 'the which is done with great change & labour of the poore slaves', who skilfully but perilously navigated the waters with their canoes. The sea was very cold, and divers were frequently expected to hold their breaths for minutes on end.[5] Divers were also found closer to home. In 1545, when Henry VIII's ship, the *Mary Rose,* sank in English waters, the Guinea-born diver Jacques Francis, in the employ of a Venetian salvage operator, led the team to recover lost weapons.

Strings of pearls could signal refined, even modest decorum, but they also offered 'a riot of tastes', as the historian Molly Warsh writes, full of 'paradoxical binaries'. In a biblical parable, pearls appeared to stand in for all the earthly wealth that a devout follower should give up for the greater gift of salvation – a moral lesson that Protestants regularly drew on to denounce earthly riches (nowhere more beautifully than in George Herbert's poem, 'The Pearl'). For Catholics, pearls could align the wearer to the immaculate Virgin Mary, or even Christ. Steeped in symbolism and the world of commerce, their bright essences were holy and earthly, evoking heavenly purity and the risky voyages provoked by the desires of the fallen. In their fragility and susceptibility to decay, they offered pious reminders of the transience of life. But they also *caused* death, 'pulled from their aqueous origins with varying degrees of violence'.[6] Pearl fishing imperilled human life and disrupted ecologies. For every pearl found in a shell, another ten bivalves might be opened and found lacking, cracked at the hinge and discarded on the shore.

In the early sixteenth century, as Henry VIII acceded to the throne, Spanish colonists received permission from their monarchs Ferdinand and Isabella to expand their pearl fisheries, subject to the same 'royal fifth' (*quinto*) tax levied against all precious goods coming from the Americas. Their grandson, Charles V, received some 34.5 million pearls from Central and South America over the course of his reign.[7] When he visited England in 1520, Charles might have gifted some of these to Henry VIII and members of his court. But Henry's connections to the Spanish Crown, and the wealth he amassed through transatlantic traffic, had come much earlier.

In 1509, Henry married Catherine of Aragon, Ferdinand and Isabella's youngest daughter. For over twenty years, before Henry divorced her, Catherine actively participated in Anglo-European political and military affairs. She arrived in England with a diverse household of her own, including Catalina, a 'Moor' from Motril, Granada – a longstanding Islamic territory that had been conquered by Catherine's parents – and several unnamed people described by the humanist Thomas More as 'pygmies from Ethiopia', possibly young Black pages.[8] In Catherine's portraits, her velvets and silks are stitched with shimmering, cream-coloured pearls. In one portrait, she holds a monkey – perhaps a capuchin brought from the tropical forests of the Americas. Henry's marriage to the daughter of these powerful monarchs signalled the burgeoning Tudor dynasty's connections to Atlantic wealth and colonial splendour.

In 1554, Henry and Catherine's daughter Mary I married Charles V's son, Philip. The prince presented her with a table-cut diamond set in a large, pear-shaped pearl pendant – a jewel so lustrous and exorbitant that it appeared in multiple portraits of the queen during her short reign. For a long time, the enormous pearl was believed to be La Peregrina, a notoriously expensive and brilliant gem that eventually ended up in the hands of Hollywood royalty. The English node in the story of its provenance seems unlikely, but Mary's pearl still ranks among the largest ever found. It is likely that it, too, was sourced in Panama or on the Pearl Coast. Through her husband, Mary had again tied England to a royal family with claims to huge stretches of land across the Atlantic. Her access to such an unparalleled gemstone made a bold statement about her own political ambitions.

The memory of such megapearls from the Americas loomed large in the Elizabethan imagination. Writing about the 'expert [African] swimmers and great divers' who harvested oysters and hunted for pearls, the privateer Richard Hawkins claimed to have opened many oysters with his own hands on Margarita Island in 1583, 'and tooke the Pearles of them, some great, some lesse, and in good quantitie'. Even in the midst of the costliest pearls, shining with 'fierie flames' of light, Hawkins could not help but recall 'la Peregrina, for the rarenesse of it, being as big as the pomell of a Poniard'. In Hawkins's revealing comparison, beauty and violence are inextricable; he compares the infamous pearl to the ornamentation on a dagger. His description reinforced just how closely pearls had come to be associated with Elizabethan courtliness. Pearls lay under many pleats and folds, he wrote, nestled in a part of the oyster 'called the Ruffe, for the similitude it hath unto the Ruffe'.[9] In the anatomy of an Atlantic shell lay the intricate folds of a collar.

Elizabeth I's obsessive use of pearls brought them to the height of fashion. What they lacked in rarity they made up for in intricate variety. In a single year, 1586, an 'Account of pearls delivered to the Queen' revealed a delivery of pearls of different sizes and qualities to the value of £644, a sum far surpassing what a wage labourer might make in a lifetime.[10] Gone was the grave, unforgiving sternness of Mary and her singular oversized pearl. Pearls were affixed to pendants, strung onto ropes of necklaces, and sewn into embellished velvet gowns, flickering and glowing in nearly all surviving images of Elizabeth and her courtiers. Pearls on clothing were detachable and could be given as secret tokens of love or favour, incorporated into an earring or a glove. One can imagine them snagging on furniture or armour, rolling down tiled floors and across corridors, lost or exchanged in wagers.

In alehouses, sailors newly returned from the Americas might take out an illicit pearl to offer physical evidence of their Atlantic adventures. But in aristocratic portraits, pearls were given heavily symbolic, often political meanings. In their brilliant whiteness and their associations with chastity and purity, pearls were fitting gems to decorate the body of the Virgin Queen. For Elizabeth, the milky sheen of pearls invited associations with Diana/Cynthia, goddess of chastity and the moon. Ralegh played with this conceit in a portrait of himself that depicts the moon guiding the tide (Walter/water) in the top left corner. For other aristocratic ladies, pearls were associated with fertility through pregnancy. In Marcus Gheeraerts's *Portrait of an Unknown Lady* (*c.*1590s), a visibly pregnant woman is encrusted head to toe with thousands of pearls, her pale fingers tangled in the many strings around her neck. She has become a pearly encasement for the treasure she grows within her own body – an heir.[11]

Against a stark black background, the unknown lady's pearls seem to shine all the brighter. At a time when ideals of beauty were equated with paleness or fairness, poems and paintings often used colour contrasts – alabaster and pearls, blackness and jet – to make aesthetic and moral judgements, ones that increasingly mapped on to ideas about skin colour. Portraits of white aristocrats, frequently women, with African servants served to enhance the sitter's paleness. One French writer of the time specified that the beauty of a white lady in a portrait would be enhanced by including a Black figure in a painting, their blackness giving 'greater lustre and brilliance to her great beauty and fairness'.[12] Depicting the attendant Africans as wearing or offering gleaming pearls simultaneously emphasised their own dark skin and positions of servitude.

Pearls continued to arrive from Asia and Africa, entering English ports along with calicoes, spices, and porcelain. But portraits and documentary evidence from the later Elizabethan era suggest a consistent link between the wealth of pearls and English aspirations in the Atlantic, particularly at the height of war with Spain.[13] They proliferated in visual renderings of navigators from John Hawkins to Thomas Cavendish, commemorating sitters who had demonstrable interests in transatlantic piracy and colonisation. In Nicholas Hilliard's miniature of a man who may be George Clifford, third Earl of Cumberland, the nobleman wears a finely embroidered shirt of blackwork and lace, and three pearls at his ears. When he wasn't engaging in court pageantry as Elizabeth's official champion, Cumberland conducted privateering voyages to the West Indies. In 1588, in the aftermath of the Armada, Walter Ralegh commissioned a portrait of himself in a pearly white doublet, each button sewn with dozens of variously shaped pearls. Waves of pearls undulate from his fur-lined cloak. Pearls encrust his breeches. His dainty hand rests on a table, wrist decorated with a double string of pearls. Even amidst all of these, the double-pearl earring dangling from his ear stands out, glowing next to his flushed cheeks.

There is a chance that some Elizabethan pearls also came from North America – perhaps even those in Ralegh's portrait, painted at

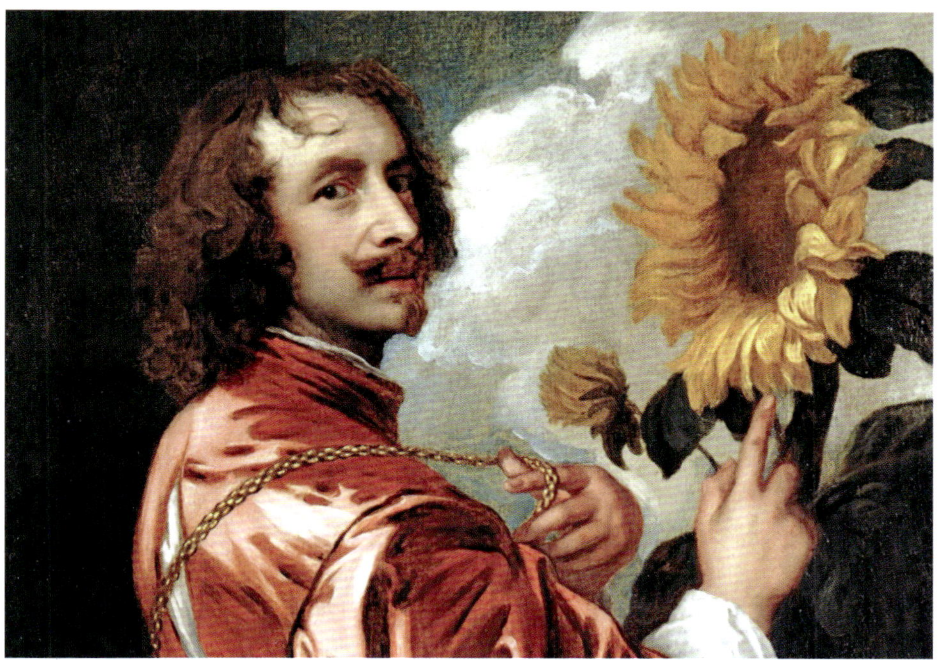

In *Self-Portrait with a Sunflower* (*c.* 1630s), Anthony van Dyck shares the composition with a plant first cultivated thousands of miles from the English court.

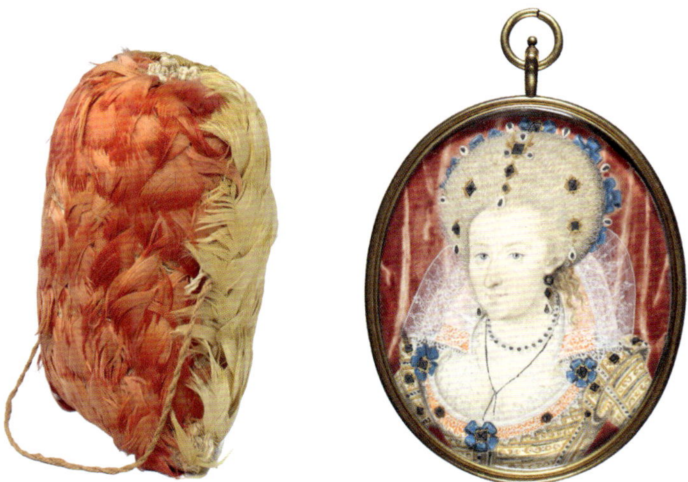

Above, left: Elizabethan travel books from South America mention bags used to carry sacred plants, perhaps like this Inca feather bag (circa the fifteenth to sixteenth century) containing traces of dried coca leaves.

Above, right: Anna of Denmark, wife of James VI and I, was a patroness of colonial literature and Atlantic venturing, as were other powerful court ladies.

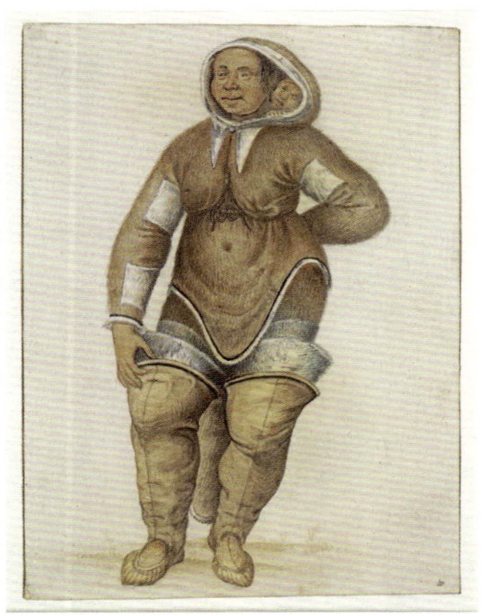

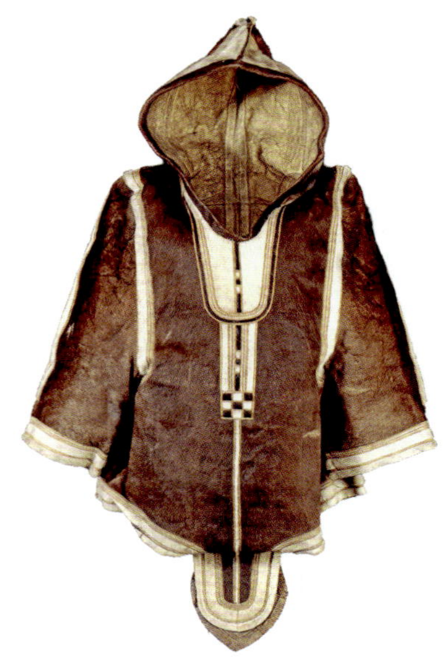

Above, left: Arnaq wears an *amauti*, a parka specially designed to carry an infant – Nutaaq ('baby' or 'new one' in Inuktitut) peers out from the hood.

Above, right: A caribou skin parka (likely nineteenth century) gives a sense of the marvellous craft of Inuit clothing that so fascinated the Tudors.

Right: Copy after copy, the Inuit and their garments found their way into different media, including *The Allegory of America* (c. 1590s).

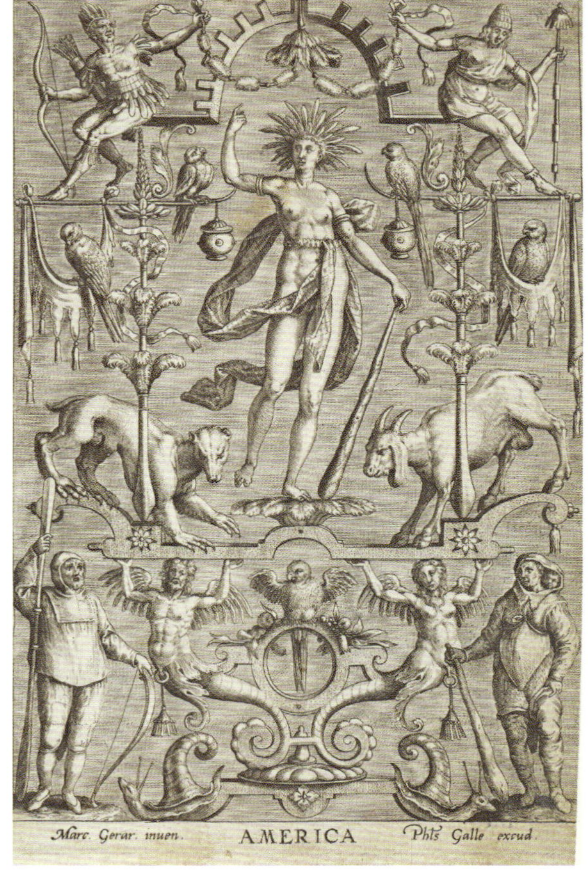

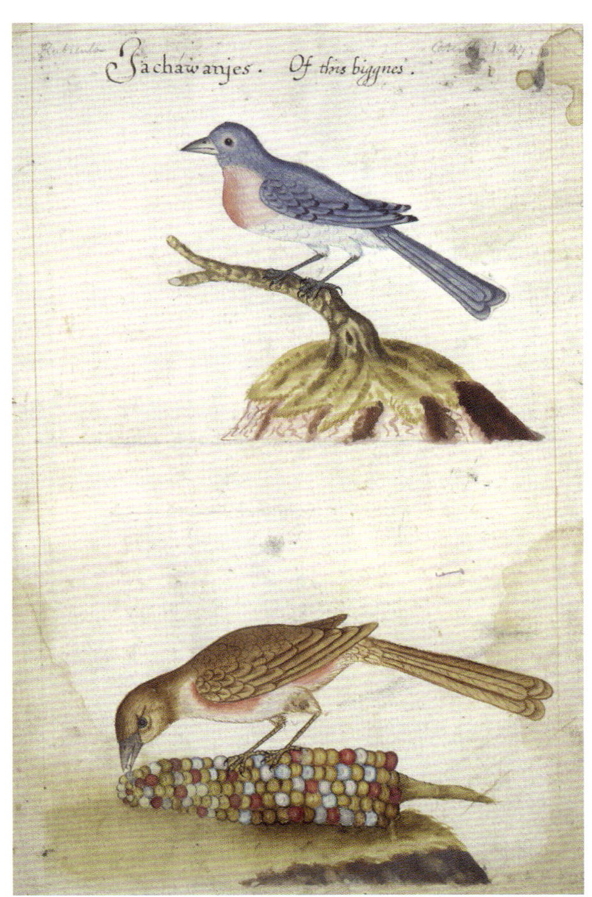

Left: Watercolour drawings of North American birds, flying fish, milkweed, and cobs of maize circulated alongside Nicholas Hilliard's exquisite portrait miniatures.

Below: Both the Roanoke drawing and this portrait (probably of the queen's favourite, the Earl of Essex), are limned with gold and contain inscriptions – Algonquian in one, Latin in the other.

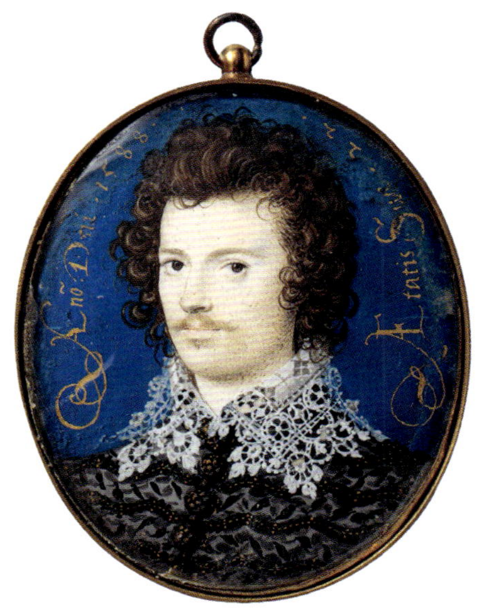

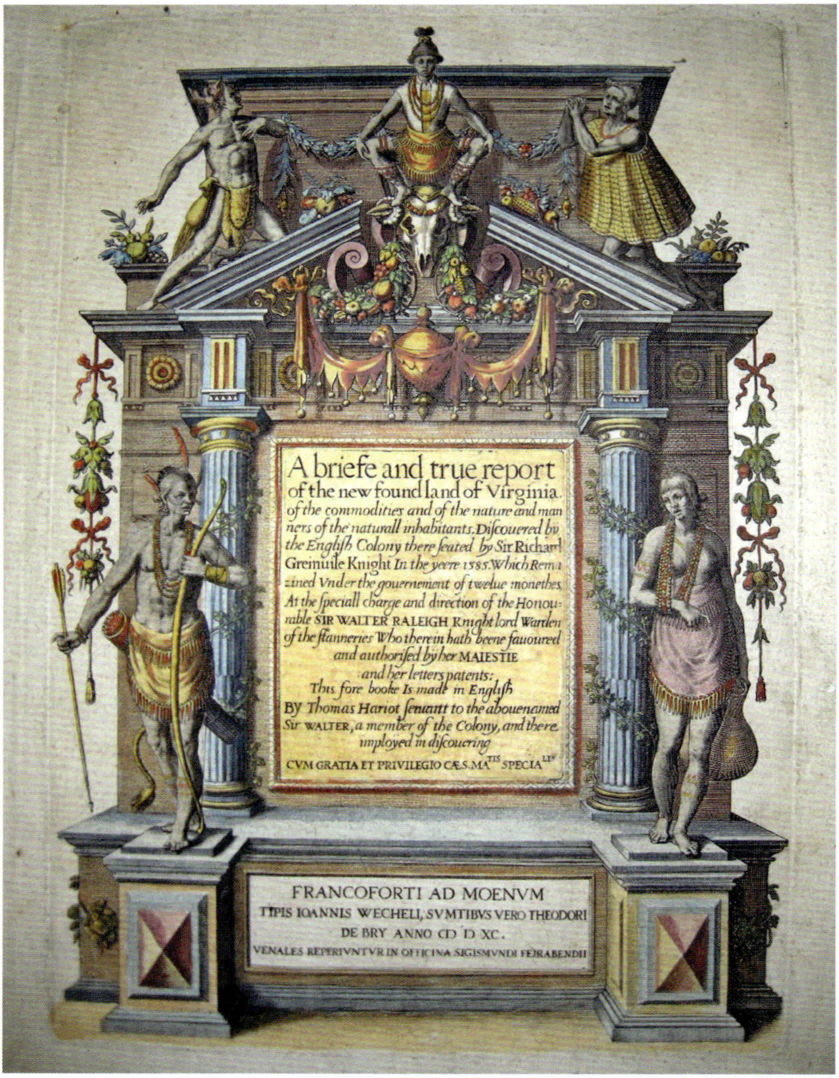

Beyond its classicised figures, Thomas Hariot's *A Briefe and True Report of the New Found Land of Virginia* (1590) became a dwelling place for words intimately connected to Algonquian lands.

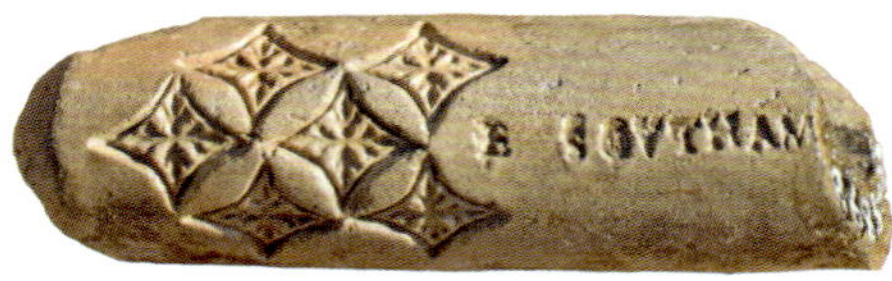

Terra cotta tobacco pipe from Jamestown, made in direct imitation of Algonquian styles. It reads: *E. Southam* – Earl of Southampton, Shakespeare's patron.

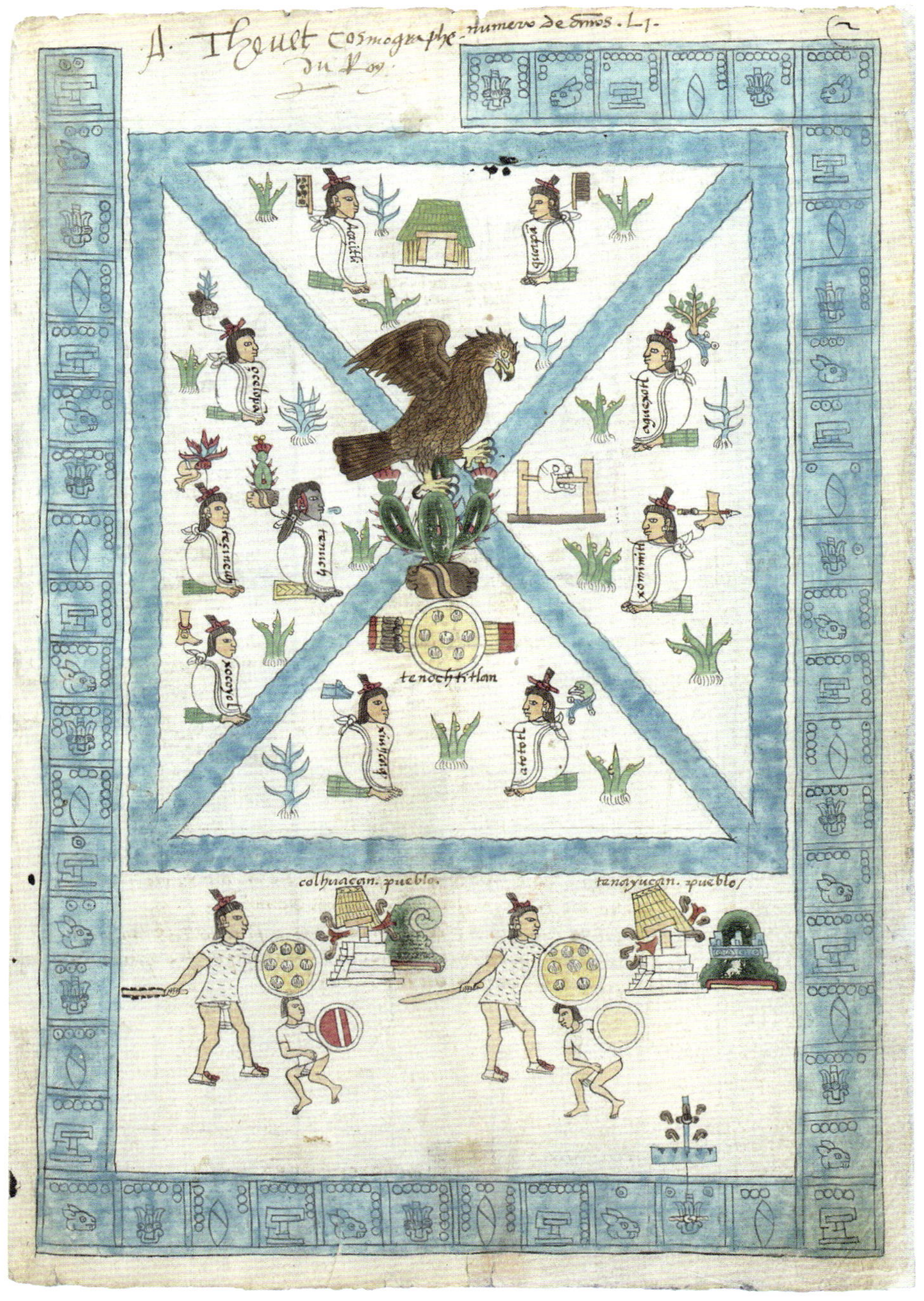

A 'painted book' of Mesoamerican pictorial writing (*c.* 1541) brought Mexica history, tributary practices, and life cycles into England.

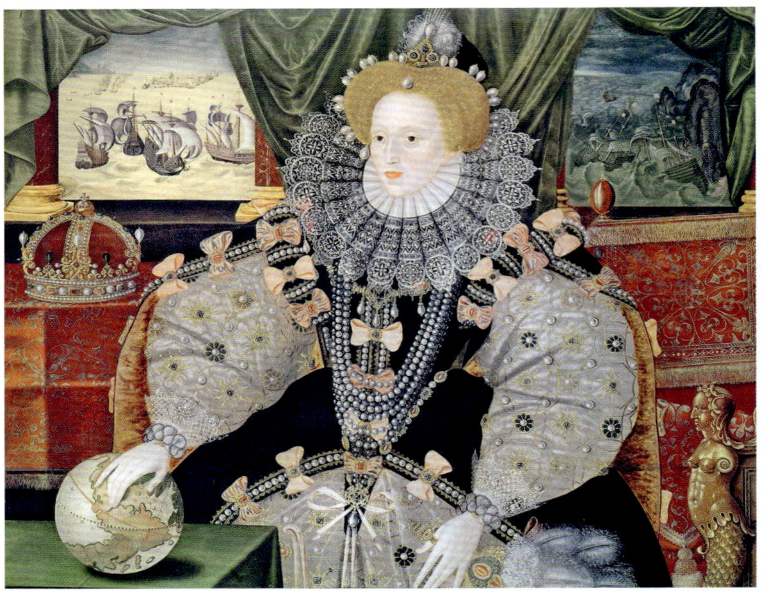

That most quintessential of Elizabethan paintings, the 'Armada portrait' of 1588. The queen's hand rests on a globe, her fingers tapping the Americas.

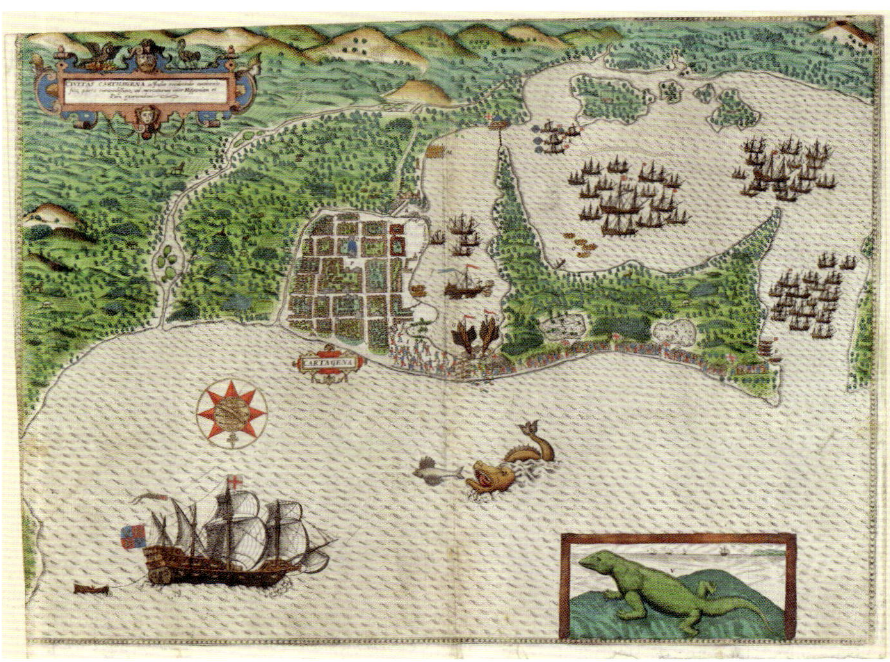

The English attack on Cartagena, part of a series of maps by Baptista Boazio celebrating Francis Drake's 1586 raids on Spanish settlements.

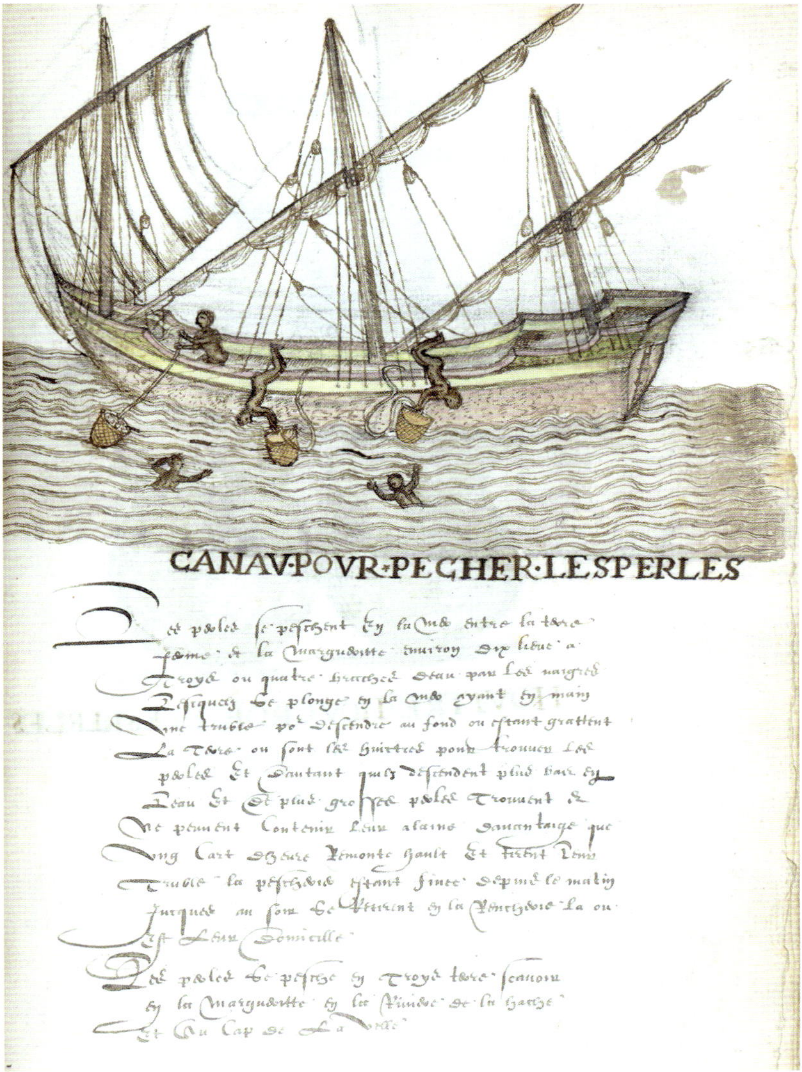

CANAV·POVR·PECHER·LES·PERLES

Above: Near Venezuela, enslaved pearl divers lean over the edge of their boat, a rare visualisation of the labour that lay behind Tudor pearl mania.

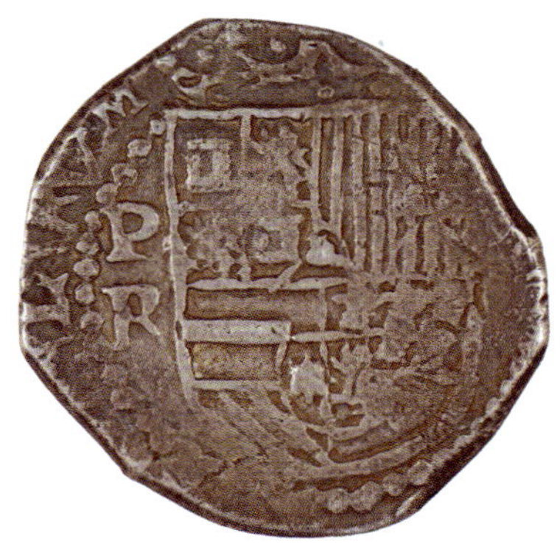

Right: A piece of eight coin, minted in Potosí. Tudor and Stuart writings are rife with references to the Americas as the source of the most covetable gold and silver.

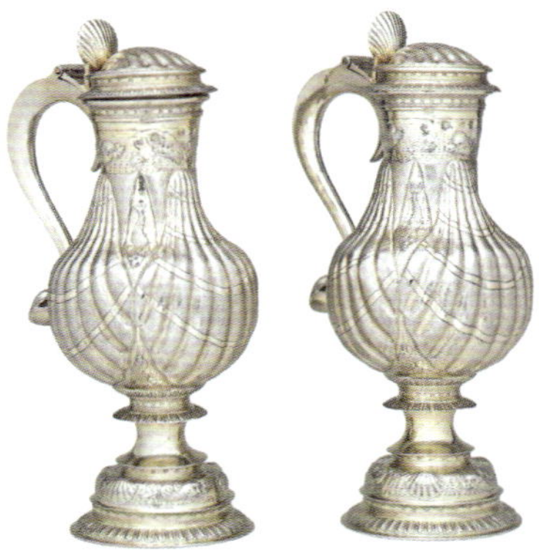

Silver flagons with maritime imagery from the 1590s, believed to have been part of the Paston family treasure – some of which appears on the cover of this book.

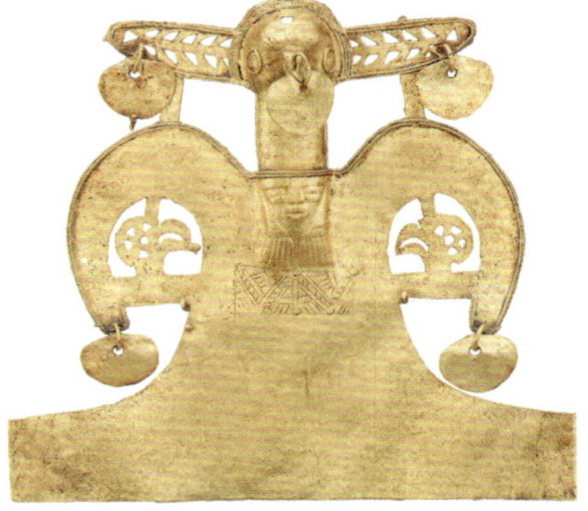

A Muisca bird pendant made in the Colombian Andes, circa the tenth to sixteenth century. Ralegh and other travellers returned with copper-gold alloys, including ones shaped like birds.

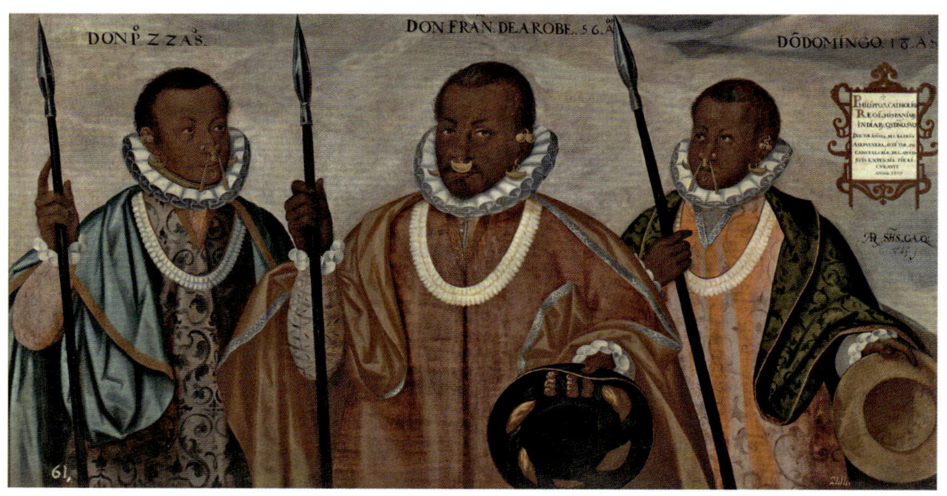

Francisco de Arobe and his sons Pedro and Domingo, painted by the Quito artist Andrés Sánchez Gallque in 1599. Drake conducted negotiations with African and Indigenous 'maroon' communities during his travels.

the time of his Roanoke project. In 1588, Thomas Hariot had written about a necklace made for Queen Elizabeth from Carolina oyster pearls. Hariot described how the settlers occasionally found pearls when feeding on mussels, but these were scarce. One colonist, however, 'had gathered together from among the savage people aboute five thousande: of which number he chose so many as made a fayre chaine'. Picking out the pearls with the roundest shapes and most brilliant hues, the craftsman made a 'very fayre and rare' necklace to present to the queen.[14]

Algonquian knowledge of the seashore and estuaries was, as Hariot admitted, crucial to creating such presentation items. He reported that leaders in Roanoke wore earrings and necklaces strung with pearls. Like Hilliard's miniatures, whose colours have tarnished and altered with time and whose pearl earrings have faded to grey specks, John White's drawings of Algonquians in Roanoke may originally have portrayed them wearing freshwater pearls.[15] By the first few decades of the seventeenth century, colonists in the Chesapeake openly documented how soldiers 'ransacked [Powhatan] Temples, Took downe the Corpses of their dead kings from their Toambes, and Caryed away their pearles, copper, and bracelets wherewith they doe decorate their kings funeralles'.[16] Whether gained through violence or more peaceable exchange, the pearls in Hariot's necklace never reached Elizabeth. A storm at sea scattered the gems into the Atlantic on the way home, along with Hariot's travel journal. Nonetheless, this lost artefact indicates how the value of jewellery might be enhanced by its connections to the Americas. Hariot's chain of pearls threaded its origins into its gift.

Like other English travellers and readers, Hariot knew that pearls did not just come from the Americas as raw goods, but as cultural belongings that reflected Native cultures and political economies. After his travels to Guiana, Ralegh recounted rumours spread by

Spanish soldiers about the inhabitants who wore *tumbagas* and hung pearls in their ears. Aztec/Mexica codices recorded female healers who used the shells of pearl molluscs for their divinations. 'It is white, translucent,' reads the Nahua inscription for the *epiollotli* (pearl, translated as 'oyster heart') in the Florentine Codex. 'It is translucent, ever translucent, crystalline, like crystal, clear . . . Some are large, some small. They are really longed for.'[17] In his account of Florida, Richard Hakluyt wrote of the 'huge quantitie of excellent perles, and little babies and birds made of them, that were found in *Cutifachiqui*'.[18] Criticising the ostentatious fashions of English gallants in the early 1650s, John Bulwer drew on earlier travel accounts to compare English codpieces to the sheaths worn by inhabitants of Trinidad, who 'before the Spaniards came into the Country . . . wore such kind of Codpieces bordered with Gold and Pearle'.[19]

This moment of colonial venturing and Anglo-Spanish rivalry led to that most quintessential of Elizabethan paintings, the 'Armada Portrait' of 1588. The pale queen appears at the centre, imperial crown at her side. She wears an assortment of gold-set jewels, gold-embroidered suns, and rich shades of her favoured colour combination, black and white. Her large ruff exhibits remarkably intricate lacework. Commissioned by an unknown courtier to commemorate the defeat of the Spanish Armada, a fleet of sun-kissed English ships set sail in the background, while Spanish ships to the right of the composition are tossed by a storm and dashed against rocks. Amidst all the dazzling finery, our eyes fall to the queen's hand, resting on a globe, her fingers tapping the Americas. This sparkling composition conveys a whole shift in English aspirations in the Atlantic, captured through the body and riches of England's monarch, refulgent in hundreds of pearls.

The 5,000 pearls from Roanoke would have made a pleasing courtly gift. But the queen's finger in the portrait rests closer to the

Pearl Coast, suggesting the Elizabethans' continuing interests in South America and the Caribbean.[20] Years later, a Jacobean merchant wrote of the high estimation of 'West-India Pearles' in Elizabeth's reign. He recalled purchasing large quantities from Francis Drake, as well as 'great unproportionated Pearles called *Barocos*' from France. In the aftermath of Ralegh's execution, the Vice-Admiral of Devonshire, Lewis Stukley, recounted how Ralegh had cheated him and his family out of their rightful profit from a ship returning from the Caribbean. Ralegh had shrugged it off, blaming the queen. Despite her seeming favour towards him, he insisted, sometimes Elizabeth was 'unjust and tyrannous' in her desires. In a fit of envy, she had taken all the sea gems in a cabinet for herself, 'without ever giving him so much as one pearle'.[21]

After the English established colonies of their own, they fruitlessly scoured the seas for pearl beds that might rival those found in the lands occupied by imperial Spain. In August 1613, six years after the establishment of Jamestown, the news writer John Chamberlain complained that few commodities were coming from the Chesapeake. He was more optimistic about Bermuda, however. Pearl and ambergris from the island, valued at £900, had recently reached the realm.[22] Ambergris, a waxy sperm whale secretion used in perfume, might not look like much, but it fetched a high price. Soon after, colonists found a clump of ambergris worth an astonishing £12,000, enough to keep London investors enthused.

In 1609, the crew of the shipwrecked *Sea Venture*, initially bound for Virginia, had staggered onto Bermuda's shorelines. In the crack of thunder and the flash of divine providence, the English had stumbled onto their second American colony. The island was unlike anything they had tried to colonise so far. It had a temperate climate, but one that was frequently disrupted by storms (the 'still-vex'd Bermoothes', Shakespeare wrote soon after). The island reefs were the notorious site of wrecks. Tropical plants, brought by European sailors over the previous century, grew alongside the endemic palmetto. One Cavalier poet would later imagine resting under the palmetto's broad branches, dreaming pleasing thoughts about his mistress in the company of sweet liquor.

In ensuing years, investors in London formed the Somers Isles Company to direct island affairs. London councillors ordered colonists to develop a whaling industry, grow cassava and sugarcane, and acquire Africans to work as pearl divers. A diverse island society soon developed. In 1616, the year of Shakespeare's death, an English ship stopped in Bermuda from a voyage to the Caribbean with one African and one Indigenous passenger, 'the first thes[e] Ilands ever had'. These two individuals were chosen as skilled labourers, able to offer specialised knowledge that would help colonists develop lucrative industries such as pearl fishing and tropical agriculture. It was through African and Indigenous expertise that colonists likely grew and prepared food, learned to thatch roofs with the palmetto, and knotted rope into the hammocks that settlers slept in.[23] Although Robert Rich (later second Earl of Warwick) and his supporters saw Bermuda as an ideal base for attacking Spanish treasure ships, these ships also brought enslaved Africans whose experience on Spanish plantations was useful to English colonists.

Despite investors' optimism, hopes for a pearl industry in Bermuda were quickly dashed. Only small numbers of pearls could be sourced, their colour cloudy and 'somewhat defective'. Other plantation goods, such as tobacco, proved more immediately profitable. The planter Robert Rich, a cousin of the Earl of Warwick, took advice from an African man named Francisco, whose excellent 'judgment in the curing of tobacoe' helped the plantation industry take off. There were at least fifty African or African-descended women and men working as tobacco cultivators on the island by 1619. The Governor of Bermuda admitted that, were it not for Africans on the island, 'I wer[e] not able to rayse one pound of Tobacco'; nor did he shy away from expressing his opinions on their place on the island: 'Slaves are the most proper and cheap instruments for this plantation.' In the early 1630s, the English captured sixteen Spanish ships with a reported loss of several thousand enslaved people.[24] A decade later, Warwick would attempt to establish pearl fishing on another island – Providence, in the Caribbean Sea – instructing captains to bring only those Africans who were skilled in pearl fishing, and to sell the rest to Bermuda.[25]

By then, the pearl mania that had accompanied the rise of Pearl Coast fisheries was beginning to wane. Pearls remained covetable luxuries, their allure and symbolism secured by the colonial surge of the sixteenth century, but fashions changed.[26] When Elizabeth I died, many of her pearls became part of Anna of Denmark's royal wardrobe. The Stuarts retained the Elizabethan love of pearl necklaces, although they ditched some of the more intricately embellished clothes in favour of chunkier baroque jewels and heaps of strings wrapped around necks or wrists. In a 1625 portrait of the Duke of Buckingham by Michiel van Miereveld, Buckingham wears a pearly leather doublet and ropes of pearls, hanging from his neck and tucked to one side. These hundreds of perfectly rounded gems are a dizzying display of the duke's prominence and favour. The year before, while Buckingham was in France to negotiate Prince Charles's marriage to Henrietta Maria, courtiers avowed that the duke's immense pearls were a thing to behold. Buckingham strutted around Paris in a large pearl earring with a heavy diamond and a pearl chain, long enough to be looped six times around his neck – perhaps the same chain that appears in his portrait the following year.[27]

During Charles I's reign, clothes softened and became more pared back. Lustrous satins, lace, and billowing gowns with voluminous sleeves replaced wide farthingales and heavy embroidery. Ruffs wilted into falling bands – collars that rested flat around the shoulders. Like her queenly predecessors, Henrietta Maria loved pearls, but a handful or two of these oversized gems could make as much of a statement as the swathes that had once decorated Tudor fabrics. In a 1638 painting by Anthony van Dyck, the Catholic queen is awash in a sheen of white silk and large baroque jewels, bulbous pearls hanging from her neck, ears, waist, and diamond crucifix. Pearl necklaces were among the jewels that she would pawn while in exile in Holland and France, to raise financial support for the royalist cause. When Charles I mounted the scaffold at his execution in 1649, he was rumoured to be wearing a pearl earring he had possessed since he was a teenager. Underneath style, personal memories and attachments lingered in the objects that were worn and passed down.

If Tudor and Stuart pearls were so ubiquitous, then where are they now? The visual aesthetic of the era, and our understanding of early modern fashion, is linked to the sea gems that those divers off the coast of Venezuela or Panama gathered in baskets and carried to shore in their canoes. Yet the story of pearls is a strangely ghostly one. They have vanished on us. Damaged by air, degraded by touch, they exist as copies and representations in daubs of paint. They have deteriorated and dissolved, like Cleopatra's earring, in the vinegar of time.

The ghostliness of pearls returns us to their alien beginnings in the depths of the sea. They are tied to oceans, and to all that oceans yield and swallow up. Long before they appeared on globes and ribbons, they came into being amidst the sound of waves and the spray of salt. Before pearls could be cultured and mass-produced, they were the natural phenomena of those liquid realms that so enthralled and terrified early modern travellers. Pearls bring us back to the force of the sea, in all its mystery and fear, and to the countless lives lost in search of them. Off the shores of Central and South America, Indigenous and African divers with whole histories and migrations of their own leaned over the edge of their boats, listening to the sounds of oysters grazing. The fates of many met in these small vessels. The sale of a pearl canoe in 1590 revealed the presence of people from Sierra Leone, Senegambia, Cape Verde, as well as 'three black women in the service of the said canoe'.[28] Perhaps, as with later enslaved communities who used canoes to escape from plantations, these boats were regarded as companions or collaborators by those who helmed them. Carved from sacred wood, they carried their navigators across vast expanses, offering protection from the harmful spirits that might reside in unfamiliar waters.[29] Not far from the pearl divers, Native groups such as the Warao of eastern Venezuela used canoes to navigate the mangroves and waterways of their forest landscapes. These wooden vessels carried them through their daily lives and sustained their livelihoods. The Warao, the English knew, 'are for the most part Carpenters of Canoas', their identities inextricably linked to boats and to the marshlands they dwelled in.[30]

It was of these lands that pearl-adorned gentlemen dreamed as they led fleets across the Atlantic towards the Orinoco Delta. They carried willing and unwilling passengers, people whose names we know and others we never will. In nearly all these vessels, pearls were there too. But before there were ships, there were the canoes, and the divers who steered them. They woke before dawn and extracted the pearls that might, if they were lustrous enough, hang from a boy's earring in a palace somewhere in England.

Feathers and Fakes

In June 1596, a gentleman named Nicholas Saunders wrote a letter to Elizabeth's State Secretary, Robert Cecil, to report an unusual sight. Saunders had noticed a pedlar wandering about with 'an Indian hatt', decorated with a jewel that appeared too valuable to be in the hands of an itinerant seller. Saunders speculated that this rare object must have belonged to a ruler in the West Indies, brought into the realm following Francis Drake's recent voyage to Central America and the Caribbean.[1] This venture had brought an influx of pearls and other lucrative goods into England, as well as the shocking news that both Drake and John Hawkins had died at sea, buried in the same ocean that had made their fortunes.

There is a good chance that Saunders associated the hat with the Americas because it contained feathers. When Francis Bacon compared the quality and colour of Mesoamerican feather art to cut diamonds and emeralds, he was admiring a practice of feather-working that Europeans had praised since their earliest encounters with Indigenous cultures. Saunders's speculation about the hat's origins may have drawn on a knowledge of costume books or travel accounts, which frequently depicted Arawakan, Kalinago, and Tupi leaders wearing brightly hued feathers. In a world map printed in Amsterdam in 1594, 'Mexicana' straddles an armadillo, adorned in gold jewellery and a feathered mantle, while 'Peruana' sits on a yellow jaguar in the company of tropical birds, feathers encircling her head. Such stylised depictions were copied and plagiarised across artists' studios and different media. Though they flattened the liveliness and ceremonial significance of feathered garments, they also solidified European understandings of feathered garments as key markers of Indigenous sovereignty.

On maps and cosmographies produced across Europe, Tupi warriors stood in feathered headdresses in territories marked 'Brazil'. Maps gave the illusion of sparsely populated regions in South America, but a huge population of Tupi-speaking peoples, estimated to number around a million, lived on the coast of Brazil in 1500, in a land they called Pindorama, Land of the Palms. The first Portuguese to arrive encountered diverse societies, each with their own political alliances and enmities.[2] European travellers relied on Tupi women, whose knowledge of the cultivation of cassava and other roots, gourds, and legumes sustained both Indigenous and settler communities.[3] Among Tupi groups, political and spiritual authority was often accessed through brilliant matter such as burnished metals or feathers, and through the songs and dreams that connected such items to cosmic power and realms beyond. Feathers from macaws, blackbirds, and other species were used at assemblies and councils in moments of celebration and commemoration, or to restore spiritual relations after violence. The capes made from scarlet ibis feathers served as connections to the ancestral realm in funerary rites, and as symbols of prestige during assemblies and captive–captor ceremonies.[4] These ceremonies, and the Tupi leaders who performed them, were vital to the life of the feathered garment. In religious and political ceremonies, they were transformed by wearing feathers, engaging with powerful, other-than-human agents. Birds were important because they offered a bridge between earthly knowledge and the heavenly realm.

Far from the forests of Greater Amazonia, Saunders's encounter with an Indian hat in the port town of Plymouth raises intriguing questions about the acquisition and distribution of Indigenous or

Indigenous-inspired objects in late Elizabethan England. His speculation about Drake's connection to the hat shows that Indigenous cultural belongings were known to travel directly into English ports, even as other travelling objects arrived via cities such as Seville, Lisbon, Amsterdam, or Rouen. The seeming incongruity of a pedlar possessing a rare American object attracted government interest, relating as it did to the regulation of global goods within the realm. But what is also clear from Saunders's letter, cutting through his sense of duty and responsibility, is the allure of the artefact itself. Above the social privilege Saunders sought to convey is the dazzling brilliance of the item that had inspired him to put pen to paper. Shimmering in the candlelight, this tantalising thing had brightened a darkening summer night with its promise of faraway places, connecting a local gentleman to an imagined West Indies king.

For a century, Europeans had been fascinated by the biodiversity of South America's tropical forests, and by the artistry of those who created things from birds. Cortés brought feathered ceremonial garments, along with feathered artworks, shields, and wall hangings, from Mexico to Europe, where they were publicly displayed and incorporated into court performances. These belongings showcased some of the many distinct feather-working traditions across the Americas, which included the making of headdresses and chequered tunics as well as figures, shrouds, and bags for storing coca, tobacco, and other plants gathered by healers. The sight of featherwork had a palpable effect on Europeans, whose emotional responses often grappled with the insufficiency of language to describe what they saw.

The celebrated artist Albrecht Dürer had spent his whole life recording the astonishing strangeness of everyday life (walruses and lilies, castles and a piece of turf). He was dazzled, almost stunned, by the sight of Nahua craft. He had been a young artist of twenty-two when Columbus returned from his first voyage across the Atlantic. As Columbus introduced captured Caribbean peoples and their flora and fauna to Spain, this German artist had been drawing a portrait of himself with a cocked cap and steady hand. On the same page, he tried capturing the plumpness of a crinkled pillow, rendering to paper the private life of the self and the bedroom, even as the world beyond him seemed to be opening up to Europeans in unprecedented ways. In 1520, nearly three decades and thousands of drawings and watercolours later, Dürer found himself gazing directly at Aztec/Mexica belongings at the imperial court of Charles V. 'I have seen the things, that one has brought to the king from the new land of gold,' he wrote. They were so beautiful that 'all the days of my life I have seen nothing that rejoiced my heart so much as these things'.[5]

Across Europe, feathers from American birds were appreciated partly because a market for complex techniques of feather-working already existed. People were surrounded by feathers all the time. The gentry flew their hawks, servants plucked birds for meals, and secretaries sharpened quills to scribble letters. When it came to decorating the body, artisans trimmed, dyed, fluffed, and embellished feathers for headwear and military accessories. Craftspeople compared feathers to velvet, a sumptuous fabric ever in peril of being damaged. They knew that bird matter, however vibrant, could fade when exposed to light or water, and that low humidity made feathers brittle.[6]

Wealthy Tudors wore plumes in their caps and incorporated African ostrich feathers into jewelled fans. Portraits from the 1570s of Elizabeth I's favourite, Robert Dudley, Earl of Leicester, seem incomplete without a feather curling from his hat. In *Urania* (1621), a romance penned by the writer Mary Wroth, feathered accessories are part of the visual language of courtly civility and its associated gestures and codes. Footmen and horses wear dyed plumes as part of their livery. A queen coyly licks her lips so that they look 'like cherries after raine, red, and plumpe, and [totters] her head, which made a feather shake she had on it'. A cruel lord, dressed in red to match his bloody disposition, rejects feathers, dismissing them as frivolous, proper only to feasts and young men who 'thought more on fashion th[a]n busines'. Feathers at the Tudor and Jacobean courts were flashy and a bit impractical, drawing admiration for the creativity and manual skill that lay behind their charm.[7]

Surviving feather garments in English museums give a sense of the incredible iridescence that stirred the Elizabethan imagination. Macaw, quetzal, and parrot feathers offer flares of electric greens, blues, and yellows, so intense that they seem to diminish the colours around them. In the toucans fastened with fibre cords, in tufty midnight-black feathers clustered into tassels, and in parakeets the colour of cashew fruits and peppertrees, the ecosystems of Greater Amazonia converge with Native knowledge and ways of making.

In the decades after Vespucci's voyages to Brazil and the Caribbean, feathers began to materialise at the court of Henry VIII in various forms. Featherwork appears in an unlikely English source from 1516, one that predates Dürer's glowing impression. In Thomas More's *Utopia* (1516), the traveller Hythloday describes how the priest of Utopia wears a multicoloured robe, 'wonderful for its workmanship and decoration'. Unlike European vestments, it contains no gold embroidery or jewels, but 'is decorated with the feathers of different birds so skilfully woven together that the value of the handiwork far exceeds the cost of the richest materials'. Had More read about feather garments in the Latin accounts of Vespucci's travels, or seen some himself? In *Utopia,* the priest's garment absorbs symbolic mysteries that are hidden in the feathers' distinct patterning, 'the meaning of which is carefully handed down'.[8] For this humanist at Henry's court, divine mysteries could be accessed through the patterns and knowledge-storing capacities of feathers.

In 1526, ten years after *Utopia* and far from the domain of courtiers and humanists, the Bristol merchant Roger Barlow travelled with Sebastian Cabot to Río de la Plata (the 'river of silver') in what is now Argentina and Uruguay. He recounted seeing men along the Paraná River who wore crystals in their lips and strung the teeth and claws of fierce animals into necklaces to absorb the beasts' power. Tupi-Guaraní warriors affixed feathers to their bodies with liquid gum and killed their enemies with clubs that were painted and dressed with feathers. Barlow admired the parrot feathers, 'like diadems which the grete men of the countrey do we[a]re upon the[i]r hedes', 'of so pure colours and so well wrought that it is [a] marvel to beholde'.

We don't know if Barlow brought featherwork to England, but he did bring feathers. Barlow wrote of tiny birds no bigger than the top of a thumb – the earliest known English description of a hummingbird. They were covered in 'the goodliest fethers that ever man might se[e], [and] the colours wo[ul]ld chaunge in moving of them', undulating like silk rolled out on a tailor's table. The crew captured a humming-bird and kept it in a cage. When it died soon after, they stuffed the bird with dried moss to preserve it on the journey home, where it scented the coffer with a sweet musk.[9]

Iridescent birds and feathered artefacts may already have been in Whitehall, therefore, when a Brazilian 'king' spent a year in London, travelling across the Atlantic on a voyage led by one of Henry VIII's principal sea captains, William Hawkins. On his second voyage to Brazil, according to his son, Hawkins befriended a Brazilian (likely Tupinambá) man, left unnamed in the English account. The man travelled to Henry's court, causing a sensation. Henry and his court-iers 'did not a little marveile' at 'all his apparell, behaviour, and gesture, [which] were very strange to beholders'. Next to nothing is known of the man's time on foreign shores. He was a resident in the city while the English king ordered his ministers to manufacture a legal justification to divorce Catherine of Aragon, paving the way for his marriage to Anne Boleyn. In 1532, the man began his journey home, but did not survive the passage. Instead, ships returned 'furnished with the commodities of the Countrey', bringing an influx of South American goods to the realm.[10]

When he wasn't holding a blade to Henry VIII's throat, Edmund Harman might have been thinking about this Indigenous man and all those commodities from Brazil. Harman was the king's barber, occupying an important and intimate role in the king's small group of trusted attendants. Born into a merchant family, Harman was also a packer at the Port of London, meaning he had opportunities to see, handle, and buy or confiscate covetable goods arriving from overseas. It may have been through these connections that Harman was inspired to build one of the most cryptic church monuments of the age. In the late 1560s (he died in 1577), he erected a stone monument for himself in St John the Baptist Church in Burford, Oxfordshire. At the base, sixteen children kneel in prayer, seven girls and nine boys – little ruffed figures that remind us of the continuous labour of pregnancy, childbirth, and care that took up so many decades of Tudor women's lives. But the monument is dominated by the four figures above, their bodies looping through the ornamental scrolls around the monument's inscription, flanked by clusters of fruits. Their angular features look jarringly modern, a kind of Renaissance art deco. All of them wear feathers on their heads.

These mysterious stone figures are widely accepted to represent Tupi people, but little is known about the monument or what it intends to convey.[11] The four men are modelled on the Italianate grotesques by the Flemish engraver Cornelis Bos, although the semi-human figures he created in the 1540s and 1550s, with their feather-like crowns, did not depict Indigenous cultures. Did these feathered figures relate to Harman's mercantile interests? Was there a connection to Hawkins's voyages, and the Brazilian king? Whatever the case, for centuries, any who have entered the church have been met with a fantastical combination of the surprising and the more familiar – small hands joined in dutiful prayer, ancient Corinthian columns and friezes modelled after classical civilisations, plump stone fruits, and those tumbling feathered figures.

Tudors and Stuarts marvelled at featherwork, but how much did they know about Indigenous techniques? By 1568, at the same time as the captive Mary, Queen of Scots wrote to the Queen of Spain, asking for foreign aid to restore her power in England, readers could take a break from domestic politics and delve into a newly translated account of life in Brazil by the French geographer and chronicler André Thevet. Birds, 'some as red as fine scarlet', produced feathers that the Tupinambá wove into 'hats, and garments, either for to cover them or for beauty', or worn into war. Others made gowns or mantles, which Thevet demonstrated by bringing one to Paris. Richard Hakluyt likely saw this garment or other Tupi belongings when he met Thevet in France in 1583.[12]

Thevet's account described the way Native people dyed and painted feathers, braided cord from plant fibres, and wove different species' feathers together according to their qualities. His description of feather-working took readers across time and space, from the Kalinago in the Lesser Antilles to feather-workers in the Aztec/Mexica and Incan empires. It was because the Portuguese had been so enamoured with the red the Tupinambá used to paint their feathers, he claimed, that they had been led to brazilwood dye, now a highly coveted commodity. In markets in Mexico, a significant trade was 'fethers of byrds, with the which they [the *amanteca,* or feather-craftspeople] made divers and sundry things, as go[w]nes fashioned after their maner, [and] Tapistry woorke.'[13]

Portuguese and French sources recognised that, in addition to masterful weaving, the Tupinambá altered the colour of feathers on live birds, a lengthy colour modification process known as *tapirage*. This caused the colours of birds' feathers to change into lighter hues that differed from those they had been genetically programmed to produce.[14] Plumes with cool colours were plucked from live birds, their skins rubbed with plant dyes or animal secretions and fats, before the new feathers grew and could be harvested. With the melanins in the feather suppressed, new feathers grew back in warmer shades of yellow and orange-red, shimmering like the golden light of the sun. Extant Tupi mantles in European collections show that some yellow feathers from the scarlet ibis (*guará*) were modified through *tapirage*.[15]

As English colonial ambitions expanded, feathers became more visible in English collections. Elizabethan and Jacobean cabinet collections, such as those in Walter Cope's Holland House in Kensington and John Tradescant's Ark in Lambeth, displayed featherwork that drew adulation. Along with a canoe and dyed skins, a visitor to Cope's cabinet in 1599 saw 'beautiful Indian plumes' and 'a Madonna made of Indian feathers', a reference to the exquisite Catholic devotional images made by Mexica artisans, often using hummingbird feathers.[16] By 1685, a catalogue of the rarities in the Royal Society's collections – some of which had likely been in England for decades – included an 'Indian bracelet' with tufts of blue and black feathers, several mantles, a feathered headdress made of black, yellow, and red feathers, and a gold-embellished hummingbird.[17]

Alongside 'girdles', 'aprons', and armbands made by Tupi or Kalinago craftspeople, English travellers to North America commented on the importance of feathers to Algonquian ways of life. They wrote of the feathers worn by Powhatan shamans; the turkey-feather mantles made by women, 'so prettily wrought & woven with threads that nothing could be discerned but the feathers'; and lustrous feathers worn in the manner of coronets for diplomatic exchanges. The wife of Pepiscunimah (Pipsco), the leader of the Quiyoughcohannocks, met the English dressed in copper, feathers, and flowers, including a resplendent blue feather mantle.[18]

Remarkably, a Tupi headdress also appears in a 1612 collection of emblems by the writer and illustrator Henry Peacham. Emblem books were a patchwork of quotations, mottoes, stories, and images, each page containing a picture accompanied by explanatory verses that entertained the reader and nudged them towards moral reflection. Peacham used featherwork to guide his readers into a consideration of honour and false appearances. 'We pick from others praises here and there,' he wrote, 'So patch herewith an Indian Diadem / Of Parrats feathers'.[19] But wearing borrowed feathers, plucked from others, created a counterfeit self. True glory did not come from imitating followers of fashion or puffed-up conquerors, but from pursuing virtue.

The use of feathers as a stand-in for borrowed finery came from a well-known fable in England, adapted from an ancient Greek tale. A crow or jackdaw decorates himself with the fine plumes of other birds, only to be viciously brought down to his proper place by his disapproving peers, who band together to retrieve their feathers. Robert Greene famously alluded to this tale when he took a dig at Shakespeare in 1592, dismissing the 'upstart Crow, beautified with our feathers' who dared to suppose he could contend with London's accomplished wits.[20] In Peacham's rendering, a patched feathered diadem of unearned accomplishments were 'plumes indeede, whereto we have no right'. His accompanying image was a multi-coloured headdress, complete with a base of plaited fibres. In its unexpected presence in a Jacobean emblem book, Tupi material culture exists as part of a distinct tradition, one the English can only observe. The headdress floats over unsettled waters, between two shores. In the ornamented border, nestled among the grotesque figures and clusters of fruit, is a turkey.

In his letter to Cecil, Saunders assumed that the pedlar's hat had been acquired through violent contestation over land, taken 'in action' against a king. The wonder of featherwork was bound up with English fantasies of conquest and possession. In Theodor de Bry's popular visual renderings of Euro-Indigenous conflict across the Americas, battles were often fought between armoured Europeans and Indigenous warriors in feathered headdresses. Describing Drake's voyage to California, de Bry wrote of how a Miwok ruler put feather crowns on the sea captain's head to communicate his intention 'to make his entire kingdom subject to Francis Drake'.[21] The feathered headdress signalled political power: while accounts detailed how the Miwok offered strings of feathers to the English in exchange for linen shirts, and used red feathers to decorate their baskets, only rulers wore feathers on their heads. The crowns were 'made of knitworke, wrought upon most curiously with feathers of divers colours, very artificially placed, and of a formall fashion'.[22] Visual renderings of this so-called crowning reappeared in later English texts to reinforce English claims to 'New Albion'.

On the other side of the continent, during the First Anglo-Powhatan war (1609–14), the Algonquian leader Nemattanew, a close advisor to Powhatan/Wahunsenacah's brother, Opechancanough, became known for wearing feathered clothing into battle. The English described how 'he used to come into the field all covered over with feathers and Swans wings fastened unto his showlders as [though] he meant to flye'.[23] The colonists dismissively called him 'Jack-of-the-Feather', but Nemattanew seemed otherworldly, emerging unwounded from skirmishes in spite of English guns. In his 'courage and policy', John Smith admitted, he was viewed as 'immortall from any hurt could bee done him by the *English*'.[24]

In 1623, Jamestown's Governor, Francis Wyatt, wrote to the Earl of Southampton to report that Algonquians had returned some twenty prisoners who had been captured in the attacks against English plantations the year before. 'Mrs Boys, the chief of the prisoners, arrived home within a week, apparelled like an Indian Queen,' Wyatt reported.[25] If they did adorn her in high-status materials, Algonquian tribal leaders may have dressed this Englishwoman in feathers, as well as beaded adornments or animal skins. The Cherokee author Betty Booth Donohue has speculated about how seventeenth-century Algonquian groups further north, such as the Nausets, used clothes to make lasting impressions on the young Englishmen they rescued or adopted in New England. Through their contact with beads, bracelets, and other Indigenous belongings, they were 'sung over' and reinscribed into 'an Indian story'.[26] Mrs Boys's presentation as an 'Indian queen' became a stark visual message against English assimilation efforts, at a time when English authorities vehemently insisted that too much cultural mixing threatened the colonial endeavour. As James I put it, 'counterfeiting the man[n]ers of others' by smoking tobacco, or preferring feathered adornment to precious metals, corrupted the English body politic and put the whole colonial project at risk.

As Nemattanew's feathered clothing and Mrs Boys's 'Indian' apparel suggest, English power on the ground looked nothing like the narratives that propagandists insisted on presenting. Alongside more overt political resistance, Indigenous tricksters were also at work. Tricksters were mischievous characters, often following paths of mayhem and disorder. They were 'everywhere working against [English settlers],' Donohue writes, 'duping them, selling them out . . . constantly offending their sensibilities'.[27] De Bry recorded a humorous incident near Río de la Plata, where an Indigenous man leapt from a dance and stole the hat on Drake's head. He offered the gold lace band to a companion, keeping the hat for himself. In the humid climate of a tropical basin, an English hat is snatched from the head of a famous captain, at a time when hats and the gestures associated with them – doffing hats to show deference, for example – were important markers of status. The story offers a small antidote to English obsessions with 'Indian hatts' and grand claims of ceremonial crownings. Drake might ostensibly receive feathered headdresses from the Miwok as tokens of submission, but he cannot even keep his own hat on his head.

De Bry's images of Indigenous societies, like accounts written by travellers to the Americas, brimmed with birds and their feathers. Brought into new contexts of use in England, however, featherwork operated very differently. Then as now, these garments were flattened and rendered lifeless by separation from their places and communities of making. As the Tupinambá artist and activist Glicéria Tupinambá (Glicéria Jesus da Silva) conveyed when she created several new mantles using historic weaving techniques, a mantle cannot exist without Indigenous stewardship and expertise. It cannot be made in a diminishing forest whose species are driven out by the encroachment of outsiders. The weave of a mantle is a network, a composition of vibrant materials that are inseparable from Indigenous land.[28]

Elizabethans who visited Cope's cabinet may have intended simply to enjoy the vivid colours of a headdress, brushing their hands across the feathers on display under the shadow of the canoe hanging from the ceiling. But such belongings, so revered by the English for their colours and craft and their close associations with Indigenous political power, offered a mystique that fuelled imperial longings. The spangled feather ruffs made for the costumes of 'Virginian princes' in *The Memorable Masque* (1613) are a testament to the artistry of Jacobean artisans and guilds, who supplied the feathers and assembled the outfits. Nonetheless, the gentlemen who wore these costumes did so to enact the fantasy of Indigenous submission to James I:

> Virginian Princes, ye must now renounce
> Your superstitious worship . . .
> Descend, and to [the king] all your homage vow.[29]

This elite appropriation of Indigenous featherwork almost always involved some conscious element of dressing up – of stepping into a role that must, ultimately, highlight the refined sensibilities of the person underneath. The performance of submission was therefore key. In 1620, Bermuda's Governor delivered a speech to colonists in which he evoked the perils of dressing up without remembering the civil Englishman underneath. Pure imitation became foolish spectacle, inviting ridicule, 'as if one of you should walke through Cheapeside [in London] at noone day, all to be bepainted and stuck with feathers like an American, wher[e] he may be sure [not just] to be looked at, but laught at'.[30]

By the late 1650s, at three o'clock each afternoon, Londoners could go to see an opera near Drury Lane about the Spanish invasion of Peru. In the din of the theatre, a symphony would begin, filling the hall with 'a wild air suitable to the region'. The curtain opened, revealing Incan nobles in feathered habits and headdresses, carrying woven baskets filled with ingots of gold. Palmettos and parrots surrounded them, valleys of sugarcane visible in the distance. In the opera, England's poet laureate William Davenant rescripted history. Between various diversions, including two apes descending from the clouds and walking a tightrope before retreating into the tropical forest, the 'Natives of *Peru*' and other dancers banished the gold-hungry Spanish and ushered in a harmonious new Anglo-Peruvian alliance, where the 'English shall sit and rule as our guests'.[31]

Were the mantles in the performance real, or fakes? A cosmography published several years later recorded that Incan cloaks were present in England. Further on in the century, featherwork from Suriname would appear on the Restoration stage, brought to England by travellers including the playwright Aphra Behn. The 1656 catalogue of Tradescant's collection contained a 'variety of Indian Crowns made of divers sorts of feathers' and multiple 'attires and ornaments made of most beautifull feathers'.[32] Whether the outfits were Indigenous-made or counterfeits, the context of the performance is significant. Davenant wrote his opera during the Interregnum, when Puritan authorities kept public theatres closed. But for Oliver Cromwell, it made sense to encourage public enthusiasm for English interventions in the Americas. *The Cruelty of the Spaniards in Peru* supported the anti-Spanish agenda that the Lord Protector was pursuing in the Caribbean. The following year, in 1659, Davenant wrote another transatlantic musical for the stage, recounting the deeds of Francis Drake, and his alliance with the African and African-descended *cimarróns* of Panama. In both performances, the playwright harked back to the Elizabethan age as the moment when English colonial ambitions had truly emerged.

In 1596, when Saunders glimpsed the 'Indian hatt', English aspirations of sovereignty in Peru and the Amazon had reached new heights. It was the year Ralegh published *The Discoverie of Guiana*, making much of that mythical Peruvian–English alliance. Perhaps courtiers still remembered the Earl of Essex's 1595 entertainment for Elizabeth I, where a blind, feather-wearing Amazonian royal burst into the court and bowed before the queen, before revealing himself to be none other than Love himself, winged Cupid in disguise. That summer, Thomas Hariot, like Saunders, was writing to

Robert Cecil, offering information about maps of the Amazon and Orinoco rivers created by English pilots with 'intelligence from the Indians'. Cecil also received secret dispatches of news about the Indies, including cargoes of pearls and silver that were carefully stored in locked cabinets and guarded by soldiers.[33] In 1596, too, Edmund Spenser published a new and expanded edition of *The Faerie Queene*. Readers could reacquaint themselves with the scene of Cupid's masque in Book III, where Fancy, 'a lovely boy, / Of rare aspect', danced in a garment of painted plumes inspired by Indigenous craft, as 'the sunburnt *Indians* do array / Their tawney bodies, in their proudest plight.'[34]

And yet. Like the feathers in Fancy's decadent dance, the 'Indian hatt' in Saunders's letter wasn't quite what it seemed. His description of the criss-crossing plates of silver and flower-shaped pearls stitched onto a velvet brim might alert us to something that Saunders himself did not at first realise: that this object was not as authentic as it seemed. In a follow-up message penned to Cecil a few weeks later, Saunders's confident tone had been replaced by one of humility. Having questioned the pedlar and examined the hat, he was disappointed to find its beauty faded. The object looked shabby, covered in little flaws and fractures in the cloth. What Saunders had initially believed to be an Indigenous headdress, 'taken in the action of an Indian king', was a counterfeit, crafted in a workshop on London's Lombard Street.[35]

It was just Saunders's luck, raving about a fake to one of the realm's most powerful political players. He was having a miserable and tedious summer. Instead of joining the Earl of Essex and Ralegh as planned in the raid on Spain's Potosí silver, docked in Cádiz, he was detained in Plymouth for a dispute over a cargo of sugar that involved allegations of theft.[36] Knee-deep in shipping affairs and itching to join English captains in their attack on the Spanish treasure fleet,

Saunders had been beguiled by the promise of the real thing – a glimpse of authentic Indigenous handiwork, something alive with a potency that came from elsewhere. All those thoughts of trans-atlantic voyages and silver fleets had primed him to see something that wasn't there.

Even if the headpiece *had* been from Indigenous homelands, it would have lost its connection to its community once it was trafficked across the Atlantic. By then, the birds' feathers would have been sundered from the land they came from, a place of jaguars, red heartwoods, and cacao. It would have ended up in the hands of those whom the Yanomami of the Amazon rainforest call earth-eaters, 'people of merchandize'.[37]

In Peacham's emblem, the parrot-feather headdress hovers over water, serving as a bridge between two lands. The featherwork in Tudor and Stuart inventories, cabinets, and travel books is witness to the presence of American birds and the work of Indigenous makers in Renaissance libraries and shopping stalls. They 'become landmarks of occupation and territorial reach, witnesses to the fact that the Tupinambá also occupied Europe'. These landmarks of Native presence existed alongside fakes and imitations – theatre costumes and Indigenous-inspired objects that allowed English women and men to draw on the imagery of Native peoples while disregarding the legitimacy of those peoples' claims to sovereignty. Feathered garments are among the 'artefacts in the Old World' that need a relationship with 'the peoples of the New World', as Glicéria Tupinambá put it. When they do, the work of past makers and the lives of their particular communities will not be displayed in inert spaces of 'extinguished memories, paralyzed memories', but will become part of 'a new story, with another shade of history'.[38]

Colombian Emeralds
in the Cheapside Hoard

In June 1912, workmen tasked with tearing down a timber-frame building in Cheapside stumbled on a treasure that brought Elizabethan life spilling from the surface. The building near St Paul's Cathedral had sat on the site since the seventeenth century, its crumbling cellars even older. As their pickaxes hit bricks and chalky soil, the workers struck a wooden casket. When they broke it open and washed away layers of clay and mud, hundreds of colourful gems began to sparkle through the grime. This treasure is now referred to as the Cheapside Hoard, the greatest single collection of Elizabethan and early Stuart jewellery ever found.[1]

It was the stuff of fable. Rubies, diamonds, sapphires, and turquoise, cut and uncut, loose and mounted, all hidden under a bustling London street in the heart of what had been the Elizabethan commercial district. The hoard offers a sample of luxury goods sold and worn by the merchant elite in that 'chief Emporium or mart of Great Britain'. Just beyond St Paul's Cathedral, jewellers and goldsmiths displayed their treasures in shops that lined the long medieval street. Perhaps, like the merchant Salarino at the start of *The Merchant of Venice,* traders and financiers sat anxiously in church, the vaulting stone ceiling reminding them of the towering rocks on which their vessels might break, the raging waters scattering the silks and gems intended for the shops across the way.

A hoard is something hidden away, or put aside for preservation. As treasures and storehouses, they are often assembled in desperation, or out of caution; created under conditions of secrecy. The Cheapside Hoard has retained this quality of mystery. The question of who would part with such riches, and under what circumstances, remains unsolved. But the jewellery was likely buried in the 1640s, perhaps by a Cheapside jeweller in the turbulent times of the civil wars.[2] The owner may have fled the city, intending to return for their goods, or may have died in battle. Many kinds of violence accompany the seductive brilliance of a gem.

Among the hoard's stones from Sri Lanka, Russia, Africa, and Afghanistan, emerald objects flicker in flames of green. A stout, parrot-shaped pin, tapering into a pointed tail. An enamelled cross pendant, each end marked by two emeralds. A brooch in the form of a sinuous salamander, its body a row of ten polished emeralds, its tail a curling string of diamonds. A pendant formed like a grapevine, yielding bundles of polished grapes carved from seven green stones. And the showstopper: a pocket watch, expertly cut from a sizeable hexagonal emerald. Gazing into the object is like peering into a pool of dappled light in an otherworldly sea.

The jeweller who made the watch, perhaps a 'stranger' or migrant artisan from France or the Low Countries, was a master gem-cutter. As they carved the emerald to set the watch and embellish it with gold, they kept the crystal's prismatic structure. Emeralds are notoriously brittle and softer than rubies or diamonds. The pressure applied to carve and decorate the jewel could have shattered the stone in the hands of a less skilled craftsperson. Whoever commissioned the object was fabulously wealthy, willing to hazard a weighty gem, mined in a rainforest on the other side of the Atlantic, to achieve this level of sparkle and finish.

All of the emeralds in the Cheapside Hoard were formed in deposits found in what is now Colombia. They were transported from the Muzo and Coscuez mining districts near Bogotá, crystallised by the Andean mountains' tectonic movements. 'The emerald mines are in the ground, and the soil contains certain sticky, clay veins, which turn the colour of sky blue,' one conquistador wrote in 1545. 'Inside the veins the emeralds grow.'[3] Before the sixteenth century, emeralds had been mined on a smaller scale in other parts of the world, including Egypt. They circulated in trade networks that spanned the Red Sea and the Mediterranean, carried on camels and ships through Silk Road routes. In Greek, Roman, and Byzantine jewellery, the vibrant green colour was associated with fertility and health.[4] But the clarity, size, and distinct blue-green lustre of emeralds excavated in the tropical forests of Colombia came to be most highly prized in European courts.

Emeralds were found in the flourishing homelands of the Muisca peoples, which stretched thousands of miles across savannah flatlands and alpine scrub. Muisca lands were abundant with emeralds and gold, but also rock salt, copper, and agricultural crops. Villages of *bohíos*, circular houses with thatched reed roofs, and temples built from the *guayacán* tree dotted the landscape. A longstanding mining tradition was part of the reason emeralds were found as far away as Peru or Mexico, where the Inca and Mexica acquired them by trading cotton and feathers. The Muisca were also skilled goldsmiths. Pouring molten gold into obsidian moulds, artisans made *tunjos,* anthropomorphic votive figures used to communicate with powerful deities.[5] Scatterings of emeralds were found alongside *tumbagas* in temples and at grave sites, ransacked by conquistadors who had so far failed to find their source. The acquisition of emeralds involved negotiations with Native women, since powerful peoples like the Panches, wrote the Spanish, 'send only women to make peace or to negotiate settlement terms with their enemies . . . They consider that these women possess greater strength and fortitude with which to make their pleas.'[6]

In 1537, the Spanish heard rumours of a centuries-old mine at Somodonco, which they renamed Chivor, deep in the eastern ranges of the Andes. Following a trail of hearsay, misinformation, and forced confessions, the Andalusian soldier Gonzalo Jiménez de Quesada led his soldiers through the highlands, launching a sustained military campaign against the Muisca. In the years that followed, Jiménez de Quesada met repeated resistance from men like Sagipa, the ruler of Bacatá. The Spanish had yet to locate the mines, but one scribe recorded some 1,815 emeralds that Jiménez de Quesada had collected through coercion and theft. Spanish accounts chronicled the discovery of what they called 'household idols' (the *tunjos*) buried or interred in water, made of fine gold and sometimes filled with emeralds.[7]

In the early 1540s, the Spanish turned their focus to the Province of Los Muzos, named after the Cariban-speaking Muzo, who had long been in conflict with their Muisca neighbours. The Muzo had extracted emeralds in the region for generations. Operating a system of dams and aqueducts made with hard tropical woods, they used water to dislodge the soil and reveal the embedded stones. The work was conducted in the sacred presence of the Fura and Tena mountain peaks, where ancient stories of love and betrayal were embedded in Muisca understandings of their homelands and the stones within them. Emeralds were the remorseful tears of Fura, the first woman, whose unfaithfulness to Tena led to the lovers' loss of immortality. Taking pity on their plight, the god Are turned them into mountains.

For two decades, the Muzo fiercely resisted the Spanish interlopers, using surprise attacks and poisoned arrows to prevent European encroachment. But, over time, diseases spread; and the Spanish cut off food supplies and brought vicious war dogs to destroy Muzo opposition, finally establishing a more secure presence. Exactly how the Spanish found the mines is not entirely clear, but by the mid-1560s, emeralds were no longer just the product of spoils and raids: they were now being shipped to Europe on an industrial scale. Settlements were populated by soldiers, Muiscas, and small numbers of enslaved Africans. After travelling to Guiana in 1595, Walter Ralegh praised the riches of 'Mozo [Muzo] where the Esmeralds are founde'.[8] Miners worked in perilous conditions, navigating steep, narrow paths and thick vegetation, striking through limestone and fossils to find the quartz. Muzo uprisings continued, but the Spanish offered severe reprisals.[9]

And so emeralds came to glisten in England during the gloomy and uncertain days of the mid-sixteenth century. When Mary Tudor became queen, in the summer of 1553, Lady Jane Grey was imprisoned in the Tower of London, awaiting execution after having ruled England as queen for a mere nine days. Edward VI had proclaimed her as his successor in his will, but Mary and her Catholic supporters had quickly defeated her. Among the record of the objects delivered to 'Lady Jane, usurper, at the Tower' was a 'sable skin, with a head of gold', garnished with turquoise, rubies, diamonds, pearls, and four emeralds. This was a *zibellino*, a fashionable, highly decorated sable pelt, made to be worn around the waist or carried as a warming accessory. Jane also received a coronet with an emerald, and a clock 'standing upon a mine of silver'.[10]

Might the emeralds in the imprisoned queen's sable pelt have come from Colombia (or the Kingdom of New Granada, as the Spanish called it)? It is impossible to know, but courtiers had access to trade networks in Seville or Antwerp that made acquiring such stones possible. Inventories of Henry VIII's gemstones listed multiple emerald jewels and rings. The emperor Charles V visited England in 1522, in the aftermath of Hernán Cortés offering him the treasures of the Mexica/ Aztec ruler Montezuma. Charles brought and distributed jewels as gifts and tokens, and emeralds may have been included in these exchanges. By the time Mary I married Charles's son, Philip, in the summer of 1554, conquistadors fighting in Charles's name were leading campaigns in the misty vegetation and river valleys of the Río Itoco and regularly sending shipments of emeralds across the Atlantic. Privateering also brought emeralds from Spanish ships to English coffers. In August 1545, Charles himself reported on the ships that the English had captured coming from Santo Domingo.[11] The cargo was undocumented, but the same letter referenced the 'emeralds and precious stones from Cartagena' that were already being used in political negotiations back in Europe.

What attracted the Tudors to these gems? In addition to being admired for their rarity, precious stones were financial assets, signalling status and allowing the rich to carry their wealth on the body. Gems were considered to hold medicinal properties; wearing them close to the skin allowed a person to absorb aspects of their healing, even magical, powers. Since emeralds had circulated in classical and medieval Europe, then known as *smaragdus*, they already had a place in pharmacopoeias and natural histories. Aristotle wrote that emeralds might bring good luck in business transactions, and could enhance the coveted gift of eloquence. They were believed to soothe the eye and promote better eyesight, restoring and sharpening one's ability to appreciate the verdant marvels of the world. Emeralds might also reveal betrayal, exhibiting strange alterations in the vicinity of an adulterer, and losing their brightness if they came near poison.[12] The salamander brooch in the Cheapside Hoard may have been created to play with these associations. In alchemical writings and emblems, amphibians represented regeneration and resurrection, moving between realms of water and land, rumoured to be able to withstand fire.

Emeralds added something vital to the kaleidoscope of colours at the Tudor court. Green was a difficult colour to make artificially. Wealthy Tudors put shades of pine and pear everywhere, bringing something of the garden or the forest into interiors and onto the body – clothes, bed furnishings, tapestries, cushions, crowns, and livery. For classical authors and their Renaissance translators, the best emeralds contained a deep, vivid colour that existed within itself, not 'uncertain & changeable' like a peacock's tail. Like the Roman naturalist Pliny the Elder, the painter Nicholas Hilliard would call emerald 'the most perfect greene on earth growing naturally, or that is in any thinge, or that is possibly by Arte to make'. The longer a person glanced at emeralds, the fairer and bigger the stones appeared, bathing their surroundings in light. Emeralds were a kind of portable Eden, seeming to carry the fertility and brightness of nature itself. 'We take great delight to behold greene herbes and leaves of tree,' Pliny wrote, 'but this is nothing to the pleasure wee have in looking upon the Emeraud, for compare it with other things, be they never so green, it surpasses them in all pleasant verdure.'[13]

In 1578, the merchant Thomas Nicholas presented Elizabeth's spymaster, Francis Walsingham, with *The Pleasant Historie of the Conquest of the Weast India*, a translation of Francisco López de Gómara's history of the Spanish invasion. In his picaresque beginning, Nicholas described chance meetings with elderly Spanish men who had been on campaign with the era's most famous conquistadors. During his time as a merchant in the Canary Islands, a convenient meeting point for voyagers coming from all parts of the world, Nicholas had spoken to a soldier who had 'served in the Conquest of the west India' under Cortés. The man had assured him that Gómara's account was accurate, and would provide a mirror or guide 'for all such as shall take in hande to governe newe Discoveries.'[14] During a long trek from the municipal town of Toledo to Castile, Nicholas joined the retinue of another aged gentleman. As they rode past mountain ranges and the ruins of Islamic gates and bathhouses, vestiges of Spain's centuries under Muslim rule, the man recounted tales of his youthful forays into the Americas. His participation in Spanish imperial expansion had brought many earthly rewards, from hoards of metals stashed in Seville to land in South America.

Nicholas's book sparkled with the promise of minerals and stones purloined from ancient civilisations, offering intriguing green glimpses of Indigenous wealth. Aztec/Mexica palaces and temples were filled with gold-worked emeralds. In places of mourning, bodies in colourful mantles might be buried with 'a fine Emerald' in the mouth. Among the jewels Cortés brought to Spain were 'five moste riche and fine Emeraldes', including 'a fishe with the eyes of gold, which was a marvellous peece of worke, beyng wrought among *Indians*'. Cortés gave the emeralds to his wife, 'the lyke never Lady had in Spayne'.[15]

Nicholas wrote as a merchant looking to foster lucrative connections between England and Spain's Atlantic empire. His publication came at a good time. Walsingham had just backed Humphrey Gilbert's plans to 'annoy the King of Spayne' by targeting Spanish and Portuguese ships passing Newfoundland from the West Indies.[16] Written in the months after Gilbert's voyage, and in the aftermath of Frobisher's own search for gold in Nunavut, Nicholas's book enticed patrons with the precious, scintillating stones the Americas promised.

In *The Naturall and Morall Historie of the East and West Indies*, the Jesuit José de Acosta wrote that emeralds attained their green flush through exposure to extreme heat and light, ripening like trees. He, too, acknowledged that emeralds were woven through Indigenous cultures. Rulers of Mexico pierced their bodies to affix 'an excellent Emerald'. The greatest store was in New Granada, towards 'the Land of Emeraldes'.[17] Acosta returned to Spain from Mexico at Philip II's behest in 1587, on a fleet that brought millions of pieces of silver, twelve chests of gold, and two chests of emeralds to Seville, along with cochineal dye, ginger, and hides. The treasure was so abundant that it helped fund the Spanish Armada against

England the following year. One Jacobean merchant called it 'the greatest Treasure that ever came at one time', and later histories recalled those same 'Chests of *Emeralds*' that offered proof of their abundance in the Americas.[18]

At the English court, where gift-giving was a blood sport, South American emeralds made a fitting gift for a queen. Francis Drake offered Muzo emeralds to Elizabeth after his Atlantic raids on Spanish colonial cities. Bernardino de Mendoza, Philip II's Ambassador in London, disdainfully recounted the spoils that Drake showcased when he returned to court after his circumnavigation of the globe in 1580. Silver from Mexico and Potosí was minted in the Tower, and now Elizabeth publicly proclaimed her support for Drake's ventures by wearing the crown he had given her during New Year's Day festivities. Over the years, Elizabeth had been presented with countless luxuries for New Year's, from candied fruits and quince pies to a velvet cap embroidered with ships, but Drake's crown surpassed these delights. It contained five emeralds, the Ambassador noted, 'three of them almost as long as a little finger', and the two others valued at thousands of pounds, 'coming, as they do, from Peru'.[19]

Over the years, Drake's purloined and paraded wares included the expertly cut emerald and gold jewels worn by the Andean Catholic aristocracy. In 1586, he led English soldiers in a raid against the Spanish colonial city of Cartagena, a thriving port grown rich through its silver exports and trade in enslaved Africans. The English spilled through the streets in the aftermath of the surprise attack, ransacking merchants' houses, workshops, and churches. In the weeks that followed, Drake set himself up in the city while his prisoners negotiated their release. The town's noblewomen offered 'a very faire jewel set with Emeralds and a ring with an Emerald & another Emerald set in a pendant', in addition to pearls and a 'fair [emerald] jewel' and a 'fair [emerald] ring'. Drake turned down the pearls, which he believed were overvalued, but he did accept the 'Jewells, which were al Emeralds'.[20] In all likelihood, crew members took additional emeralds illicitly when they looted the town.

As emeralds travelled from sacred Muisca and Muzo lands to the English court, to be polished and reworked in jewellers' shops in Cheapside, associations with South America lingered for a while. In the 1580s and 1590s, travellers' tales and printed books continued to recount stories of emeralds found in Incan Peru, the result of trade networks with Muisca and Muzo nations.[21] In anti-Catholic rhetoric, emeralds featured in discussions of Iberian cruelty. A popular source for the Black Legend was the Seville-born friar Bartolomé de las Casas's narration of the destruction of the Indies, which had first been published in the 1550s but regularly resurfaced in anti-Spanish propaganda. Las Casas wrote of how New Granada had been 'full of infinite people, kinde hearted like the rest, and very rich as well of Gold as of precious stones, which they call Emeralds'. Evidence of governors robbing and killing to find the stones, he insisted, remained hidden away in government offices in Seville, in chests with complicated locking mechanisms intended to keep out prying critics of imperial power.[22] The loss of Indigenous lives, however, did not lessen English demand.

The 1604 Anglo-Spanish peace treaty put a halt to the ostentatious display of colossal Andean spoils at court, but a continuous influx of emeralds were still incorporated into coronets and rings, of exactly the sort found in the Cheapside Hoard. In Jacobean portrait miniatures, emeralds dangled from earrings, brooches, and ribbons, casting a blaze of green across pale skin. Miniatures became jewels themselves, locked into gem-encrusted cases. A watch case made around 1620 featured the royal coat of arms on the reverse, encircling this emblem of the Stuart dynasty in the distinct blue-green glimmer of emeralds. James I owned a large looking glass studded with costly stones, including diamonds and at least a dozen emeralds.[23]

Seeking to showcase their own technical expertise, gem-cutters in Tudor and Stuart London developed complex shapes that heightened the mirror-like sparkle of jewels to dizzying effect, capturing the desires and fancies of prosperous consumers. Francis Bacon wrote that emeralds were among the gems most capable of bringing solace and beauty through expert cutting, glimmering like '*Pictures of Indian Feathers*'.[24] Sketches for pendants and aigrettes (ornamental hair jewels), set in table-cut emeralds like those in the hoard, survive in the design book of the jeweller Arnold Lulls and his associates, the pages teeming with sketches of vines and foliage made with green gems. Anna of Denmark, who inherited many of Elizabeth I's jewels after James became king, may have acquired the emerald pendants fashioned into earrings that the late queen had received in 1575. A clock at Anna's court at Somerset House, silver-gilt and shaped like a tortoise, used emeralds to imitate the animal's rough green skin: a 'great Emeralde' for the head, and nearly two dozen more for the neck, body, and tail.[25]

As the English developed their plantation industries and the East India Company increased its trading operations under the Stuarts, emeralds became useful currency in exchanges between England and eastern powers. In Mughal and Safavid cultures, emeralds were integrated into sacred art, used to depict the pastures and palms of paradise, and incorporated into Islamic displays of piety and magnificence on everything from daggers to inscribed jewellery.[26] English visitors to the Mughal court quickly recognised the value that emeralds had in the Islamic world. Thomas Roe, the first English Ambassador in India, listed emeralds among the goods that English factors traded in Surat in 1618, along with velvet, armour, and embroidered purses.[27] Captain William Hawkins noted that large, hexagonal emerald drinking cups were used in the social and diplomatic rituals of Mughal banquets.

After pilfering emeralds from Spanish treasure ships in Atlantic waters, English merchants increased their efforts to sell the stones in Asian markets because of this demand. Where emeralds had once been symbols of South American wealth and abundance, they were becoming a useful commodity, sent elsewhere to secure cloves, calicoes, and indigo. Over the course of the seventeenth century, emeralds brought America and Asia together, sweeping the gems 'into an Asia-centred world-system'.[28] By the 1670s, a history of jewels sought to dispel the 'ancient error of many to believe that the *Emerauld* is found in the East'. This had been the case 'before the discovery of *America*', but now they came 'from the source of the West Indies'.[29] Even 'orient' emeralds had begun life elsewhere. Before it had been sold to a court official in India, an emerald had been mined from the earth by Indigenous or African hands, carried by mule across wetlands and cloud forests – perhaps even taken at sea by pirates, sold in London, and pawned by a lady at the death of her husband a decade later, before it came to be acquired by East India Company merchants.

While merchants sought emeralds to traffic across the Indian Ocean, the seedy underside of the gem trade came to light in a dramatic dispute between agents of the East India Company. In 1631, Gerhard Polman, a Dutch gem merchant and jeweller, had boarded an English ship leaving Persia, carrying a fabulous collection of precious stones. Polman entrusted several members of the crew to help safeguard his goods, but the bags and boxes filled with gems did not stay secret for long. Sailors overheard him describing 'a great diamond about his necke which cast such lustre of candles burning' and openly admitting that he wore many precious stones in secret compartments close to his body. Polman died during the voyage, perhaps murdered, his treasure disseminated among members of the crew despite the captain's best efforts to keep them hidden away. Soon, these gems sparkled in pockets, taverns, and workshops across London.

In the years that followed, Company agents attempted to find the scattered gems. The privy councillor Robert Bertie, Earl of Lindsay, searched out jewellers' shops in Cheapside and questioned eye-witnesses and Company associates. Christopher Adams, who had used his skills as a carpenter to break open the chests that contained Polman's treasure, ill-advisedly boasted of these objects and showed them to admirers, revealing them in taverns with a drunken flourish and soliciting friends to stash them away. When Adams was finally caught, he relinquished an emerald, about three inches long and three inches wide. After some time in prison, he provided further intelligence that led Lindsay to a Susan Bradaye's house in Hockley in the Hole, where a seven-inch-long green stone had been hidden among old shoes.[30]

Could the Cheapside Hoard contain some of this dispersed cargo, buried to keep meddling government agents away? Some think so. The premium placed on emeralds would have made East India Company councillors keen to track the rarest specimens that crossed English borders, like the one used to make the watch. Large emeralds were the subjects of illicit and underhand dealings in Stuart London, as when a jeweller came before the council in 1633 to admit that he had 'lost the Company's great emerald', believing it to be the same that had recently been found by a maid and 'since come to the hands of an Italian'.[31] Just as likely, a shopkeeper, not a potentially murderous thief, had buried the chest to protect their goods. But, beyond the mystery of the treasure and who possessed it, the emeralds testify to their availability and desirability in early modern London. They offer a glimpse of the wide variety of quality, colour, and cut available to English consumers.

Although the emeralds were quite literally entangled with other globally sourced stones and metals, from Persian turquoise to Sri Lankan sapphires, they connect English culture to colonial mining and Muisca and Muzo homelands. In lamenting the plight of those living in Spanish-invaded lands, Protestant writers both acknowledged the effect of such extraction on Indigenous nations, and subsumed a multiplicity of lands, peoples, and practices under the word 'Indian'. But Indigenous peoples had long resisted colonisation in the tropical forests where emeralds were taken, fighting to retain their ancestral connections to the land, refusing to convert or to make life easy for those who had come to steal from the mountains Fura and Tena. One eyewitness in Puerto Viejo wrote in 1552 that, 'in order that nobody shall find [the mines], the Indians, who knew where they were, closed the road and let it become lost so that the Spanish should not make themselves owners of them'.[32]

Most of the emeralds to have survived from the time of the Tudors and Stuarts have found resting places in museums and heritage sites; but salvaged shipwrecks have resurfaced stones that, like the gems in the hoard, lived beyond the grasp of human hands for centuries. In 2017, twenty loose emeralds and a dozen pieces of emerald jewellery went to auction at Sotheby's and Christie's. These pieces, including an 11-carat emerald necklace with gold links, had been recovered from the *Nuestra Señora de Atocha*, a galleon wrecked by a hurricane off the coast of Florida in 1622. In 2022, a 5.27-carat emerald ring from the same wreck went to auction at Sotheby's, selling for $1.2 million.[33]

In 2024, Indigenous communities in Bolivia contested Colombia's plans to excavate a shipwreck that Colombian authorities have called 'the biggest treasure in the history of humanity', believed to be carrying precious stones and metals valued at £13 billion. The *San José* had been laden with gold, silver, and emeralds in Cartagena when the British sank it in 1708, in the very waters Drake had navigated over a century earlier. The survival of so many precious objects – silver from Potosí, emeralds from Chivor – opened up international debates about

Indigenous labour, colonial power, and the memories and histories that become bound with material goods. A public letter by members of the Caranga, Chicha, and Killaka peoples stated: 'We think that extracting important fragments from that era from the bottom of the ocean is like discovering an island, and on that island live our memories and the objects that the work of our ancestors created.'[34]

As islands of living memories, the emeralds that found their way to England in European galleons carried histories of their own, before they were fashioned into silver clocks or sent to the Mughal court. English writers often compared the green of emeralds to meadows and fields – beautiful tapestries of light, 'the Ey[e]'s Favourite', surpassing nature itself – but they ignored that the colour had always been important to the Muisca and Muzo, too.[35] The flicker of a green gem revealed sparks of the cosmos and embodied the saturated glow of their homelands and the earth's resources, which had to be respected to maintain balance. The deep vegetable landscape that flashed in an emerald captivated the Tudors and Stuarts who gazed into it. But the surface, like a mirror, reflected the gaze of the beholder. More than the lagoons and mountains of Colombia's ecosystems, they saw pastoral landscapes and other Indias reflected back.

A Gold Mine at Whitehall Palace

On a wintry night in February 1613, Londoners navigating the lanes and alleys between the Inns of Court and Whitehall could have caught sight of something extraordinary. Dozens of Virginians, dressed in sun-embroidered clothing and colourful feathered ruffs, rode horses from Chancery Lane to the royal palace in a dazzling spectacle of astonishing expense. Their black hair waved down to their shoulders, their heads topped with feathered crowns. They carried cane darts dipped in gold. All along the Strand, past the elaborate facades and walled gardens of aristocratic residences, the metallic spangles of the travellers' attire sparkled in the night, brightening what had been a gloomy and tempestuous season.

The Virginian 'priests' and 'princes' who processed to Whitehall on horseback were not Indigenous Americans, but wealthy English gentlemen enacting an elaborate scenario of make-believe. They were flanked by torch-bearers and a string of performers dressed as ruff-clad baboons. Two of London's legal institutions, the Middle Temple and Lincoln's Inn, had commissioned *The Memorable Masque* as their contribution to the festivities celebrating the marriage of James I and Anna of Denmark's sixteen-year-old daughter, Elizabeth Stuart, to Frederick, Count Palatine of the Rhine.

The forces behind the masque were leading members of the Virginia Company. Unlike the Atlantic flora and fauna collected in cabinets or kept in the domain of the home, the act of dressing up brought Indigenous imagery into the realm of imperial spectacle.

The whole parade, at least on the surface, was a glowing endorsement of English colonialism, bringing diverse and inconsistent fantasies about Indigenous peoples to the archways and public streets of London. Performed six years after the establishment of Jamestown, the masque combined longstanding associations of the colonial Americas with English imperial ambition – pearls, silver, and feather headdresses, sun worship and divine right.

The procession was only the beginning: once the masquers arrived at the palace, the pageant would become a more private affair. But before that, for one winter's night, perhaps warmed by a roasted apple or buttered parsnips, laundresses and watermen gazed upon an unparalleled exhibit of the English colonial imagination. No known entertainment had staged English transatlantic aspirations on such a scale. The effect left people breathless with exhilaration. It was in 'all parts so novell . . . and glorious, as hath not in this land . . . beene ever before beheld'.[1]

The Inns had a reputation for being the heart of literary London. The organisers hired the dramatist and poet George Chapman to script the masque. Seventeen years before, Chapman had written the poem 'De Guiana' to endorse Walter Ralegh's voyage to South America. Then, he had framed Guiana and Queen Elizabeth as sisters, bonded together through love and amity, and urged Elizabeth to send ships across the Atlantic to 'create / A golden world in this our iron age'. With honour, the English might acquire 'theft-free treasures with gold', not spoiled and stolen through bloody conquest, but willingly offered as gifts of friendship. *Golde is our fate*.[2]

The centrepiece of *The Memorable Masque* was a large gold mine, sitting on the stage as a rather unsubtle shrine to excavated wealth. But Chapman was more cynical than he had been in 1596; he had spent the last two decades writing plays that explored humankind's follies, and translated two epics, Homer's *Iliad* and *Odyssey*, that probed the grim realities of war and voyaging. Like any joint-stock company, chartered by the Crown but managed by its investors, the Virginia Company was rife with factions, its members unable to agree on any single coherent vision for what colonisation might look like. And although masques were forms of courtly entertainment that largely served to proclaim the virtue and splendour of the monarch, the Inns of Court were full of outspoken parliamentarians who had offered vociferous public opposition to royal prerogative in recent years. The gold-drenched dazzle of the Virginia masque was an articulation of English colonial desire, but an ambiguous one, reflecting the vanity of Jacobean projects back onto their aristocratic audience.

For years, Chapman's principal patron had been the young Prince Henry, who promoted Virginia colonisation as a pious project of conversion and settlement. The masque seemed designed with Henry in mind. The prince's court at St James's Palace was a centre of transatlantic activity, drawing together soldiers, captains, and writers whose passion for cartography, navigation, and warfare aligned with the young royal's. In 1610, the prince had helped to finance both Henry Hudson's search for a north-west passage to Asia, and Thomas Roe's voyage to the Orinoco Basin. His keen interest in Jamestown meant that many settlers reporting on the settlement in the first few months of its foundation wrote to Henry, not James.

Tragedy had struck three months before the show. In November 1612, Henry died after a swim in the Thames, possibly from typhoid fever. He was eighteen, and his unexpected death triggered widespread mourning. In Henry, 'a *glimmering light* of the Golden times appeared,' his chaplain wrote.[3] The prince's demise was a political blow for the nation's more militant Protestants, who were frustrated by James's relative tolerance towards Catholics. Many of these were colonial promoters who regarded Henry as indispensable to safeguarding

Protestant expansion in the Atlantic. Elegies and songs of mourning lamented a prince whose 'care had beene / Survaying India'. Encouraging settlement and conversion on the shores of America, Henry had been armed 'with all the arts / That sute with Empire'.[4]

In the aftermath of Henry's death, grim tales of uncanny weather were scribbled and published in cheap pamphlets, linking these events together. After a hot, arid summer, bitter blasts of wintry gales toppled buildings and ravaged Britain's coastlines, causing shipwrecks. In London, a silk dyer's house had blown down close to Christmastime, and timber frames had crashed onto the bed of a sleeping couple, though they survived.[5] The unruly winds, coupled with the 'darts of death' from recent plague outbreaks, '[give] us an outward calamity to our inward griefes'.[6]

The masque set off a flurry of preparation, offering a welcome distraction for those involved. Revels and other courtly festivities were as elaborate as they were whimsical. The final production was a momentary flash of colour and sparkle that had taken months to prepare. The royal household even had a Master of the Revels, responsible for overseeing its panoply of plays, masques, mock battles, and other 'devices' or entertainments. Account booklets of the Office of the Revels record payments made to tailors, embroiderers, and painters for costumes and set pieces. These give us a sense of what artisans made and decorated – ivy crowns and wild men, enchanters and Greek goddesses, griffins and dragons, chandeliers and a Roman senate house. Mountains and forests were painted on canvas and stretched over frames, or pasted together, to transport viewers into other times and realms.[7] When James I's banqueting house burned down in 1619 (possibly because of those flammable props), he spent over £15,000 building a new one. Inigo Jones's neoclassical masterpiece, the Banqueting House, is the only part of Whitehall Palace that remains visible today.

To contend with the royal performances, gentlemen at Middle Temple and Lincoln's Inn spared no expense. They hired Jones, already the kingdom's 'most Artfull and Ingenious *Architect*', to create the set design, which included the large mechanical gold mine, as well as a hollow tree around which the baboons danced in the topsy-turvy antimasque. The total cost of the production for the two Inns was an eye-watering £2,255 – enough to furnish multiple ships to Jamestown.[8] The Inns paid Chapman £100 for his service, Jones £110. To recuperate some of the costs, Lincoln's Inn charged its members between £1 and £4, about the cost of a custom portrait miniature.

Onlookers often raved about the lustrous clothes in court masques, and this performance was no different. Satins offered a 'glorious shining', like sparks of fire. The 'chiefe Maskers, in Indian habits' wore silver garments embroidered with gold suns. This design referenced the common reports, in English travel lore, of sun worship among peoples ranging from the Inca to Powhatans. Around each sun, a 'traile of gold' was made to '[imitate] Indian worke'. The masquers' feathered ruffs were spangled with seed pearls. On their heads, they wore 'high sprig'd-feathers' wrought into coronets. The motion of the feathers, no less than the gilt thread, 'shew'd exceedingly delightfull, and gracious'. While riding on horseback, the masquers wore buskins over their silk stockings, laced with rows of feathers, 'altogether estrangefull, and *Indian* like'.[9]

What inspired the artisans who had made the 'Indian-like' clothing? The response of various eyewitnesses makes it clear that the costumes struck viewers with awe, but details about the outfits remained vague. They were nothing like the clothing of Algonquian shamans or *werowances* that English colonists saw in Roanoke or Tsenacommacah. Travellers to North America noted that wealthy Algonquians decorated their bodies with shells and pearls, and might wear feathers to mark honours that had been bestowed on them. But beyond pearls and feathers, the masque costumes seemed to collapse geographies and iconographies together. There was a motley assemblage of influences, from the feathered headdresses of the Brazilian Tupi, to the classical breastplates and buskins of imperial Roman soldiers. The outfits equally served to differentiate gentlemen of the Inns based on their own highly calibrated understanding of social status. The 'civillest gentlemen' played Virginian princes. The torchbearers, though in 'Indian garb', wore showier, more ostentatious clothing that signalled their less graceful positions. The baboons were dressed as harlequin figures 'like fantasticall Travailers, in Neopolitane sutes, and great ruffes', looking as ridiculous as the rest did elegant.[10]

The horses clopping down the Strand, their saddles decorated with suns and jewels, were accompanied by two 'Moores, attir'd like *Indian* slaves'. In this brief description, things get even more confused. The sight of multiple priests and princes from the Americas might have seemed novel to many Londoners, but African or Muslim figures, often conflated in terms such as 'Moors' and 'blackamoors', would have been more familiar. Depictions of 'blackamoors' had long circulated in English visual art, emerging from European encounters with the Mediterranean and Africa through the Crusades, Spanish military campaigns in North Africa and Spain, and long-standing trade networks. Black characters appeared on the popular stage and in City processions. *Othello* (1603) is the best-known example, but Shakespeare had also given the stage to Aaron the Moor in *Titus Andronicus* (written in the late 1580s or early 1590s). In 1605, Queen Anna and her ladies had dressed up like African women and blackened their skin for a masque. Thomas Middleton's City procession, *The Triumphs of Truth*, performed in the same year as *The Memorable Masque*, included a 'King of the Moors' who had converted to Christianity due to friendly commerce with English merchants. 'I see amazement set upon the faces / Of these white people,' the king spoke to the crowd,

> Is it at me? do[e]s my Complexion draw
> So many Christian Eyes, that never saw
> A King so blacke before?'[11]

The 'Moors' in *The Memorable Masque* were not presented as kings, however, but '*Indian* slaves'. Transatlantic trafficking and enslavement were reshaping older stereotypes. The Venetian Ambassador, Antonio Foscarini, must have had this in mind when he contrasted the magnificence of the 'Princes of Virginia with crowns of feathers and pearls on their heads, and their hair down to their shoulders as in the custom of the country' against the 'hundred blacks dressed in gold and blue, the dress of Indian slaves'.[12] Behind the stylised depictions of African or 'Indian' people, meanwhile, living, breathing individuals from places ranging from Angola to the Caribbean moved in and out of English houses, parish churches, and the residences of Spanish or Italian merchants and ambassadors in London – some might even have caught sight of the procession themselves. Dederj Jaquoah, the 'sonne of Caddi-bian King of the river of Cetras … in the Country of Guinny', sent 'by his father in an English ship', was baptised in 1611. Black servants lived in households near Cheapside and St Paul's Cathedral, including an Isobel, a Peter, a Fortunatus, and an unnamed 'blackamore gerle'.[13]

Eventually, the crowd lost sight of the performers. The masquers passed under the chequered towers and griffins of the gothic Holbein Gate and paraded around the tiltyard at Whitehall before streaming into the Great Hall. The palace had undergone a transformation under the Tudors, enlarged with new galleries, long porticoes, and decorated chambers overlooking the Thames. Henry VIII had spent a colossal amount on renovations and refurbishments. A visitor to the palace at the end of the sixteenth century had noted its tennis courts, intricate carvings, and pattering white deer.[14] James had then helped to transform the landscape of the adjacent St James's Park, adding ponds and islands, and improving the marshy grounds through drainage projects.

In addition to the animals kept in the Tower, the king established a second menagerie in St James's, which contained camels, birds, a beaver, and two Hispaniola crocodiles. A few years after the masque, around 1615, a Continental traveller would include a watercolour scene of St James's Park in his *album amicorum,* or friendship book. An Algonquian man stands at the centre in fringed deerskin, his hair worn long over one shoulder, a woven bag tucked at his side.[15] This is believed to be the Powhatan traveller Eiakintomino, who was present in London around this time along with a companion named Matahan. On the masque's doorstep, Indigenous North Americans were there to remind onlookers of the gap between those feathered costumes and real Powhatan people.

After processing through the tiltyard, the masquers entered the Great Hall to begin the performance. A craggy 'artificiall Rock', nearly as high as the hall itself, dominated the stage, its surface covered with veins of gold. The prop was so large that performers climbed up and down its facade via two winding staircases. A silver temple stood to one side, flanked by silver statues and pillars. The mountain and temple were some of the first things that audience members noticed when they took their seats. The Venetian Ambassador offers a singular view of Jones's stage mechanics:

> When the King entered the Hall one saw a mountain all
> full of crags and on the top the Temple of Honour, made of
> silver . . . Hardly had the King appeared when the crags came

forward five paces towards his Majesty; clouds gathered, the mountain split, and there appeared a rich mine of gold with all the Masque[rs] inside and a vast number of torches; it all took place in a moment.[16]

The entertainment began with a humorous exchange between Plutus, god of wealth, and the foolhardy traveller Capriccio. The vain Capriccio irks Plutus by attempting to intrude into the golden mine, but he also heralds the impending arrival of the Virginian princes and priests. He announces that, on his fantastical travels, he has seen the inhabitants of an island in the orbit of 'the Virginia continent' making their way to the shores of Britain, soaked in gold and coming to pay their homage to the royal marriage now taking place. Plutus is wary of the ostentatious Capriccio, who puffs around with too much confidence in his own wit. Capriccio and the other antimasquers' crude desire for wealth had 'cut out the skirts of the whole world, in amorous quest of . . . gould and silver'. The baboons from the procession join Capriccio for the antimasque, or comic dance, where they prance around the barren tree, a reminder that pure avarice is never fruitful. Plutus banishes Capriccio, hurling a single wedge of gold at him as a party favour to send him on his way.[17]

After Capriccio's exit, the masque can truly begin. Plutus calls on a personified Honour and Eunomia, goddess of the law, to be his guides. The mountainous rock rumbles forward and breaks open, revealing its 'rich and refulgent' gold mine. The Virginian princes spring out, greeted by Honour, who calls on those 'Princes of the Virgine land' who have crossed 'the Britan Ocean / To this most famed Ile, of all the world, / To do due homage'.[18] The radiating gold and silver costumes hit the gleaming surface of mine and temple, beaming the light of metals to the furthest end of the hall. In the background, 'certaine white Cliffes' can be spotted beyond the mine.

The props and painted scenes on the stage compact vast geographies together, transposing Virginian mines onto the White Cliffs of Dover, creating a fiction of proximity.

Over the course of several songs and dances, the troupes of 'Virgine Knights' and 'Priests of the Sun' are transformed into loyal subjects of King James, their grace and sparkle channelled towards the most accepted form of idolatry: fealty to the Crown. 'Virginian Princes,' Eunomia says, 'you must now renounce / Your superstitious worship of these Sunnes, / Subject to cloudy darknings.' Already prone to worshipping the sun, the princes can instead channel their adoration to the king, who is likened to Phoebus, god of light.[19]

As goddess of the law and good governance, it shouldn't surprise us that Eunomia was chosen to guide the masquers to virtue. The masquers, after all, were students of the Inns of Court. When they weren't smoking tobacco and writing racy poetry, they spent their days reading law books, debating legal matters, and participating in mock trials. In banishing the foppish Capriccio at the start of the performance, the gentlemen of the Middle Temple and Lincoln's Inn were not renouncing their hopes for gold mines, but rather proclaiming the value of their involvement in colonial projects. It was wealth *with* honour and good governance that would make England the imperial power it wished to be. This vision wasn't so unlike the one Chapman had presented in his poem for Ralegh way back in 1596, when he imagined '*riches* with honour, *Conquest* without blood'.

Still, much had changed in seventeen years. After the long reign of the Virgin Queen, the Stuart dynasty celebrated the role that women played in dynastic security. The gold mine became incorporated into the magnificence of kingly imperial power, but women and marriage had a role to play in empire-building, too. The earth's 'wombe of gold' shone out in celebration of Princess Elizabeth's marriage to Frederick, and she was celebrated for continuing the golden line of the Stuart dynasty. The masque ended with 'A Hymne to Hymen', or marriage song, encouraging the princess to embrace Frederick on her wedding night. The union of two youthful royal bodies ushers in a new era of prosperity, for 'the blessings of the golden age, / Swimme in these Nuptials.'[20] It wasn't the only moment during her wedding festivities when Elizabeth would sit through a masque explicitly encouraging fruitfulness and increase. Shakespeare's *Tempest* included a masque engineered by Prospero to bless the political marriage of his daughter Miranda.

Courtiers liked a sumptuous party, and masques were often the prelude to many more hours of merriment and sanctioned disorder. Plutus' final address to the Virginia knights was an invitation for revelry. As the speech drew to an end, the performance concluded with a ballet that brought the revellers streaming into the crowd. The Indigenous figures moved into the audience, taking the ladies of the court in their arms and spinning them around the candlelit room.

What was it like to dance with a 'Virginian'? What did it mean for those up-and-coming gentlemen of the Inns to gain access to the royal court for a night of fantasy, and to choose to do so through a transatlantic theme? This was a momentous occasion for many of its young participants. Their own sense of civility was polished through the gleaming embers, the 'refulgence', of the performance. Masques were events where women and men came of age, stepping into society to see and be seen. When Dorothy Unton commissioned a portrait of her recently deceased husband, Henry Unton, in 1596, she included a court masque alongside other scenes depicting key moments in his life, from university to diplomatic service in France. On the night of Chapman's masque in February 1613, its performers, and those spectators who joined their hands to dance the closing ballet, came of age under a scintillating vision of empire.

In a masque performed several years before, Queen Anna and her ladies had moved across the stage in sea-coloured silks, playing water nymphs adorned with shells and other maritime decorations. The poem scripted by the writer Samuel Daniel for that performance honed in on this strange, suspended world of performance, in all its momentousness and effervescence:

> *Are they shadowes that we see?*
> *And can shadowes pleasure give?*
> *Pleasures only shadowes bee . . .*
>
> *When your eyes have done their part,*
> *Thought must length it in the hart.*[21]

We can imagine how it felt to feast in the banquet afterwards, dizzy with wine and confections that could well have been sweetened with sugar grown on Brazilian plantations. Masques were notoriously raucous; those in attendance nursed hangovers and wrote tale-bearing letters to friends the following day, commenting on who had made intoxicated fools of themselves. Back in their chambers near Holborn, those Virginian princes and priests laid down their olive-coloured masks and unfastened their shimmering costumes, having promised to return them to the organisers the following day. Although they had twirled in those feathered clothes for only a night, the performance must have lingered in the minds of many, lengthening 'in the heart' this experience of exhilarating refinement as a memory that came back to them when they sat in chambers not far from Whitehall, deciding on Virginia Company affairs.

In that blustery winter of 1613, in the wake of dead princes and collapsing timber-frame ceilings, the success of the English colonial project hung by a thread. Both Prince Henry and Robert Cecil

– James's Secretary of State and a savvy proponent of Atlantic intervention – had died within six months of each other. To prevent English imperial ambitions from becoming mere shadows and vanished hopes, one needed action – to invest funds, build ships, and encourage artisans, servants, and farmers to undertake odysseys of their own.

Meanwhile, far from Inigo Jones's manufactured gold mine and its wonder-inducing mechanisms, John Rolfe experimented with West Indies tobacco specimens, planting them in Chesapeake soil with the help of Powhatan seed-bearers, sowing the crop that would change Virginia's fortunes. Laws and ordinances published the year before forbade colonists from blaspheming against God or uttering seditious words against James or his royal authority, on pain of death. Those who slandered His Majesty's Honourable Council for the colony would be whipped and forced to ask forgiveness on bended knee. Matoaka, or Pocahontas, was still living among her people, unaware that she would soon be kidnapped and held prisoner at Henrico, a town named after England's now-dead prince.

While the gold mine at Whitehall offered a materialisation of all those dreams of rich America that had seduced English patrons for so long, the fleeting promise of a mine became the means for one Wampanoag man to find a way home. As a newlywed princess blushed (or perhaps rolled her eyes) at being publicly encouraged to succumb to the 'scorcht phantasies' of love in her new husband's embrace, an Indigenous man in London named Epanow plotted a way back across the ocean.

In 1611, Epanow had been captured in Capawak/Noepe – the island that captain Bartholomew Gosnold rechristened Martha's Vineyard – along with a man named Coneconam. In the same voyage, Captain Edward Harlow took three other men: Sakaweston from Nohono (Nantucket), and Monopet and Pekenimme from

Monhegan Island off the coast of Maine. Six years before, English captains had captured five Abenaki – Tahanedo/Nahanda, Amoret, Skicowaros, Maneddo, and Sassacomoit – in the region of Mawooshen (Maine). Maneddo, Skicowaros, and Sassacomoit lived with Ferdinando Gorges, a seasoned soldier and administrator who had fought against the Spanish in the Netherlands before taking charge of harbour defences at Plymouth. 'We have brought them to understand some English,' the sailor James Rosier wrote of the Algonquians the crew had brought to England in 1605, 'and we understand much of their language; so we are able to aske them many things.' These men were 'merry; and so kinde', disinterested in material trappings, so that if 'you give any thing to one of them, he will distribute part to every one of the rest'.[22]

Epanow became widely known and recognised in England in the years that followed, being 'shown up and downe *London* for money as a wonder'. He and his companions' presence in the metropolis may have inspired Trinculo's dark comment, in *The Tempest*, that callous and entertainment-hungry Londoners would 'not give a doit to relieve a lame beggar', but would 'lay out ten to see a dead Indian'.[23]

Meanwhile, he conjured up a mine as counterfeit as the wedding masque's stage props. He circulated a rumour that Capawak was home to a rich gold mine. Gorges was sceptical about this potential source of wealth, and his journal entry about Epanow's information is vague and secretive. Lodging Epanow in his residence with Sassacomoit in Plymouth, Gorges spent time observing the two men speaking among themselves, eventually deciding that Epanow's promises were sound. He approached a fellow colonial enthusiast, the Earl of Southampton, to plan the voyage and assemble a crew. In the summer of 1614, 'Epenow, Assacomet, [and] Wenape, another native of those parts', accompanied English captains and sailors across the Atlantic.

In a story that so often involves loss and broken connections, here is a small moment of relief. In a ship under the command of Nicholas Hobson, Epanow and his companions reached Capawak. After years of being prodded as a curiosity in the vicinity of Whitehall Palace and the Globe Theatre, he was back among white cedar and sweetgrass, birchbark canoes and blue heron feathers, moose-hair shoes and fireflies.[24] His friends and kin crowded around the ship to greet him. Gorges had assigned several guards to prevent Epanow from escaping, even specifying that he should be clad in long, cumbersome garments to hinder any nimble attempt at wriggling away. In the excitement and activity, however, Epanow arranged a plan with his kinsmen. The following day, a group of Wampanoag in a large assembly of canoes provided a distraction. Epanow leapt overboard and swam ashore. 'Thus,' Gorges wrote, 'my hopes of that particular [mine] made void and frustrate . . . [the crew] returned without doing more.'[25] The conflict wounded and killed English and Wampanoag fighters; but Epanow had made it home.

That same spring and summer, in the months leading to Epanow's escape, two more ships had travelled to North America, looking to profit from whale-hunting and to make trials of rumoured gold and copper mines. John Smith was on board, expressing reservations about the venture. 'Whale-fishing' was costly; 'we saw many and spent much time in chasing them, but could not kill any'. As for the gold, it had been 'the Masters device to get a voyage that projected it'. Patrons knew that the promise of gold might incite a journey, but fish and furs were more dependable commodities. Even so, the voyage wasn't particularly lucrative. Smith traded for beaver and otter skins to supply the realm's growing beaver hat industry; but, though the English 'ranged the Coast both East and West much further . . . our commodities were not esteemed'.[26]

Smith's choice of words stands out. The elusive gold, he wrote, had been a '*device* to get a voyage'. A 'device' can be something contrived; 'an arrangement, plan, scheme, project, contrivance'. But it is also 'something devised or fancifully invented for dramatic representation, as in a mask played by private persons'. In the early 1610s, masques, revels, and transatlantic schemes were fused together, like the metals in a banqueting cup. In 1611, the Lord Mayor of London was a goldsmith. At his inauguration, an entertainment involving ships returning from 'the rich and Golden *Indian* Mines' brought with them a king and queen riding on golden leopards with a host of 'Indian' pages, laden with ingots of silver and gold.[27] The gold mine in Whitehall Palace set the scene, in a crudely literal way, for Jacobean England's most feverish hopes. During this time, there were plans to 'discover' gold mines in a Virginia that spanned the length of North America's eastern seaboard, from Florida to Martha's Vineyard. Gold was the binding agent in *The Memorable Masque,* colonial propaganda, and Epanow's plan.

In *The Memorable Masque,* many of the realm's aspiring lawyers, writers, politicians, and colonists participated in a performance that both lampooned the avaricious, foolhardy traveller and presented English civility as the model for an idealised transatlantic empire. But this was no straightforward triumph. Chapman had scripted a warning into the story through the vain Capriccio and his wedge of gold. And if the stage taught one anything, it was that appearances were deceiving. Costly apparel, wrote one seventeenth-century traveller, was like a masquing suit, 'wherein wee act, not what wee are, but what we seeme to be . . . and by a jug[g]ling tricke makes us take that for a brave man which is a piece of shreds, a meere thing of the Taylors fashioning'.[28] Civility was a veneer, displaying a confidence that exposed corruptions and moral failings underneath.

*

For a moment, in the flickering glow of the candles, the darkness overtakes the light. For a moment, all is shadow, as in Daniel's poem. The dancers are in limbo. The mine is not a mine, but a towering prop. It does not signal the reality of gold, but the figments of one's own desires, vanishing fast. The insubstantial pageant faded, Prospero would say. Beyond the gold mine, there aren't the cliffs of Dover, but Epanow, running home.

Tobacco Leaves and
Laurel Crowns

As a rich and beautiful young man with a vigorous love of poetry, the Earl of Southampton graced the dedications of countless books of Elizabethan verse. 'What I have done is yours,' Shakespeare professed to him at the start of his erotic poem, *Venus and Adonis* (1593). But the most remarkable instance of Henry Wriothesley's name in print is not found in a book, but on a tobacco pipe. This extraordinary object was created thousands of miles from England, in lands the Powhatan called Tsenacommacah. It was made by the pipe-maker Robert Cotton in the aftermath of the establishment of Jamestown, moulded from local terracotta clay in direct imitation of Algonquian styles. On a fragment no bigger than a finger, next to a cluster of tiny imprints of fleur-de-lis, you can just about make it out: *E. Southam*.

Southampton was an investor in the Virginia Company. Later, he would become its treasurer, and a powerful advocate of colonialism in Parliament. The pipe connects tobacco and fledgling colonial projects to poets and literary patrons in London. It is fairly well known that tobacco became a popular pastime in Shakespeare's day. But how related was smoking to the Americas? And what role did it play in the development of English literary culture?

Before chocolate, tea, and the rise of coffeehouses, there was tobacco: the first foreign intoxicant of mass consumption in England. In the sixteenth century, it had come into the realm on a relatively small scale. Decades before the settlements in North America, tobacco entered English ports in sailors' pockets and merchants' cargoes, during the privateering voyages of the 1560s. By the 1630s, the plant had become a recurrent feature in recipe books, household accounts, diaries, herbals, plays, satires, and port records. Women, men, and children consumed it.

Four-hundred-year-old fragments of characteristic white-clay pipes can still be found on riverbanks and scattered in fields as waste from kilns. Pipe-making industries developed across England, though the official company for their manufacture was the Worshipful Company of Tobacco Pipe Makers of Westminster, incorporated by a royal charter in 1619. While seemingly commonplace, these pipes signal an important shift in English practices of consumption. Unlike glass and earthen vessels for eating and drinking, clay pipes were disposable objects. They were functional, but not made to last. Smoking left clouds of vapour and the lingering scent of slightly sweet, sharp tobacco, but also a scattering of broken clay – a new kind of waste, caused by the whims of consumers across a range of social groups.

In its meteoric ascendance, it can be easy to forget that tobacco came to the English as an artefact of sorts. To be successfully cultivated and packaged for consumption, each pinch of tobacco bore distinct characteristics based on the knowledge and practices of various Indigenous groups, as well as how long it had travelled for, or the climate's effect on particular crops. Tobacco cultivated in Trinidad, such as the *Nicotiana tabacum* plant, came to the English via Spanish merchants and physicians, and had such an influence on the English palate that North American tobacco (*Nicotina rustica*) initially seemed distasteful and too bitter for colonists in the Chesapeake.

Thomas Hariot's *A Briefe and True Report of the New Found Land of Virginia* (1588) offered an early English description of the pleasures of smoking. Translations of medical books, such as the Spanish physician and botanist Nicolás Monardes's *Medicinall Historie of Things Brought from the West Indies* (1565), contained detailed images of herbs and flowers filling the page. But whereas medical books removed the plant from its Indigenous contexts by turning it into a specimen, Hariot related smoking to Algonquian ceremonies. He introduced tobacco as *uppówoc*: 'The leaves thereof being dried and brought into a powder, they use to take the fume or smoke thereof by sucking it through pipes made of claie.' In addition to its health benefits, he acknowledged that *uppówoc* played a spiritual and social role in Indigenous communities.

Hariot specified that the English learned their method of smoking directly from Algonquians. The Spanish tended to smoke cigar-like rolls of tobacco, a practice adapted from Carib, Arawak, and Tupi peoples in the West Indies and South America. André Thevet, the French cosmographer who travelled to Brazil, noted that the Tupi had a 'secret herbe' that they dried and wrapped in the leaf of a palm tree, making rolls the length of a candle and receiving the smoke through their nose and mouth.[1] When Hariot smoked, he did so through the elbow-shaped stem pipes made by Carolina Algonquians. 'We our selves,' he wrote, 'during the time we were there used to suck it after their manner, as also since our returne, & have found manie rare and wonderful experiments of the vertues thereof; of which the relation would require a volume of it selfe.'[2]

Even in this very early period of colonisation, Anglo-Algonquian exchanges had a substantial influence on English culture. This is partly why archaeologists find so many clay pipes in their excavations of early seventeenth-century theatres, taverns, and country houses. In 1605, the Artois botanist Carolus Clusius cited the 1585 Roanoke expedition as the founding moment of English pipe manufacture: 'The colonists reported that the inhabitants often used certain pipes made of clay to take in the smoke of burning tobacco. The English, upon their return from there, brought with them similar pipes for taking tobacco smoke. Thereupon the use of tobacco spread even throughout the whole of England, especially among the courtiers.' Though he didn't mention Hariot by name, Clusius seemed familiar with *A Briefe and True Report*. He noted the significance of Ralegh's Roanoke project for the spread of smoking among the upper classes especially. While sailors who had accompanied privateers on their transatlantic voyages had been bringing tobacco into the realm for decades, Hariot and his affiliation with Ralegh's circle of aristocrats helped turn tobacco into a civil pastime for the elite, or, as Hariot put it, for 'men & women of great calling as else'.[3]

In turning tobacco into a commodity of mass consumption, the English departed from the value systems of Indigenous peoples. Surviving codices, ceramic vessels, and woven bags from across the Americas tell us of the importance of tobacco to countless Native groups throughout history. Whether smoking or chewing leaves, scattering plants or infusing them, tobacco served sacred social, medical, and diplomatic functions. One anonymous traveller to the Chesapeake in 1607 observed that Algonquians offered tobacco to the sun and sprinkled its leaves into rivers in the mornings before washing. Sunrise ceremonies involving mixtures of healing and sacred plants, such as tobacco, cedar, sage, and sweetgrass, are still practised by some Algonquian groups today. Among the Tzeltal and Tzotzil Maya in the highlands of Chiapas, pink-flowered *Nicotiana* plants continue to be used for protective or medicinal purposes, considered to be a helper and guardian, and carried in gourds that hark back to the ancient Maya.[4]

Tobacco could increasingly be found in English kitchens and gardens, where women and men conducted botanical experiments to find effective remedies for ailments ranging from headaches to surface wounds. In early seventeenth-century Gloucestershire, the writer Elinor Fettiplace included tobacco in her manuscript of recipes and medical remedies. The book was a work in progress, a place where she could test and modify her recipes, note her impressions, and make alterations to assist future readers, drawing on the advice of friends and on material she gathered from printed books. Among instructions for making rose syrup, meringues, and sweet-potato dishes, Fettiplace listed 'tobacco water' and 'syrup of tobacco' – two recipes she had received from Walter Ralegh himself.

Physicians and moral authorities, meanwhile, fervently debated the properties of tobacco in pamphlets and medical books. Scrappy arguments broke out between those who believed the plant corrupted the body and the soul, and those who subscribed to its healing properties. In London's Lime Street, botanists and other members of the scientific community, many of them migrants with strong ties to Europe, nourished Atlantic seeds and plants along the city walls. Travellers returning from their voyages brought roots and flowers from the Strait of Magellan or Caribbean islands to the botanist John Gerard and the physician Matthias de L'Obel. These transplanted specimens shared soil with roses and garlic. The deep green leaves and small, trumpet-shaped flowers of tobacco's long-blooming plants dotted the landscape of country estates and physic gardens, turning domestic ecosystems into Atlantic microcosms.

Tobacco's hot and dry properties were considered beneficial in countering afflictions that might accost the denizens of a cold and rainy island, from sluggishness to melancholy. The medical advice was often to bind the leaves against the skin, or to steep them in liquid, rather than inhale their vapours. John Frampton's *Joyfull Newes Out of the Newfound World* (1577), a translation of a treatise by the Sevillian doctor Nicolás Monardes, explained that 'stamped leaves' would unlock 'mervellous medicinable virtues'. In Edmund Spenser's chivalric romance, *The Faerie Queene* (1590), the huntress Belphoebe heals the wounded Timias by powdering and bruising 'divine Tobacco' and squeezing its juices into the squire's wound. In 1595, a pamphlet that praised the many uses of tobacco's velvety leaves included the story of a woman who saved her poisoned cat by forcing a little ball of tobacco, mingled with butter, into the feline's mouth.

Cut green leaves, or tobacco distilled into a syrup, could be applied to most parts of the body that needed healing. In this way, tobacco was employed for health reasons, while avoiding more direct associations with the smoky rituals of 'savage' or 'pagan' America. The physician John Cotta, who also wrote about the power of witches, attributed the profusion of new discomforts and diseases gripping England to 'the riotous use of this strange Indian'. James I's silkworm expert, the Huguenot John Bonoeil, expressed the belief that 'there is some sorcery in this weed', relating its intoxicating qualities to the fact that it had been 'first sowne (it seemes) by some Indian Enchanters hand, with spells and Magicke verses'.[5] A safer remedy, less perilous to the soul, was crushing leaves to release their scent, followed by a restorative walk.

In 1571, an image in Pierre Pena and Matthias de L'Obel's book of plants, *Stirpium Adversaria Nova*, starkly conveyed the realities of the labour involved in tobacco cultivation. As was common in herbals and medical texts, the book contained detailed images of flora to help the reader identify local and global plants, from primroses to cactuses. Unusually, the page for tobacco also contained a human figure: the head of an African man with a large roll of tobacco in his mouth. In the mid-Elizabethan period, while the queen was strengthening her commitment to Protestantism after excommunication by Pope Pius V, her subjects could open a printed book by European physicians living in London and find evidence of the enslaved labour and Indigenous smoking practices that underpinned their own access to tobacco plants.

But English smokers were addicted. Medical discussions sought to disassociate tobacco from its origins, but its connections to the Americas were also part of the plant's appeal. As an intoxicant, smoking brought with it the heady pleasure of indulgence and excess. The Swiss traveller Thomas Platter commented on just this when he wrote about the ubiquity of tobacco in London alehouses and taverns in 1599. The English regard smoking as a medicine, he wrote, but also 'a pleasure'. In playhouses and taverns – basically, anywhere they could also get a drink – men and women pulled out the pipe. Platter keenly observed that, beyond the rhetoric about the benefits or ills of medical tobacco, the English smoked abundantly because it was gratifying, even though 'their preachers cry out on them for their self-destruction'.[6] There was something subversive about puffing your way through the public spaces of the city, spending your cash like a prodigal son or daughter, when you then had to sit in church and hear grave Protestant preachers warn you about the sins of vanity and pride. The emptiness of vapour was a favoured conceit: how did it feel, moralists asked, to watch your fortunes drift off in a cloud?

Yet the leaf prevailed. It wasn't just vapour, after all, but a tangible thing, wrapped in little papers or stored away in rounded boxes that were becoming common presences at dinners and drinking parties. In university plays and theatres, young men dressed as Tobacco appeared onstage in russet-coloured suits, their skin dyed brown, acknowledging tobacco's migrations across the Atlantic:

> *Tobacco is a Travellour*
> *Come from the Indies H[i]ther;*
> *It pass'd Sea and Land*
> *Ere it came into my hand.*[7]

The figure of the tobacco smoker was often depicted as a swaggering gentleman, obsessed with travel and fashion. In John Donne's 'Satire I', penned during his years at the Inns of Court, the speaker pokes fun at members of the young gentry arriving in London, eager to enjoy the vices of the city and striving to exude an aura of refinement by learning to 'excell / Th'Indians, in drinking [their] Tobacco well'.

Women, like the rambunctious pickpocket Mary or 'Moll' Frith, might also inhabit such personas. In 1611, Moll Cutpurse was notorious enough to become the subject of a play called *The Roaring Girl*, which depicted her as a cross-dresser, strutting around in masculine fashions with a sword in one hand and pipe in the other. Two gallants in the play, hanging around a tobacco shop looking to seduce women, observe her sense of independence, gained partly through her economic self-sufficiency. 'She's a Gentlewoman borne I can tell you, tho it be her hard fortune now to shred Indian pot-hearbes,' Laxton says. 'Oh sir tis many a good womans fortune,' Goshawke responds, 'when her husband turns bankrout [bankrupt], to begin with pipes and set up again.'[8]

As Platter reported, the English accessed tobacco from the Indies on a large scale. Until they successfully established their own plantation industries in North America, their tobacco largely came from the West Indies. Tobacco was sometimes referred to in English sources as 'Trinidado', reinforcing its distinct connection with the Caribbean. By the time it got to an English port, it had likely travelled from Brazil or Trinidad to Seville and then across the Channel. Clay pipe bowls in Platter's time were only about the size of an acorn. Even a pinch of quality tobacco came at a high price. Over time, as tobacco got cheaper, the bowls grew larger. To know 'what state Tobacco is in towne, better than the Merchants,' wrote the pamphleteer Thomas Dekker, 'gain Gentlemen no meane respect'.[9] Social embarrassment awaited the gentleman who knew his Rhenish from his Spanish wine, but couldn't make distinctions between Trinidado and English garden-variety tobacco.

Protestants were all too aware of how the economic dependence on Spanish and Portuguese tobacco stood at odds with their fierce denunciations of Catholic activities in the Americas. Essentially, their dependence on Iberian plantations meant they were pouring money into the very empire they were intent on challenging, and sometimes at war with. Increasingly, English taste-makers in London condemned such tobacco as inferior to what came to them from the fledgling English plantations in the Chesapeake and then Bermuda. West Indian tobacco, wrote one anonymous author in 1615, was crudely mixed with juices and syrups that masked the rotting taste of that 'filthy leafe'. These tricks included using annatto – the crushed achiote seeds that Indigenous peoples used as body paint and dyes.[10]

After tobacco leaves were cultivated and packaged, shipped across the Atlantic, and sold by apothecaries, tobacco-induced fancies could begin. In 1602, a teenager named John Beaumont wrote what is one of the first known English poems dedicated entirely to tobacco. Beaumont was studying at the Inner Temple, becoming part of a coterie of accomplished writers who orbited in and around the Inns of Court. He wrote his poem in smooth rhyming couplets, lending an air of comic heroism to his tale of tobacco's grand entrance into European civilisation. *The Metamorphosis of Tobacco* riffed off Ovid's *Metamorphoses*. It offered a retelling of classical myths, with their tales of desire and transformation, for a new generation growing up in the wake of colonial expansion. The poem celebrated debauched intoxication and elevated artistic style. Beaumont's extravagant praise of tobacco seems almost avant-garde, as he yearns to imbibe the pagan essence of the drug:

Avant base Hypocrite, I can not thee,
But thou great God of Indian melodie,
Which at the Caribes *banquet govern'st all,*
And gently rul'st the studiest Caniball . . .

Infume my braine, make my soules powers subtile,
Give nimble cadence to my harsher stile:
Inspire me with thy flame.[11]

Beaumont doesn't want the tainted smoke of cheap tobacco, contaminated by dyes and syrups. He sees himself as a connoisseur, a cut above his foppish peers who access the corrupted drug and believe it's the real thing. He wants the tobacco that he imagines cannibals to smoke at their most anarchic banquets. Mixing stereotypes and stories of various American spaces, he wants to tap into the source, and access the stuff 'by whom the Indian Priests inspired be'.

For Beaumont, tobacco is responsible for the literature of the Golden Age. It comes into the world when the supreme god, Jove (or Jupiter), pursues a nymph, which his vengeful queen Juno turns into a tobacco plant. Impelled by love to bestow on the plant all the best qualities, Jove invests this 'glorious bud' with mystical powers that trigger the Golden Age. It is thanks to this blessed moment that the muses can truly inspire human interlocutors. Tobacco reigns so supreme, Beaumont wrote, that the era's epic quests for gold lose their lustre by comparison. Next to its vivid green leaves, even Apollo's garland of bays – the laurel crown that sits atop the head of the accomplished god of poetry and prophecy – looks a little rumpled.

The *Metamorphosis of Tobacco* is whimsical and inventive. But it also brought political debates about colonialism into the most seemingly fantastic expressions of literary wit. Assigning tobacco such a prominent role in English literary culture escalated demand. The tobacco leaf

– that 'nymph', a term used repeatedly at the time to personify American landscapes – was not fossilised into a remote classical past, but a conduit to changing ideas about civil refinement. Like rhetoric – an essential component to any civil society by classical standards – tobacco persuaded and elevated. It graced the lives of those who knew how best to smoke it. The poem's persona may take a deep breath of the herb and get a whiff of cannibals and Bacchanalian nights, but it also gives him a fluent tongue. Language and colonialism went hand in hand; who yet knew, as another author wrote around the same time, where the 'treasure of our tongue, to what strange shores . . . / What worlds in th'yet unformed Occident / May come refin'd with th'accents that are ours'?[12]

Towards the end of his poem, Beaumont linked Jove's nymph to 'our more glorious Nymph, our moderne Muse', Queen Elizabeth herself. It was through her sovereignty that the English asserted power over '*Virginia*, and the *New-found-land*, / And spread the Colours of our *English* Rose / In the farre countries, where Tabacco growes'. Pure literary fancy mingled with fictions of supremacy and superior European knowledge. The pursuit of tobacco under the banner of refinement would allow the English to 'tame' the 'savage nations of the West, / Which of this jewell were in vaine possesst'. Centuries-old Indigenous knowledge about the plant was swept aside in a verse. Tobacco, and the land it grew on, was a suitable prize for the spread of civility.

A year or so later, shortly after ascending the English throne, James I published a little pamphlet that denounced the behaviour of exactly the kind of gentlemen Beaumont wrote for. *A Counterblaste to Tobacco* (1604) was a vehement rejection of tobacco smoking, revealing the king's deep personal dislike of the habit, linking the corrupt human body to an imperilled body politic. James drew on one of his favourite political metaphors, of himself as a physician to his subjects. He declared tobacco to be a social and political problem, infesting merchants, lawyers, and 'common people'. But the king reserved much of his blame for the nobility and gentry; they were setting a poor example and neglecting their service to state and nation. James's bombastic rhetoric reprimanded his subjects while reducing Indigenous peoples to 'aliens from the holy Covenant of God' and 'slaves to the Spaniards', writing them out of the history of tobacco.[13]

The king's blast against smokers tends to be interpreted two ways: either as an early example of an anti-smoking pamphlet, or as a fragment of history that upholds the longstanding image of James as gauche and eccentric, prone to bookishness and tedious arguments. James's upbringing hadn't exactly equipped him with a sense of security and warmth. His father, Henry Stuart, Lord Darnley, had been murdered when James was eight months old; his mother, Mary, Queen of Scots, was executed by the very Crown that he eventually inherited. But beyond any personal aversion to tobacco, and alongside a deep-rooted desire to foster peace and propagate royal prerogative, James seems to have written *A Counterblaste* as a conduct book, laying out idealised masculine behaviour in the context of imperial ambitions. For the king, transatlantic encounters were intimately connected to his subjects' changing manners, and he believed their behaviour had an impact on British identity and political stability. He was very conscious of the fact that tobacco had come into the realm through contact with Indigenous nations. Shall we, James asked, 'without blushing, abase our selves so farre, as to imitate these beastly *Indians* . . . ? Why doe we not as well imitate them in walking naked as they doe? in preferring glasses, feathers, and such toyes, to gold and precious stones, as they do?'

In addition to being harmful to one's personal health, James believed smoking was bad for a budding empire. You couldn't acquire the gold that was necessary for displays of princely magnificence (or pay your own prodigal private expenses) if you adopted Indigenous values or ways of seeing the world. You couldn't successfully export English civility and Protestantism if you were constantly falling from the vanguard to smoke tobacco with your companions. Delicacy, James wrote, had led to the eventual fall of the Persian and Roman empires. And yet 'so many smoke-buyers, as are at this present in this kingdome, I never read nor heard'. To imitate such a fashion was to be 'counterfeiting the man[n]ers of others, to our owne destruction'.[14]

But if James was a physician seeking to cure a polluted body politic, he was coming to the problem too late. Tobacco use had already become pervasive, infecting his subjects beyond repair. As another anti-tobacco Jacobean pronounced, the reason was simple: 'Men like and love this *smokie* kind of life'.[15] To complicate matters, it was becoming even more apparent that tobacco might be the only means of ensuring the survival of English colonies in North America. The English needed an industry that would bring profits in and keep the ships sailing out. They tried silk-weaving, glass-working, and iron forging. Wine-makers and women skilled in embroidery were sent to diversify Jamestown's economy. But it was the planter John Rolfe's experimentation with West Indies tobacco seeds, combined with cultivation techniques he had learned from Algonquians, that enabled him to set up a lucrative industry the English could really benefit from.

The Mattaponi oral history of Matoaka or Pocahontas's life recounts how the Powhatan primarily used tobacco for spiritual and ceremonial activities. It was the *quiakros*, or religious men, who held the secret knowledge to successfully process tobacco. In order to access this guarded knowledge, Rolfe used his marriage to Matoaka in 1614 to foster kinship ties, acquiring the skills and practical understanding he needed to cure tobacco in the distinctive landscape of the Chesapeake. When Matoaka crossed the Atlantic in 1616, she travelled on the ship that brought Rolfe's first crop to London's investors. The success of this crop came at a critical moment in the colony's history. By 1621, heated debates in the House of Commons would force MPs to admit that the estimated 4,000 English subjects in Virginia had no means to survive without it.[16]

A decade and a half after *A Counterblaste*, the king sat for dinner in one of his royal hunting lodges in the company of the planter George Yeardley. The king loved to hunt; perhaps a crisp December day among the stables and porticoes of his lodge at Newmarket had put him in an especially indulgent mood. It was 1618, and the recently knighted Yeardley was preparing to return to Jamestown in all the glory of his newly elevated status to serve as its governor. John Ferrar, a merchant and Virginia Company councillor, eagerly reported that James had spent over an hour and a half talking to Yeardley solely about Virginian affairs, asking questions about the behaviour of his subjects there, and whether the Powhatan were open to conversion.

Supporters of colonisation were immensely excited by the royal favour bestowed on the occasion. Prince Charles and leading members of the nobility had also been present, and the king's enthusiasm spurred on their own renewed promises to support the Virginia project. Over glasses of wine, the king had even admitted that, although he felt a natural antipathy to tobacco, he understood why the crop needed to be planted, at least in the short term. His love of the plantation would make him overlook tobacco, James decided, but Yeardley should make a plan to phase out its cultivation and focus on more refined and lucrative commodities, such as silk. He was confident that, in coming years, colonists 'might growe into contempt, & so into disuse of that fantasticall herbe'.[17]

What savvy, pro-colonial gentlemen did was to yoke their enjoyment of tobacco with the rhetoric of political necessity. They could have their cake and eat it – indulge in the pleasure of intoxication and call it patriotism. In the years after James's dinner with Yeardley, Rolfe's strain of tobacco spread across the plantations dotting the James River. Smoking Chesapeake tobacco became a means of supporting English political expansion and economic self-sufficiency. The English no longer relied on Spanish-grown tobacco to fuel their habit. When they smoked Virginia-grown tobacco, they were putting their money towards English colonialism, rather than Catholic Spanish endeavours.

Within the Virginia Company, however, disagreements over colonial management and trading operations worsened. Quarrels between factions reached a fever pitch around 1623, the same year Prince Charles gallivanted to Spain with the Duke of Buckingham in an attempt to woo the Spanish Infanta. Company members challenged each other to duels, and brawled outside the Royal Exchange. Following a series of imprisonments and investigations, the king brought the colony under direct royal control in 1624.

The gentlemen who debated plantation affairs in the fiercely divisive arenas of Parliament and Virginia Company meetings were part of convivial fraternities with complex rituals of sociability, played out in private chambers and taverns. On the first Friday of every month, at the Mermaid Tavern on the Strand, members of the 'Sirenical fraternitie', including Ben Jonson and John Donne, were joined by those who had spent the day reading up on affairs in Bermuda or New England, or maintaining correspondence with agents in the fledgling colonies. Many of them had contacts with those councillors and courtiers who might have been present in the room when James had asked Yeardley about life in the Chesapeake.

As candlelight flickered in sugared cups of wine, gentlemen took what they knew about the Americas – information that had already been embellished and twisted to varying degrees in letters and reports – and transformed it further. They took their inspiration in part from Greco-Roman symposia, where intoxication and literary production went hand in hand. Plato had used drinking parties as a literary device, one that opened up philosophical dialogues about virtue, manliness, and desire. Writing poetry, like taking tobacco, was a means of accessing truths and possibilities beyond immediate reality. For the likes of the Sireniacs, writing under the influence allowed fantasies of imperial control to unfurl before them, long before the English had any actual empire to speak of.

In their verses, the 'Indian weed' became linked to a burgeoning sense of their own civility as something that involved, for the first time in their history, a sophisticated interest in transatlantic affairs. Like Beaumont's *Metamorphosis,* their poems brought the old world of classical myths and heroes together with the new possibilities of colonial projection. Revelry became a notable part of their conception of *translatio imperii,* the transfer of power and civilisation from east to west.

Bacchus, god of wine, was a recurrent figure. In one Latin poem that circulated in the 1610s, Bacchus leads his wine-sodden companions to the West Indies as a conqueror, teaching Indigenous Americans to smoke 'in civil fashion', subduing cannibals with good husbandry.[18] Like his Jacobean brethren, Bacchus became a rather good figurehead for masculine conviviality because he is a traveller and a conqueror. He brings prosperity, fertility, agriculture: all those things that transatlantic planters celebrated when they imagined exporting English civility to the Chesapeake, or New England, or the Caribbean. The spade triumphs over the sword; settlers are not conquerors, but reframed as honest yeomen.

Colonisation was debated at court and in Parliament, but it was also rooted in the dinner party and the tobacco shop – less official but equally formative spaces where politicians, merchants, and financiers gathered to imagine a world where they were imperial contenders, even as empire remained an aspiration more than a reality. The English gentlemen who travelled to the Chesapeake in the 1610s and 1620s often came from this environment of rakish urban sociability. George Sandys, younger brother to the prominent MP and Virginia Company member Edwin Sandys, had studied at Oxford and the Inns of Court before travelling across the Mediterranean and as far as Constantinople, where he wrote about *coffa* (coffee) and *sharbat* (sherbets flavoured with dried herbs and spices such as saffron, violets, or peaches). In Tsenacommacah, he experimented with distilling maize into liquor and began a translation of none other than Ovid's *Metamorphoses*. It begins, 'Of bodies chang'd to other shapes I sing.'

The culture of politics, drink, and smoking fostered white sociability across the Atlantic, far earlier than we tend to think. Colonisation was now pitched as a political necessity, but also as fashionable for the civil gentleman and his self-styling. By connecting tobacco leaves to the vine and the laurel leaf, gentlemen began to imagine their own place in the colonial project in this 'golden age' of refinement. In the drinking culture of the Renaissance elite, intoxication involved transformation: from mortals to gods, kings to beasts. It promised liberation, but also dangerous licence, as if drinkers were the slippery and subversive characters in Ovid's myths. With their access to the royal court, joint-stock company meetings, and Parliament, gentlemen who supported empire in their clubs and societies were well placed to know of the brutalities and complications of what was happening on the ground. Their fantasies of refinement allowed them to leave bloodshed and resistance out of the narrative they told themselves about imperial greatness. Not all were convinced by such rhetoric, however. 'Alas, poore Indians!' the poet Joshua Sylvester lamented in 1616. The English 'carried

Avarice, and Gold they got: / They carried Bacchus, & TOBACCO brought.' This pitiable exchange, he wrote, came when the English were led by the dangerously licentious 'cup god' Bacchus, one intoxication fuelling the insatiable desire for another.[19]

In the end, the fantastical herb that the king so detested made Virginia's fortunes. The plant remained vital to Indigenous ceremonies and practices, 'sang . . . out from the earth' and carried knowledge in its leaves, but the English turned it into a commodity to be extracted on a large scale. Fuelled by the increasing demand for the intoxicant back home, which was stoked by its associations with Native peoples and places, tobacco plantations encroached on Indigenous villages and sacred spaces. Enslaved Africans were commodified, too, purchased to provide the labour that escalating demand required. Across North America, Bermuda, and the Caribbean, European colonisers modified, industrialised, and commercialised tobacco on an unprecedented scale. From the moment Columbus stumbled on Taíno and Kalinago lands in the Caribbean, colonisation, as Indigenous peoples have put it, 'altered – and continues to alter – the culture, language, and traditions of the original inhabitants of this land', impacting how tobacco is still regarded and regulated today.[20] The English imagined tobacco coming into the golden world of the Renaissance, but their own hunt for their nymph and muse disturbed people's relationships with their environments and communities. Four hundred years later, the work of repair has hardly begun.

And so we return to Robert Cotton's tobacco pipe, stamped with the Earl of Southampton's name. Over 1,500 fragments of Cotton's handmade pipes survive. A small number bear names, all of them men, all of them involved in Virginia Company affairs, perhaps intended to be sent across the Atlantic as gifts. There's Walter Ralegh, so often credited with making smoking popular among the elite;

Matoaka's kidnapper, Captain Samuel Argall; William Faldo, a member of the Society of Mines Royal who committed himself to finding silver in the Chesapeake; and Thomas West, the third Baron De La Warr, who invested a staggering amount of capital in early Virginia Company voyages.

In an era when the English all too often coveted and appropriated Indigenous practices and resources while emptying them of their original meanings – an era that became enamoured with tobacco, but held little real regard for the communities they took it from – Cotton in fact appears to have worked closely with Algonquians to understand their methods of making. In the contact zone of James Fort, some years before Rolfe sent his first crop across the Atlantic, Cotton experimented with the earthy clays of the region, producing pipes the colour of pecans and dried leaves. Unlike long-stemmed, white-clay pipes with their circular bowls, created in London and exported to the colonies, Cotton's pipes were thicker, with a more angular bend between bowl and stem, similar to those made by his Algonquian neighbours. In the Cotton pipe, we get a glimpse of what has always been there, but can be difficult to see – an entanglement between England and Indigenous America marked by some level of reciprocity. The pipe brings together the histories of Algonquian technologies and ceremonial practices, colonialism, manufacture and industry, even print-making. It contains the name of a somewhat flamboyant earl, whose reckless youth gave way to a zeal for Protestant expansion, but it simply wouldn't exist without the Algonquians of Tsenacommacah moving through and outside of James Fort, bringing sustenance and knowledge about their plants.

At Jamestown, archaeologists have unearthed a tiny tobacco seed, barely visible to the eye. Under a microscope, it is shaped a bit like a black walnut. It might even be one of the seeds of South American *Nicotiana tabacum* that Rolfe picked up during his travels and used in his experiments with local varieties in the Chesapeake. Tobacco's migrations and transformations left behind a range of surviving objects – Nahua tobacco gourds, Caribbean seeds cultivated by Indigenous and West African peoples, Chesapeake plants (its leaves dried, or juiced), terracotta pipes, fragments of Dorset clay, engraved silver boxes, and even poems, printed in berry inks and read in libraries and dining rooms. These objects transmit stories of care, desire, capitalist extraction, and endurance beyond anything even Ovid could have conjured up. In the imperial imagination of the English, there was no Golden Age without the divine leaf. But in the hands of those who cherish them as ancestors, these seeds might awaken to a different song.

Duchesses and
Pretty Pamphlets

While their husbands and fathers were gathering in London clubs to write odes to an Indigenous drug, wealthy Tudor and Stuart women studied geography and voraciously read travel books and romances that put heroines at the heart of the story. They listened to tales of cross-dressing wanderers and shipwrecked maidens while embroidering green parrots and sea monsters onto dresses and samplers, inspired by those found on the edges of maps. Stories of faraway places might have given them a moment of escape from those who curbed their freedoms. Stuck in the countryside while her spendthrift husband Richard Sackville, third Earl of Dorset, got drunk at metropolitan parties, Lady Anne Clifford kept herself entertained by commissioning an account of her father's voyages to the Caribbean some decades before. Mary, Queen of Scots stitched a series of embroidered panels in the company of her custodian, Elizabeth Hardwick, during her long years of captivity in the 1570s and 1580s – confined to country estates while Frobisher and Drake crossed oceans in the name of the woman who had imprisoned her. Along with coats of arms, flowers, and coded political messages, Mary embroidered an armadillo and two Atlantic birds, a toucan and another 'byrde of America'.

What information about the Americas could women access? And how did their involvement with colonial affairs shape travel literature, and inspire their own writing? For her embroideries, Mary used printed emblems and travel books. She based her *tatou*, or armadillo, on an image by a French naturalist who had come across these South American creatures in a crowded marketplace within the Ottoman Empire. But she may also have recalled the tropical birds and Tupi featherwork in the collection of the French cosmographer André Thevet.[1] Thevet had been to Brazil in the 1550s, returning to the French court when Mary still resided there.

Tudor and Stuart women were involved in gathering and disseminating transatlantic knowledge to a far greater extent than they have been credited with. The historian Misha Ewen has investigated how prosperous merchant women 'adventured' their purses, contributing funds for charitable acts such as building colonial chapels, and profiting from joint-stock investments that made knowledge of overseas affairs important business strategies. Then there were wealthy women of letters, such as Lucy Russell, Countess of Bedford, who wrote witty poems and helped the nation's budding poets and playwrights to find their voices. These high-ranking women who supported art and literature in England fused colonial knowledge and intellectual culture. Some of the most enduring and best-known travel narratives of the era were dedicated to women. Where there was Walter Ralegh and John Smith, patronesses were there, too.

In 1555, Richard Eden translated multiple accounts of Spanish colonisation in the Americas, dedicating his work to Mary I and her husband Philip. In 1577, the translator Richard Willes expanded Eden's work, producing *The History of Travayle in the West and East Indies*, which provided essential knowledge about life in Central and South America as well as Asia and Africa, and ending with the Spanish invasion of Mexico. The book was immensely popular. A case can be made that Shakespeare consulted it when he wrote *The Tempest*. Both texts mention Setebos, the deity worshipped by Sycorax, Caliban's mother; in Willes's *History of Travayle*, the god appears within the account of Magellan's travels through Patagonia (in Chile and Argentina).

Willes dedicated his expanded edition of Eden's work to Lady Bridget Hussey, an earlier Countess of Bedford. In his dedication, he outlined how he had brought together 'huge workes' and 'pret[t]y pamflettes' to present her with all that had been 'brought to passe in the conquest of that halfe worlde'. Willes offered the countess lively descriptions that would distract, amuse, and pique her curiosity. The 'infinite treasure' of pearls and precious metals might 'recreate and delight a mynde travelled in weighty matters, & weeried with great affayres'.[2] Willes's account of Martin Frobisher's search for a north-west passage also included a dedication to Lady Anne Dudley, Countess of Warwick. The dedication was not haphazard. Willes wrote in direct response to the countess's 'question concernyng your servantes voyage'.[3] It was seemingly her patronage that inspired Frobisher to rename Kodlunarn Island in Nunavut as Countess of Warwick Island. On the day before their departure, the crew lit bonfires at the summit of the highest mound and volleyed a farewell shot in her honour.

Women read those chronicles and pretty pamphlets in their libraries, discussed them at gatherings with friends, and had servants read them chapters at bedtime. When they did so, they would have come across colonial violence, the enslavement of captured women and children in the Caribbean, trade reports on cinnamon and sugar, and men and women in different parts of the world adorning themselves with shells or woven cottons. In a section called 'Of the colour of the Indians', Willes marvelled at the way 'God useth [colour] in the composition of man . . . which doubtlesse can not be consydered without great admiration, in holdyng one to be whyte, and an other blacke'. Within this diversity, 'some men are whyte after dyvers sorts of whitnes . . . & blacke after dyvers sorts of blackenes'. There were sympathetic portrayals of those who 'doe dayly peryshe with intolerable travayle in the golde mynes'. Anguished pregnant women, wishing to spare their unborn children the same fate, 'use medecine to destroy theyr conception'.[4]

Did women connect the brutal extraction of silver or other luxury goods with the jewellery pinned to their gowns? Was Mary Stuart interested in the life of the armadillo when she stitched its armour, in silk the colour of a candied nut? It is difficult to know. But if duchesses and captive royals flipped through the pages of *The History of Travayle,* or accounts of English privateering, they could have accessed details of the perilous depth at which the choicest pearls were cultivated in Venezuela and the Caribbean. The best were 'created, nouryshed, and increase in the deepest places of the sea', where enslaved Indigenous and African divers seldom dared go willingly, out of fear of the 'monsters of the sea, as also least their breath should fayle them in [too] long remaining in the water'.[5] Deep in Atlantic waters, sheltered from the tempests that rocked the surface, lay the greatest and biggest pearls, including the large asymmetrical varieties that elite Europeans fastened to their ears with ribbons.

In 1609, a violent storm tossed the *Sea Venture,* an English ship bound for Virginia, into the subtropical archipelago of Bermuda. The reefs around Bermuda were so perilous that sixteenth-century sailors referred to the lands as the 'Devil's Islands'. In Shakespeare's *Tempest,* Ariel calls them the 'still-vex'd Bermoothes', a place of perpetual turmoil. These islands, wrote one *Sea Venture* survivor, are 'reputed a most prodigious and inchanted place'.[6] In attempts to banish Bermuda's associations with the grim and the uncanny, the English renamed the archipelago as the Somers Isles, after the naval commander Sir George Somers. Somers had steered the crew safely onto the island after the storm, and not a single person had died. One survivor, William Strachey, wrote an account of the shipwreck that conjured the drama of the storm. His 'True Reportary' described the profound sense of dislocation triggered by the tempestuous seas.

Strachey's work is known as a likely source for *The Tempest,* but a woman may have read it before Shakespeare did. The whole report is an address to a mysterious, unnamed lady. The account begins: 'Excellent Lady, know that upon Friday late . . .' Strachey wraps her into his narrative, not letting us forget she is there. 'For surely, noble lady'; 'let me give your Ladyship a brief description before I proceed'; 'You may please, excellent Lady, to know . . .'[7] He offers her information about the quality of the soil on the island; the vines, citrus fruits, and sugarcane that might be cultivated in its Mediterranean-like climate; its flora and fauna, including prickly pears and feral hogs, and berries that could be used for dyes. The Bermuda palmetto that spread across the coastline, Strachey wrote, had branches that could be peeled off into pleats as delicate as satin or paper, used by the crew to thatch roofs and insulate cabins. The document also contained important political intelligence, including details of the disagreements between colonists, the shaky authority imposed in the colony, and the adversities brought by vanity and riot. To better understand the fortunes of the colonists when they did eventually sail to the Chesapeake the following year, Strachey recommended further reading: 'I can only refer you (honored Lady) to the book which the adventurers have sent hither entitled *Advertisements unto the Colony in Virginia.*'[8]

Who was the 'excellent Lady' who seems so present, yet so elusive, in this famous account of a Bermuda shipwreck? There are guesses. Sarah Blount, for one, wife of the merchant and politician Thomas Smythe. Smythe had served in governing positions in the East India and Virginia companies, so Strachey may have been acquainted with her through his involvement with trade and travel. Similarly, Lucy, Countess of Bedford, had an interest in Virginia and Bermuda. She would be listed as a shareholder in the combined Virginia/Bermuda charter of 1612, and on the 1615 charter when the Somers Isles

Company became its own entity. But other elite women were share-holders, too, and the mystery shrouding the unknown lady arises because there are many contenders.

Even those who were not recorded as shareholders might have been present at gatherings sponsored by investors. In one account of Frobisher's 1576 Arctic voyage, it was a woman who encouraged the crew, upon their return, to test the pieces of black stone that 'seemed to be some kinde of metal or Mynerall'. The gentlewoman, one of the adventurers' wives, had a piece of the ore which she threw into the fire. When she took it out, it glistened like gold, whereafter 'it was brought to certain Goldfinders in *London* . . . who indeed found it to hold gold'.[9] In late 1629, a Mi'kmaw *sachem* (paramount chief) named Segipt travelled to Plymouth with his wife and son to garner support for his people's fight against the French in Nova Scotia, a province that the Scottish courtier William Alexander had also recently laid claim to. The three Indigenous visitors were entertained at the estate of the politician John Poulet in Somerset, where Poulet's wife Elizabeth seemed especially taken with her guests: they were 'much made of, especially my lady to the savage queen'.[10]

When King Charles called the Mi'kmaq visitors to court, Elizabeth Poulet accompanied her guests to the coach at their parting, fastening a necklace around the 'queen' with a diamond valued at £20. Across the span of time covered in this book, snippets of evidence show how the wives of colonial investors and state administrators came face to face with resources and peoples from many places in the Americas. Their fantasies and imaginations are there in glimpses, too: from the unnamed gentlewoman's hopes of finding gold in iron pyrite, to Elizabeth Poulet's seeming affection towards the Mi'kmaw woman. The woman accepted the diamond necklace, but 'for thanks or acknowledgment made no sign or expression at all'.[11]

As projects of exploration became projects of settlement, women financed ships and helped raise money for supplies. In 1617, Elizabeth Throckmorton, Lady Ralegh, sold some of her property in Surrey to contribute funds for her husband's Guiana voyage. Ralegh wrote to his wife with updates at sea, while she mustered support for her husband back home. The original is lost, but one Jacobean newswriter noted that he had seen a widely circulated letter from Ralegh to his wife in 1618, in which he assured her that he had arrived safely and begun his search for gold mines, while reconnecting with the *casiques* or rulers of the Orinoco Basin.[12]

Other letters to prominent women were even more explicit in acknowledging their role in colonial expansion. Imprisoned in the Tower and desperate for a way out, Ralegh had written to James I's wife, Anna of Denmark, encouraging her to speak to the king about the possibilities of tapping into 'the riches of Guiana before it is too late'.[13] The most eccentric letter to cross the queen's desk came in or around 1610, when a group of anonymous petitioners wrote to Anna, referring to the aid that Queen Isabella of Spain had given Columbus. They promised that they, too, had a 'like disposition' to venture across the Atlantic. America was key, they believed, to the English achieving a wider global empire, facilitated by connecting trades in the Atlantic and Indian oceans. There were 'divers knights and esquires of the best sort and great livings, who desire this society', and they recommended Anna's militantly Protestant son, the dashing and much-loved Prince Henry, to serve as their figurehead.[14] It made a good story: a vestige of Elizabethan chivalric culture, overlapping with the merchant world of the City. Whether the queen's interest was piqued or not, Henry's death in 1612 must have extinguished the projects of these knight-adventurers.

We know frustratingly little about how patronesses responded to such invitations and proposals. We can imagine them casting a glance at a sailor or projector's letter resting on an oak table carved with grotesques, as a green Brazilian parrot flutters from tapestry to tapestry, scattering maps with the rustle of his wings. (One parrot in 1596 was reportedly fond of nestling in a gentlewoman's ruff all day, and drinking claret in the afternoons.)[15] Women might have discussed their husbands' ventures and the rumours of colonial projects as they smoked and played cards, or prayed for the success of the ventures they had helped finance as they kneeled in chapels or at their devotional cabinets. We know they were present in the high galleries that overlooked halls and chambers where Virginia Company meetings were held, leaning in to hear debates about colonial affairs.[16]

In 1624, John Smith published his influential *The Generall Historie of Virginia, New-England, and the Summer Isles*, dedicating the work to 'The Illustrious and Most Noble Princesse, the Lady Francis, Duchesse of Richmond and Lennox'. A famed and somewhat rebellious woman, the 'double duchess' Lady Frances had been a Lady of the Bedchamber at Anna's court. As a widow, she had offered the financial backing that Smith needed to print this immense chronicle of English colonialism in North America.

As a seasoned soldier, Smith both drew on his military successes and offered them up as an excuse for his own deficiencies. He apologised that his prose was not 'clad in better robes then my rude military hand can cut out in paper Ornaments'. Nonetheless, Smith boasted, he was an adventurer, less skilled in compiling information than in being 'a reall Actor' on the Atlantic stage. Framing himself as a knightly hero, he gratefully acknowledged the virtuous ladies who had long protected and assisted him in his adventures, from a Turkish noblewoman in the Ottoman Empire to 'that blessed *Pokahontas*, the great Kings daughter of *Virginia*'. The work had sprung, Smith wrote, using some rather muddled allusions, out of the '*influence* from your

Gratious hand, which hath given birth to the publication of this *Narration'*. If 'your *Grace* shall daigne to cast your eye on this poore Booke, view I pray you rather your own *Bountie* (without which it had dyed in the wombe)'.[17] Without the duchess, *The Generall Historie* – still regarded as one of the most important sources for understanding early English colonisation in North America – might never have existed at all.

The duchess could have been one of the women who met Matoaka, referred to in most English sources as Pocahontas, when she came to the English court in 1616. A character in *Henry VIII*, a play Shakespeare had written with John Fletcher three years before the visit, recalls the way women had clamoured to catch a glimpse of 'some strange Indian . . . come to court'.[18] Since the play had a historical setting, the reference may have been to the Brazilian 'king' who had visited Whitehall in the early 1530s, overlaid with women's more recent interest in meeting Indigenous travellers living in London. A flurry of fascinated activity would swirl around Matoaka, too. 'The small time I staid in *London,*' Smith reported, 'divers Courtiers and others, my acquaintances, hath gone with me to see her.' To encourage the queen to publicly receive Matoaka, Smith addressed a letter to Anna, which may have accompanied a lengthier text that no longer survives. Smith alludes in this letter to an account written in 'a little book' before Matoaka arrived in England, making 'her qualities knowne to the Queenes most excellent Majestie and her Court'. What appeared in *The Generall Historie* was a briefing of sorts, asking the queen to endorse the colonial project by treating the Algonquian visitor favourably.

Smith recognised the social barriers that might stand in the way of Anna's willingness to receive Matoaka. The Algonquian woman had married the planter John Rolfe, whose status was too humble to ensure a welcome at court. Although her husband's estate made him unfit to attend to Her Majesty, Smith insisted, Matoaka possessed the high status of a *werowance*'s daughter, a position that the artist Simon van de Passe recognised in his 1616 half-length portrait. The border encircling Matoaka tells us that this is 'Matoaka Al[ia]s Rebecca', daughter of 'the mighty Prince Powhatan Emperour of Attanoughkomouck [Tsenacommacah]'.

In Smith's telling, Anglo-Indigenous female diplomacy would be crucial to the success of English colonisation in the Chesapeake. The English were poised to 'have a Kingdome by her meanes', but the issue was delicate, and Matoaka might turn against the English if they did not treat her well. Royal favour and kindness between women would 'so ravish her with content' that the queen and the realm's subjects would gain what they 'most earnestly desire'.[19] Anna did receive Matoaka, and conceivably other members of her entourage as well. Uttamatomakkin, a trusted Powhatan shaman whom the English knew as Tomocomo, had accompanied Matoaka to London, with instructions to meet the royal family. Other members of the Powhatan delegation met with prominent religious figures in the city, leading to their presence in the homes of ministers and Puritan merchants.

Doors – slamming, creaking, locking – open and close in the corridors of time. Kitchens at midnight. Private studies and chambers. Gatehouses, pantries. What happened to Indigenous women behind their public appearances in bustling streets or banqueting rooms? We know next to nothing about the day-to-day lives of Indigenous and African women who lived in the households of merchants and MPs. Matoaka died in 1617, shortly before her planned return to the Chesapeake, and around the time when Anna of Denmark commissioned a portrait of herself in riding costume, attended by an unnamed African groom. The modern Monacan poet Karenne Wood wrote a poem that imagines how Matoaka felt in those last months, in the company of Jacobean ladies and Puritan preachers, far from the sycamores and white dogwood blossoms of her home:

> I gave up my sacred name,
> Matoaka, she who kindles,
> and I became Rebecca,
> a biblical woman who left homeland for Canaan.[20]

While Elizabethans and Jacobeans avidly consumed romances and tales of oceanic travel, real-life stories of forced marriages, abductions, and violent conflict in the Atlantic played out in the city. Two Powhatan women, rechristened as Mary and Elizabeth, lived in London for several years after Matoaka's death. Eventually, the Virginia Company made plans to send them back to the Chesapeake as 'Indian brides' who would serve as go-betweens. One of these women, likely Mary, died at sea. The voyage of the other included an interlude in Bermuda, where her marriage to a settler took place before an audience of over a hundred guests. The ensuing banquet was a deliberately flashy event, so that once in Tsenacommacah, the couple might relate the liberality of the English to the region's powerful tribal nations.[21]

Then there were the women who were left in the shadows. Even at the time, the actions of some Englishmen were viewed as stains on their civil projects. During his circumnavigation of the globe, Francis Drake left Maria, a Black woman taken from a Spanish ship near El Salvador, and two African men on an island in Indonesia. When the chronicler William Camden summarised Drake's quest for precious metals in the Americas, he listed Maria's fate as one of the few dishonourable actions committed by the renowned captain. Though he had won the admiration of the realm's subjects, Camden wrote, Drake had escaped blame 'for having most inhumanely exposed in an Iland' that 'Black-more-Maide, who had beene gotten with Child in his Ship'.[22]

In his account of Guiana, Ralegh made troubling allusions to the exploitation of Indigenous women. He swore before God 'that I neither know nor beleeve, that any of our company one or other, by violence or otherwise, ever knew any of their women, and yet we saw many hundreds, and had many in our power'. None in his company, Ralegh promised, took so much as a pineapple or potato root without giving appropriate payment, nor did any man 'so much as to offer to touch any of their wives or daughters: which course so contrary to the Spaniards . . . drew them to admire her Majesty'. In presenting Elizabeth as the Virgin Queen, worthy of adoration, and the Spanish as rapacious and licentious, Ralegh positioned the English as ideal colonisers, governed by godly temperance. 'But I confesse,' he added ominously, 'it was very impatient work to keep the meaner sort from spoile and stealing.'[23]

Maria's story and Ralegh's own admission of the hundreds of women 'in our power' leave irreparable cracks in the story of civility that colonial supporters presented to their readers. We know very little about how the Indigenous and African women who survived invasion or the perils of life on board ship experienced life in London or other port cities. Their lives exist in the historical record as fragments, if at all. We can try to read between the lines or against the grain, searching for what Imtiaz Habib called 'imprints of the invisible'. We locate part of the puzzle, only to find that all the pieces around it are lost to time. Even in the rare moments when such women are visible, they do not speak in their own words. Still, the work of recovery is vital. 'Unfortunately I have not discovered a way of deranging the archive so that it might recall the content of a girl's life or reveal a truer picture,' Saidiya Hartman wrote of searching for the enslaved in the archives. But 'it is clear that her life and ours hang in the balance.'[24]

What the Mattaponi oral history of Pocahontas's life does insist on is that Matoaka was not an exceptional spokesperson for her people. She was representative of many Indigenous women: a girl who loved her family and acted on behalf of her community in whatever ways she could. There were others like her, but their names don't survive. We will never know what they thought of the golden world they confronted, or how they responded to their surroundings in their own languages. Recounting a language class held by her own tribe, the botanist and author Robin Wall Kimmerer (Citizen Potawatomi Nation) recalls a great-grandmother reflecting on the disjuncture between Potawatomi and English: 'The language is the heart of our culture; it holds our thoughts, our way of seeing the world. It's too beautiful for English to explain.' Native women in England spoke a range of languages, vernaculars that were closely related to their lands and homes, and are essential to understanding their histories, memories, and impressions. Languages that would offer invaluable insight into our understanding of multilingual London. But any records of such impressions have vanished, or simply don't exist, a consequence of the brutal sunderings of colonialism.[25]

Did the ladies who read Smith's book in England – wealthy, but bound by the strictures of patriarchy – feel sympathy when they read about the young Indigenous girl and the military man whose lives became connected? When they gazed at Matoaka in the sparkling light of the Banqueting House, in the masque she attended in 1617? Perhaps, when they read the many commonplace metaphors in moral literature and travel books that likened ships to pregnant women – sails puffed and rounded from the wind, cargoes swelling to bursting point – they rolled their eyes. Or perhaps they recognised that the image was even truer than a male writer intended, for pregnant bodies often carried death instead of life.

In 1607, Robert Wilkinson preached one such sermon to the court at Whitehall, to celebrate the marriage of Honoria Denny to James Hay, Earl of Carlisle. The entire sermon was an extended metaphor that compared women to sailing vessels. Women should be strictly navigated, so that they did not blow off course; to venture onto an unstable ship (e.g. to marry too independent a woman) was possibly ruinous; too much 'rigging' (adornment) would deform the elegant simplicity of a polished but unostentatious ship. Ruffs, like sails, puffed the vain woman towards her own ruin, scattering slippers and silk ribbons in her wake. Ever prone to ensnarement, women must be careful not to become tangled in the reefs of their own waywardness.[26]

But those pretty pamphlets that elite women read and circulated opened up the world to them. They might contain an emphasis on piety and English civility, but they were cabinets of curiosities that one could put in one's pocket, hinting at other beliefs and ways of living. Their books contained marvels that ignited the imagination, and offered them detailed intelligence about Atlantic plantations and people. Fancy and geopolitics were blended into the genre. As the seventeenth century progressed, much more evidence emerges of women engaging creatively with what they were picking up about the world. Listening to their brothers, fathers, uncles, and husbands conducting company affairs and planning voyages, women began to draw connections between transatlantic voyaging and their own sense of literary voice.

By the time the author and natural philosopher Margaret Cavendish published her *Poems and Fancies* in 1653, she was unapologetically revelling in how the unfettered imagination allowed her to live in a world of her own creation, idiosyncratic but taking inspiration from recent voyaging. Her love of travel and science came together in her utopian tale, *The Blazing World* (1666), and in poems that compared the human heart to the West Indies, playing on 'veins' of silver and vessels in the body.[27] Earlier in her career, Cavendish wrote romances that shed stark light on the vulnerability of travelling women. 'Assaulted and Pursued Chastity' begins with the ever-present threat of rape that women, no matter their status, might face. Heaven, she wrote, does not always protect the virtuous from 'rude violences' committed by the 'masculine sex'. Rare indeed is the heroine who is 'protected from violence and scandal, in a wandering life, or a travelling condition'.[28]

The Blazing World might remind us, for a moment, of Shakespeare's *Othello*. An outsider travels to a foreign country and falls in love with a younger lady. He is a 'stranger in that nation', beneath her in birth and wealth, yet determined to win her. But Cavendish's Lady isn't destined to die at the hand of a jealous man. And, unlike Desdemona, she is allowed the light-hearted adventure that the convention of tragedy forbids its heroines. When the man abducts the Lady, their ship spirals in a tempest and is carried towards the North Pole on huge pieces of ice. Philosophical enquiry, bear-men, golden ships, sea battles, and long conversations between female friends ensue. In the Blazing World, 'there are most delicious fruits of all sorts, and some such as in this world were never seen nor tasted'.[29] Cavendish wants a world, and not just a room, of her own: 'There is more gold in it than all the chemists ever did [produce], and (as I verily believe) will be able to make.' The possibilities are endless, and women are at the forefront. 'I have made a world of my own,' Cavendish declares, as 'ambitious as ever any of my sex was, is, or can be'.[30]

To imagine sovereignty over her own circumstances, Cavendish drew on the historic 'discovery' of those other places that had seemed so wondrous and alien to the generations before her. But even as women began to carve out more of a place for themselves in the literary sphere, conjuring 'the vast *Atlantique*' and the 'furious storms and Hurricanoes' of Barbados and St Kitts, their patronage of court performances, books, and public theatres tied their flights of fancy to Atlantic economies of exploitation and dispossession. Anna of Denmark played the parts of an African woman and an imperial sea-goddess in court masques of the early 1600s, her body luminescent with the glow of pearls, silver, and emeralds that had themselves been sourced by Africans and Indigenous Americans. Women investors in public theatres in the 1630s may have earned some of their initial capital from plantation tobacco grown on St Kitts.[31] When the Restoration playwright Aphra Behn acquired a set of 'glorious Wreaths' of feathers made by Indigenous women in Suriname, she brought them to London to use as props on the stage. They had, she wrote, an inimitable beauty. Behn described beaded aprons decorated with floral designs, and woven baskets made by Indigenous hands, braided with Amazonian palm fibres.[32]

From the time when a captured Scottish queen had stitched the winding tail of an armadillo in an English country house, Indigenous women's patterns and weaves had appeared in English interiors. In the Tradescant collection catalogue, drawn up at the time of Cavendish's writing, Henry VIII's hawking glove and Anne Boleyn's silk-knit accessories were kept with embroidered North American shell-beads, or *wampum*; 'night-caps made from grasse, from the *West Indies*'; Peruvian shoes, featherwork, and Chesapeake mantles of bear, deer, and raccoon skin. This displayed the labour, skills, knowledge, and self-expression of women from Iroquois North America to Quechua Peru. A 'match-coat from Canada' from the original Tradescant collection survives today. Its fringed caribou-skin tunic is decorated with porcupine quills, flattened with tools to render them more pliable before being woven, sewn, or wrapped into place.[33] The quills appear dyed and undyed, in their natural hues and coloured ochre, brown, and red.

Long encouraged to put needle to linen or silk, the women who viewed and admired Indigenous-made weaves and embroideries might have thought about parallels in their craft. Travellers to the Americas compared Indigenous arts to a 'kind of Arras', or rich Renaissance tapestry, rife with diverse colours and forms. For one Massachusetts settler, the nimble fingers of Algonquian women working with grassy twine became mixed up with English women's embroideries, 'their fine fingers fit . . . [to depict] Rare Stories, Princes, people, Kingdomes, Towers, / In curious finger-worke, or Parchment flowers'.[34] It was to satisfy his women readers that the New England colonist William Wood described the work of women who sewed moccasins and wove turkey-feather mantles, their baskets decorated 'with intermixed colours and [portraitures] of antique Imagerie'.[35]

In reality, there were vast differences in the beliefs, practices, and motivations behind women's needlework across the Atlantic. The stringing devices in *wampum*, the use of fringing and weaving patterns, connected Wampanoag or Arawakan women to their lands and their histories in highly localised ways.[36] The travellers who compared Native embroideries to those made by wives and daughters at home did so partly to encourage white women's labour with the needle. As seventeenth-century women writers began to assert their literary voice, they disdained a patriarchal culture that forced needles into their hands instead of pens. Though 'most of our Sex are bred up to the Needle . . . yet some are bred in the publike Theatres of the World', Cavendish declared.[37]

Still, when aristocratic ladies folded deerskin into cabinets, or arranged woven feathers on the stage, they brought the lives and labour of Native women into these sites of performance and display. 'The journey of a basket is also the journey of a people,' Kimmerer writes, after observing a Mohawk Akwesasne basket-maker. It contains 'the laughter and the stories of the gathered women'. The sweetgrass used to construct the container means that 'even an empty basket contains the smell of the land', holding people, place, and identity together in its pattern.[38] The threads of baskets and garments allow the stories of those gathered women to whisper back. Their echoes remind us that, even as English women battled to assert their independence in a Renaissance whose literary culture was overwhelmingly dominated by the writings of men, the influence of other artists and storytellers could be felt in the theatres and salons where women wielded their wit.

From the Ark

In 1535, the Cornish lady Honor Grenville, Viscountess Lisle, received a humiliating letter from one of Henry VIII's ministers, informing her that Anne Boleyn had rejected her gift of a South American monkey. 'Of a truth, madam, the Queen loveth no such beasts nor can scarce abide the sight of them,' he wrote. The animal had been in Lady Lisle's care since the previous year, when she had received three Brazilian animals as gifts: two marmosets and a long-tailed monkey, 'a pretty beast and gentle', who liked to be kept near the fireplace.[1] Urbane travellers to the Continent in the time of Henry VIII could purchase Atlantic animals from cities such as Lisbon or Seville. In Antwerp, where many Tudor merchants spent their time, agents of the Fugger bank kept foreign creatures caged in a large garden near their offices, selling them to prosperous clients.[2]

When the vindictive Jewish merchant Barabas surveys the piles of treasure he has amassed, in Christopher Marlowe's *Jew of Malta* (1590), he celebrates the transoceanic traffic that makes it possible to 'inclose / Infinite riches in a little roome'.[3] But, sometimes, what the English collected weren't things at all. By the early seventeenth century, collections such as John Tradescant's famous 'Ark' in Lambeth contained beaver and otter skins, a muskrat and wildcat from Virginia, an armadillo, the skeleton of a monkey, a hummingbird, a variety of necklaces made from the teeth of wild animals, and a woodpecker from the West Indies. Atlantic animals were admired for their rarity, but they were also vividly, vitally present in a range of spaces in Renaissance England.

Merchants' houses were inhabited by feathered and furred bodies that had long held important places in Native communities. American creatures – kin, guardians, knowledge-sharers alongside humans – found themselves trying to adjust to life on a cold little island, clambering on the stone lions and unicorns that flanked stately stairs and fireplaces. Birds and marmosets occupied the interiors of middling and aristocratic chambers, often tended to and cared for by a host of less wealthy keepers and tenants. The captain Christopher Newport gave James two baby crocodiles and a 'wild boar', likely a peccary, from Hispaniola (now Haiti and the Dominican Republic) for the king's zoo in St James's Park.[4] Before these crocodiles roamed St James's, they had been part of an interconnected ecosystem in Taíno lands, two apex predators on the rise, their young ridged skin flecked by the shadows of ferns. Other animals, viewed less as individual marvels than as comestibles, were baked into pies and crystallised in sugar.

Unlike Anne Boleyn, other Tudors rather liked receiving tropical pets. Parrots were presented to family members and patrons and passed down in wills. In 1596, Elizabeth's Secretary, Robert Cecil, wrote to John Gilbert, Ralegh's half-brother, to ask why Gilbert hadn't sent his parrot to the queen after she had expressed an interest in it. A rather stressed Gilbert vowed that he had received no such request, but that Her Majesty could have anything he possessed, from the parrot to his very life, and made arrangements to send it immediately.[5]

Europeans had long delighted in parrots from Asia and Africa. Roman authors including Pliny and Martial described parrots heralding new emperors, squawking their allegiances with an 'Ave, Caesar'. In the Middle Ages, Asian parakeets and African grey parrots had been gifts for popes and cardinals. In medieval art, parrots were associated with Catholicism and the Virgin Mary. There are multiple

Madonna with Parrot paintings, drawing all kinds of mixed associations between wealth and lust, paradise and God's word. Parrots could represent both eloquence and meaningless chatter.

But when Europeans invaded Mesoamerica and the Caribbean in the late fifteenth century, they found the multicoloured brilliance of American species beyond anything they had seen before. The Italian navigator Amerigo Vespucci commented on the immense number of birds he witnessed, with their emerald- and lemon-coloured feathers. In their earliest initial exchanges, Europeans met diverse societies that had captured, tamed, and cared for these birds for centuries. Vespucci received countless birds from local inhabitants – 'a generosity of parrots', as the Taíno-descended José Barreiro puts it.[6]

Even into the mid-seventeenth century, the association between the Americas and its splendid birds remained strong. 'For their Fowl, they are all so beautiful in comparison with ours, as we may well say, Nature learnt her *colours* there,' wrote the traveller Richard Flecknoe of his residence in Brazil from 1648 to 1650. Macaws were like 'a whole Garden of *Tulips*, every Feather being of a several colour, which beheld in Sun-shine, even daz[z]le your Eyes, they are so bright & glittering'.[7] Flecknoe kept his chamber furnished with Brazilian creatures for the duration of his trip. He brought his sagoins (marmosets) everywhere, calling them his pocket lions. He tried to bring his animals to England, but they died on the voyage home. He wrote a short farewell poem to his parrots, lamenting that creatures with wings should drown at sea.

Flecknoe could have acquired other parrots once he returned home. If these birds proliferated in paintings and illuminated manuscripts during the Middle Ages, they became more physically present in urban households over the sixteenth century, gradually gaining the status of pets in a more modern sense.[8] Most royal women in England had lavish aviaries with live birds that included species from the Americas. They also collected bird parts. Mary, Queen of Scots had that beak from a Brazilian bird. Red cardinals, known as 'Virginia night[in]gales', flitted in Anna of Denmark's green and white aviary in Greenwich, their chirping met with the pleasing sound of an elaborate hydraulics system. The household accounts of Princess Elizabeth Stuart, James and Anna's daughter, include payments to maintain 'her grace's monkeys', and to a joiner for mending her parrot cages. In 1613, Elizabeth received a parrot from her friend, the ambassador Thomas Roe, who had travelled to the Amazon several years before in the employ of her brother, Henry. Charles I's queen consort, Henrietta Maria, kept parrots. Her capuchin monkey, Pug, was immortalised in one of her portraits, painted by Van Dyck in 1633.[9]

In December 1609, the Earl of Southampton wrote to James's Secretary of State, Robert Cecil, about the king's wish to obtain a flying squirrel from the Chesapeake. He had told the king of 'the Virginia Squirrills which they saw will fly, wherof there are now divers brought into England', Southampton wrote, after which James 'was sure [your Lordship] would gett him one'. Southampton was an active member of the Virginia Company, busy garnering support for its endeavours after the initial flush of enthusiasm in the venture had begun to wane. He had better things to do than to chase down a flying squirrel, and he knew Cecil did, too. 'I would not have troubled you with this but that you know so well how [the king] is affected to these toyes,' he wrote.[10] Southampton alluded to the presence of Virginia squirrels in London already, fluffy rodents that had left the branches of sugar-maple trees to leap through foliage in a very different environment, gliding against the backdrop of London's chapels and cathedrals.

In Essex, a guinea pig lived in the manor house of the courtier and diplomat Thomas Smith. Remnants of its bones were found among fragments of glassware and ceramics in a pit dating to 1574–5.[11] In one of the greatest gifts of Elizabethan portraiture to come down to us from an anonymous artist, a painting of three unknown children from around 1580 depicts a seven-year-old girl standing between her brothers, cradling a guinea pig with lustrous black, white, and auburn fur. When animals came from rainforests and grasslands to reside in English households, children had access to them, too.

Tutors could open up chronicles and maps and show their young pupils how their pets were connected to English travel, or to life in Peru. In their original homes in the Andes, guinea pigs lived in Indigenous communities, bred for consumption and used for medical and religious purposes. Sixteenth-century Spanish accounts commented on the use of guinea pigs in ritual offerings. There were rumours that the Inca sacrificed 1,000 rare white guinea pigs and 100 white llamas in harvest ceremonies. The Jesuit chronicler José de Acosta reported that guinea pigs were used in 'ordinary sacrifices' across villages, sometimes stuffed with coca leaves and other sacred plants.[12] Though Spanish authorities tried to eradicate their ceremonial use, they never succeeded.

Guinea pigs appeared as 'the Indian little Pig-Cony' in Edward Topsell's *The Historie of Foure-Footed Beastes* (1607), accompanied by an explanation of their colourful coat varieties and their love of nibbling a wide assortment of herbs and fruit. Their gentle, unassuming presence appeared in devotional and secular paintings, fitting companions for Venus and Cupid or the Virgin and Christ. Wealthy Stuart patrons collected paintings by Brueghel and Rubens, and the guinea pigs, monkeys, and parrots in these works hung in aristocratic galleries alongside other works of art. These creatures came alive again through paint, for 'pictures serve them, whose active fancy give / Spirit to paint, and make *dead Colours* live'.[13]

Beyond these painted menageries, animals from the Americas were found, alive or dead, in kitchens and dining rooms. In the 1567

Cobham family portrait, six children sit around a table with several Atlantic companions. A yellow-shouldered Amazonian parrot walks across the table, past the fruit, nuts, and sugared comfits that rest on polished silver plates. The youngest daughter holds a marmoset, who sits tuftily on a plate. Animals were symbolic presences in art, and the portrait cannot be taken as straightforward evidence that the Cobhams owned such pets. Dogs evoked fidelity, monkeys vice (in this case, vice brought under control), and goldfinches Christ or the devoted soul.[14] But in using such imagery, whether from life or inspired by emblems and artistic practice, this composition appropriates a certain tropical flair, bringing the denizens of Central and South America to the Tudor dining table. Lady Cobham even wears a large, jewel-encrusted ship pendant.

For prosperous Tudors and Stuarts, ideas about gentility and nobility had a lot to do with hospitality – with displaying, sharing, and distributing food. Less advantaged members of society, frequently forced to travel to find work, waited at the gates of country estates, hoping for kitchen scraps and leftovers. Civility manuals and travel books praised the English custom of keeping tables furnished, 'not onely prepared for the family, but for strangers and reliefe of the poore'. Charity aside, the English liked their dainties. The Elizabethan clergyman William Harrison described how a host of banqueting delicacies were seasoned with sugar – marmalades, sugar bread, florentines, and 'sundry [other] outlandish confections', sometimes sprinkled with edible gold leaf. By this time, banquets had emerged as a special category of meal – not the large feast itself, but the offering of sweet meats and liquor after the main courses, often in a separate, purpose-built room or 'house'. In 1591, Queen Elizabeth attended a banquet at Eltham where hundreds of sweet dishes, shaped like castles and mythical creatures, were presented on glass and silver platters. The quantities of sugar for these elaborate displays of wealth and culinary skill were immense, increasingly supplied by sugar exported from Portuguese plantations in Brazil. Potatoes from the West Indies, coming into English ports from Seville or Lisbon, were also used 'to furnish up our banquets', roasted with sugar and added to pies, or turned into comfits.[15]

Status-conscious hosts sought to outdo each other in their banqueting displays. The rarer and more expensive, the better. These events were extravagant in their excess and in their ephemerality. Resources and time were poured into breathtaking displays that were then deliberately thrown away or destroyed. By the early Stuart era, potatoes were out of fashion in such meals. These tubers were 'growne to be so common here with us at London,' the Royal Gardener John Parkinson wrote in 1629, 'that even the most vulgar begin to despise them, whereas when they were first received among us, they were dainties for a Queene.' The heads of sunflowers were roasted and eaten like artichokes, but Parkinson found them too strong for his liking. Sprigs of 'Indian basil' were used to flavour meats, and roots and walnuts from the Chesapeake were candied, their leaves distilled into liquids. In addition to enjoying the tart and tender fruit of a pineapple, their 'shells' or 'cones' were used by apothecaries, cooks, and bakers in their concoctions, and repurposed by City vintners for interior decoration, painted to resemble bunches of grapes.[16]

In the sparkle of sugared dainties and sprawling fruits, peacocks and turkeys made lavish set pieces. The West and East Indies were brought together on the table through these large, ostentatious birds acquired through trade, the former with Asia, the latter with Mexico and eastern North America. As they came to be acquired and bred in larger numbers, turkeys became permanent fixtures in pies and less formal dining. Civic banquets, from feasts at the Inns of Court to the dinners enjoyed by justices of the Star Chamber, included substantial numbers of turkeys along with oysters, partridges, rabbits, cream, and apple tarts.[17] In Ben Jonson's play *Bartholomew Fair* (1614), the hypocritical Puritan Zeal-of-the-Land Busy is caught raiding a pantry with a cold turkey pie between his teeth. Recipes for such pies abounded in seventeenth-century cookbooks, which also warned readers of turkeys' propensity for ravaging gardens in their hunt for leeks and corn.

Some animals were coddled, others bred for consumption. Others still were valued in parts. From jaguar claws to bezoar stones taken from the insides of llamas, animal matter frequently appeared in English cabinets. Like banquets, curiosity collections allowed influential patrons to exhibit their access to networks of colonial trade and plunder. A row of silver-gilt cabinets lined the chambers of Anna of Denmark's residence at Somerset House. They were made of marble, crystal, ebony, and walnut, often gilded with precious metals and decorated with flora and fauna. One contained jars of apothecary drugs, another a mirror and a panoply of silver boxes next to a globe, reinforcing the connections between collected objects and transoceanic trade.[18] Merchants and agents were the go-betweens who connected faraway treasures and curiosities with those little rooms, stuffed with all things wonderful and strange.

Literature of the time poked fun at 'the *Indies* in . . . mouldy Cabinets', but they were more than storage spaces. Francis Bacon loosely described cabinets as containing 'whatsoever the hand of man by exquisite art or engine has made rare in stuff, form or motion; whatsoever singularity, chance, and the shuffle of things hath produced', revealing human craft and the wonders of God's creation.[19] In addition to purpose-built furniture, cabinets could also apply to closets, private rooms or chambers, and even small lodgings such as summer houses or cabins, influenced by princely fashions and architectural innovations in Italy, Spain, the Netherlands, and France.

Entire rooms became repositories of reverie and pleasure, where tropical shells, feathers, and fossilised teeth delighted the senses.

In the 1610s and 1620s, the king's new favourite, George Villiers, future Duke of Buckingham, sought to accrue cultural capital and political power by amassing a large collection of art and naturalia. Villiers came from the minor gentry, but he climbed the Jacobean social ladder with exhilarating speed. A young, spruce Villiers attracted James I's eye during a moment of animal bloodshed – the hunt, one of James's favourite pastimes. The following year, in 1615, Villiers began to dance in court masques, beguiling the king with his easy grace and confidence. He steadily rose in rank; knight to viscount, earl to duke. To celebrate his earldom, Ben Jonson wrote *The Vision of Delight,* a masque that Matoaka and the shaman Uttamatomakkin attended in 1617. During these years, Buckingham lived a charmed life. His expenses included payments to 'Vandyke, the picture drawer' and to the keeper of his tennis courts for balls.[20] When Buckingham accompanied Prince Charles to Madrid in 1623, James asked him to return with animals for his menagerie. Buckingham complained about his lack of funds. 'If you do not send your babie jewels enough, I'le stop all other presents,' he pouted.[21]

Knowing that rarities were a marker of cosmopolitanism and prestige, Buckingham hired the Dutch-born Balthazar Gerbier as his art agent and advisor. Skilled in science, drawing, and staging courtly entertainments, Gerbier helped his patron build a collection worthy of princes. 'During the time I have been in Paris, I have not passed one hour without searching for some rarity,' Gerbier wrote to Buckingham in 1624. When he saw singular objects in aristocratic homes, he imagined how they would look at York House, Buckingham's London residence: 'We must have them,' he scribbled.[22] The gardener and collector John Tradescant, busy with his own Ark, was also in Buckingham's employ, and the duke tasked him with finding goods from around the world. Tradescant was expected to 'furnishe His Grace with all manner of Beasts & fowles & Birdes[,] Alyve or Not', including heads, horns, beaks, claws, feathers, and skins. Such creatures brought the ecosystems of Ottoman cities and 'the New plantation towards the Amazonians' to rest in aristocratic estates, alongside classical busts and tropical plants. His Grace wanted all manner of rarities, Tradescant wrote in 1625, but '[e]spetially [from] the Virgine & Bermewde & Newfound Land'.[23] Even with all the world's objects seemingly at his disposal, Buckingham was drawn to matter from the Americas: it was 'new' and in vogue.

From 1619, Buckingham occupied the role of Lord High Admiral of England, responsible for overseeing the navy. The Thirty Years War had erupted on the Continent, and Princess Elizabeth's marriage to Frederick of Bohemia connected England to those conflicts, while intensifying debates about political and religious allegiances at home. The escalating tensions played out at sea, where the English mounted attacks against Catholic powers. Buckingham's position gave him privileged access to cargoes of looted Iberian goods coming from the West Indies. These shipments later fuelled accusations of corruption against the favourite, when Parliament sought to impeach him in 1626, the year after James's death. Buckingham was accused of using his position to detain ships and goods for his own profit, having once acquired 'three hundred *Mexico* Hides' alongside sacks of ginger. From a Spanish fleet, Buckingham allegedly confiscated sixteen barrels of cochineal, eight bags of gold, twenty-three bags of silver, two boxes of pearls and emeralds, and various jewels and other commodities to the value of £20,000.[24]

But Buckingham survived the monarchical change, moving seamlessly into Charles's favour at a time of escalating tension between the Crown and Parliament. To protect him, Charles simply dissolved the assembly before the impeachment succeeded. Those who critiqued the immense profligacy of the superrich and their prestigious offices compared them to peacocks and chameleons. The court was a technicolour menagerie of trussed-up creatures ready to change their colours at a hint of danger. They were like parrots, too, uttering lofty phrases about moral responsibility with no sense of their true meaning, professing a duty to the commonwealth that contained little bearing on how they actually behaved. But using state offices for exorbitant profiteering was a common pastime at the Jacobean court, and Buckingham survived the turmoil.

In 1623, back when James still hoped to find a 'Spanish Match' for his son, Buckingham had travelled to Madrid with Charles, both of them causing a diplomatic sensation by going to Spain in disguise. At the court, Buckingham received a curious proposal from a Flemish informer, offering to help the duke carry out an expedition to the Caribbean. There were people in those islands, the Fleming swore, who had found great stores of gold somewhere beyond the reach of colonial overseers, and who hated the Spanish so much that they would only reveal their secret to another nation. If Buckingham could muster the forces, the English could acquire the island's gold and silver. During these covert conversations with projectors in Madrid, Gerbier was there with Buckingham, urging him to subscribe to a plan that might make him 'master' of the Gulf of Mexico. Displaying Atlantic riches and rarities in his London residence was not just a matter of taste-making; rare animals and Atlantic metals became exhibitions of Buckingham's political aspirations and patronage of overseas ventures.

Little came of the scheme, in the end – James was too intent on maintaining peaceable relations with Spain. But for years afterwards, plans for a West India Company were developed and discussed in Parliament and among various joint-stock company agents, with the aim of attacking places such as Puerto Rico or Cuba to intercept treasure coming from the Viceroyalty of Peru.[25] During the Interregnum, Gerbier would draw directly on the Madrid proposal to pitch a new Caribbean project to Cromwell.

In 1628, Buckingham's fortunes fell as sensationally as they rose. In the wake of disastrous military campaigns in Cádiz and the Ile de Ré, a disgruntled military officer named John Felton brought down the court darling with a knife shortly after breakfast. Felton had served in Buckingham's recent campaign in France, which had left him badly wounded and troubled with dreams and memories of the conflict.[26] No wonder Felton was upset. He was owed £80 in back pay from a man who spent more money furnishing his cabinets with Italian paintings and Amazonian flora than his soldiers would earn in a lifetime. In the vicious libels and satires that circulated before and after Buckingham's demise, the relentless, empty promises of Caribbean treasure – so at odds with the harsh reality of daily life for subjects who could barely afford bread – were at the heart of public resentments against Buckingham and the courtly vices he embodied.

At the time of Buckingham's assassination, George Calvert, Charles's diligent State Secretary, who had never really seen eye to eye with the duke, was failing to start a colony in Newfoundland. Calvert wanted to create an enclave for devoted Catholics who no longer felt that England was home. He travelled to Newfoundland several times after securing a royal charter, but soon realised that the climate was less commodious than promoters had let on. Facing religious disputes and unwilling to withstand the icy blasts of Newfoundland winters, Calvert requested permission to start a colony in the Chesapeake instead, in a region he called Maryland after the queen, Henrietta Maria. Calvert died shortly after he received his charter, but his sons Cecil and Leonard threw themselves into the enterprise. Leonard arrived at the Potomac River in

March 1634 with two ships, the *Ark* and *Dove*, vessels whose names wove the collection of creatures and the search for other lands into the biblical story of travel and salvation.

While court ministers fought for favour and prestige, the fledgling colonial settlements in the Chesapeake sent a steady influx of small-scale Atlantic animals and Indigenous belongings to London on the *Ark* and other ships. The 1632 charter granted by the king had specified that 'two Indian arrows of those parts', perhaps made by the Yaocomaco and stitched with feathers, should be sent to the Keeper of His Majesty's Wardrobe, to be stored at Windsor Castle.[27] In addition to these ceremonial objects, correspondence between Leonard Calvert and his agents recorded hundreds of beaver, muskrat, and otter skins obtained from the Yaocomaco, as well as Native-made coats.

In 1638, Leonard wrote to his brother Cecil from Maryland about the possibilities and perils of acquiring local birds, beavers, and wild-cats to send to England. He had procured a red-plumed bird, but a servant had accidentally let it out of its cage. Cecil had received the beavers, but the 'lion' (a bobcat or mountain lion) had died – though 'if I can get another I will send it you'. Catching local animals was difficult for colonists who lacked the resources and specialist knowledge. 'I have no cage to put [the birds] in when they be taken,' one of Calvert's agents insisted, 'nor none about me dextrous in the taking of them, nor feeding of them'; and anyway, he was too busy trying to survive.[28]

The patrons in England who scrambled to acquire a spotted bobcat or crested cardinal from their agents in Maryland were ultimately reliant on the Indigenous inhabitants in and around colonial settlements. The English Jesuit Andrew White wrote about his attempts to learn Algonquian after he arrived, which would help him to establish relations with the communities around him, furthering his project of conversion. Rivalries, alliances, and diplomatic exchanges with different groups, including the powerful Piscataways and Susquehannocks, influenced whether beavers and birds were transported across the Atlantic. Before a canoe came to hang in a cabinet of curiosities, English settlers went into Indigenous villages, conducting exchanges on Native terms.[29] Because the colony was Catholic, treatises about Maryland circulated among prominent Catholics at Charles and Henrietta Maria's court; others were translated into Latin and sent to Rome. In Latin versions, colonial promoters highlighted their pious aims of creating a multicultural settlement founded on the Catholic faith. For investors in London, the emphasis fell on the hickory nuts, fox coats, and crested, ruby-red birds that could be sent to fill those little rooms back home.

For many English people, the parrots, marmosets, guinea pigs, and squirrels that survived transatlantic voyages were viewed as exotic animals. In Indigenous environments, however, animals were not property or mere curiosities. Their distinct roles and contributions to Indigenous life depended on place, on the lands they came from. In the stories of some Eastern Woodland groups, such as the Haudenosaunee and Lenape, North America was formed when water animals such as Muskrat put some earth on the back of a turtle who grew and grew, giving Turtle Island its name.[30] In Mesoamerican, Caribbean, and Amazonian societies, notions of kinship and predation structured human attitudes towards a range of different species. The particular qualities of animal matter had a 'transforming capacity', as when elite jaguar and eagle warriors in Mexica society wore the pelts of animals to absorb their individual prowess and access desirable essences, such as courage. Regalia used in community events incorporated parts of other-than-human animals that could not be eaten, such as feathers, bone, or quills, enabling absorption in other ways.[31] The activist Manari Ushigua (Sápara) recalled his father teaching him about the red-eyed spirit that dwelled among the *arao*, a species of parrot, in the Ecuadorian Amazon. This 'lord of all the species of *arao*' moved through the mountains while protected by 'thousands, thousands and thousands of birds, thousands and thousands of parrots'; birds were guardians with special access to travelling spirits.[32]

While wearing raptors' feathers or claws was a means of manifesting predatory qualities, Mesoamerican communities adopted parrots as beloved pets. Their feathers were used to access other avian qualities, such as beauty and transcendence. Europeans' emerging interest in acquiring parrots as pets might owe something to Native practices of adopting birds as kin. European travellers mostly obtained parrots through Indigenous assistance and trade, relying on technologies and practices of capture and taming that had been developed over centuries by those who knew the environments best. As one historian has put it, parrots crossed the Atlantic with 'elements of the [Indigenous] mode of incorporation in tow . . . not just as tabula rasa animals, ready to be made over into European pets, but rather already tamed and trained, already made into kin'.[33]

The Atlantic animals in Tudor and Stuart England were evidence of the disjuncture that had taken place when Europeans disturbed ecosystems for their own profit, taking more than they needed.[34] When visitors entered Tradescant's Ark to witness its global curiosities, they were encountering the world in a room – but at a cost, having disrupted the equilibrium of the communities from which such flora and fauna had been taken. They viewed their access to such goods as a fair exchange for introducing English religion and customs, which would 'enrich [the Indigenous inhabitants] with such ornaments of a civill life, wherewith our Countrey doth abound'.[35] Such 'enrichment' was pragmatic. Encouraging Indigenous peoples to rely on European-manufactured goods was a political strategy. It allowed settlers to '[bind] savadge Lives, in civile Chaines'.[36] As colonial promoters insisted, making Native peoples consumers of English goods was a means of ensuring their dependence. Civility was a kind of entrapment, leading to a reliance on material things and encouraging the commodification of the natural world.

Not long after Charles I's accession to the throne in 1625, the Ferrars, a family of prosperous merchants entrenched in Virginia Company affairs, moved to a manor in Huntingdonshire, pursuing lives of rigorous study and religious contemplation. At their 'Little Academy', family members – women and men, children and grandparents – engaged in lengthy debates, coming together to discuss topics they had researched in advance. On one such occasion, John Ferrar's niece, Mary Collett, argued that the European invasion of the Americas had become a Pandora's box, unleashing an assortment of evils despite intentions for good. To her, the desire to possess and acquire lay at the heart of the whole debacle. 'We receive only strange shaped beasts & glorious feathered Birds,' Collett insisted, all at a terrible cost, for Europeans had 'compassed the whole Circumference of this Earthly Globe, & ransacked every obscure & hidden corner thereof', all for the sake of 'Commodities' – here we can imagine her pausing with a rhetorical flourish – 'or rather Calamities'. The worst example of all, she stressed, was tobacco, which the English took 'with a kind of Absolute Necessitie, as though Life & Livelines[s] were depending thereon.'[37]

Collett knew that the European fascination for collecting the Americas permeated more than princely cabinets. Those who could afford it now sought an everyday reality augmented by dizzying colours, foreign intoxicants, and gloriously feathered birds. The search for life and liveliness itself was not rooted in spiritual matters, but dependent on colonial intervention. Meanwhile, alongside the opulence and glitter of the most valued luxury assemblages, turkeys, tobacco leaves, and Algonquian earthenware trickled into Tudor and Stuart chambers. From Jamestown in 1608, Francis Perkins sent home turtle doves, two Algonquian 'pots of our ordinary earth', an 'ear of the native wheat' (a corncob), and twelve pounds of sassafras 'to use in medicines or between linnens'.[38]

Little by little, whole realms of Native practice and knowledge contributed to colours, scents, and movements in domestic spaces. Iridescent parrots, having been taken and adopted by Indigenous communities before they entered into English households, were dressed in ruffs. In medicine cabinets and closets where servants stored linens, sprigs of Chesapeake sassafras wafted through, mixing the scent of sugary spice with oak, lingering on the fabrics that people wore to bed.

Portrait of a Lady
in a Beaver Hat

Scuttering across the wetlands of North America, an industrious rodent was about to transform English fashion. When Amorphous, the traveller in Ben Jonson's *Cynthia's Revels* (1600), lays his eyes on a beaver hat, he is ravished by it. 'Good faith this Hat hath possesst mine eye exceedingly!' he exclaims. 'Tis so prettie, and fantastique; what? is't a Beaver?' The flashy Asotus assures Amorphous that it is indeed a 'beaver', a hat made of felted beaver wool, purchased that morning. 'A very pretty fashion,' Amorphous says with jealous appraisal, and 'a most novel kinde of trimme'.[1]

Before the beaver was transformed into a felt hat, flaunted onstage at Blackfriars Theatre, there was a chance it had dwelled on shore-lines in Massachusetts or the Great Lakes, in the company of oysters, lobsters, acorns and pond lilies. It had eaten birch and maple, growing into a skilled constructor, learning to make dams through observation. Muskrat and Beaver, earth-divers in numerous Turtle Island creation stories, have shared stewardship of wetlands with human and other-than-human creatures since the beginning. In some Anishinaabe stories, beavers and muskrats were sent by the Great Hare to secure a grain of sand from the water's bottom to form the first land.[2]

The story of beaver hats is a chronicle of transatlantic supply chains, sacred landscapes, and merchant rivalries. Whereas the animals displayed in cabinets were valued for their colour or strangeness, hats made of felted beaver furs – brushed, dyed, lined, decorated, traded, and stolen – were part of the everyday lives of many women and men in England. They could be turned into costly status objects, embellished with taffeta hatbands and diamond pins; but they also appeared in the portraits of merchant couples, as stage props, in pawn shops, or at second-hand markets.

Subject to the whims of microtrends whose minute variations are lost to time, beavers were continually being amended, reworked, or traded in. Wide-brim hats, with their large swathes of material, were showy markers of status, while the canonical 'steeple' shape with smaller brims were for more practical, day-to-day use, worn indoors and out. In his denunciation of this 'guilded, not golden age', Walter Cary boasted that he had purchased an outmoded beaver hat for only 5 shillings, which the year before would have cost at least 30. More expensive versions could cost upwards of £3. Because they were so ubiquitous, becoming an important part of a citizen's silhouette, hats were part of heated discourses about prodigal spending and the health of the national economy.[3]

Until the end of Elizabeth's reign, beaver pelts were mostly sourced in Northern Europe, especially Russia and the Baltic. There's a beaver in Dante Alighieri's *Divine Comedy*, and beavers were hunted throughout the Middle Ages for their *castoreum,* a secretion used for medicines and perfume. By the early seventeenth century, however, the depletion and near-extinction of beavers in Europe led merchants to turn to North America. English translators published French intelligence describing the large stores of beavers found around the St Lawrence River. As Virginia Company councillors noted in 1610, those furs that merchants 'draw from *Russia* with so great difficulty, are to be had in *Virginia* and the parts adjoining, with ease and plenty'.[4] Such arguments offered colonial trade as an obvious solution to scarcity and to old economic dependencies. At the same time, the beaver trade involved different kinds of partnerships with Indigenous nations than those of a plantation industry such as tobacco.

In 1620, James I granted the Council for New England a charter that gave councillors and their descendants the right to claim Indigenous lands and resources stretching along the eastern seaboard from Massachusetts to Maine. In 1632, his son Charles granted George Calvert a charter to begin the Catholic settlement in Maryland. When Leonard Calvert became Governor of Maryland in 1634, he relied on a captain named Henry Fleet to help him navigate the region's waterways. Fleet's account of his travels survives, offering a glimpse into the elaborate transactions between English traders and Indigenous groups that made possible the presence of beaver hats in England.

Fleet wrote of the hospitality of inhabitants along the Potomac River who greeted him 'laden with beaver'. He catalogued the skins he received from numerous communities, including 114 from the Piscataways. 'I was for years together compelled to live among these people,' Fleet wrote, 'and by that means am better proficient in the Indian language, than mine own.' Others on the voyage corroborated Fleet's claims, describing him as well versed in Algonquian dialects, something he used to ally himself with, or to trick and sabotage, rival traders.[5]

The interlopers operating in Algonquian lands and into Iroquois territories in the Great Lakes helped ensure the availability of muskrat and beaver skins in English households. These expeditions were primarily conducted to participate in the 'great Beaver trade' and to satisfy the demand of English consumers, who dreamed of 'blacke glistering Otters, and rich coated Be[a]ver, / The Civet s[c]ented Musquash smelling ever'. The colonist William Wood, describing the wetland ecosystem of the Shawmut Peninsula in 1634, described the 'musquashes' (muskrats) that emitted a sweet, vanilla-like musk, and whose skins were sent 'for Tokens into *England*'. One quality skin, transferred from pond to bedroom, could 'perfume a whole house-full of clothes'. Of beaver furs, Wood added, these were in such demand that, 'if I should at large discourse, according to knowledge or information, I might make a [whole] Volume'.[6]

And so beavers appeared in inventories, wills, petitions, satires, portraits, and plays. Hats were necessary components of one's wardrobe, worn by men and women whose daily labours might take them on long journeys across damp meadows and craggy landscapes. Merchant women presented them to friends, and family members passed them down in wills. Among his list of expenditures in the early seventeenth century, which also included tobacco, satin suits, and dinner at the trendy Mermaid Tavern on the Strand, the Jacobean gentleman William Petre owed money 'for a new black beaver hatte for [my] self' and, several years later, for a white beaver hat with a spangled band. When the Restoration merchant John Verney travelled to Aleppo on family business as a Levant Company merchant, he sent home Ottoman clothing and pistachios, asking for a beaver hat to be sent him in return. For Verney, far from home, his beaver might have held a personal meaning, but London's developing industry also made hats profitable exports. Beavers, circled with gold and silver bands, were among the goods that Charles I sanctioned for trade in the East Indies, to be exchanged for nutmegs, ginger, aloes, carpets, calicoes, and porcelain.[7]

At the royal court, courtiers met with their jewellers and hatters, discussing the width of their hat brims and inspecting the brushed felt of new models. The courtly gallant was nothing but an overdressed peacock, one satirist scoffed, 'haires curl'd, eares pearl'd', and 'on his head [a] Beaver rare'. In a single year of his reign, James I purchased nearly two dozen beavers. When Anna of Denmark's brother, the Danish king Christian IV, visited in 1606, onlookers marvelled at a grey beaver hat 'with a Hat-band of Pearle, and Diamonds set in Gold-smiths worke, and a Jewell of Diamonds, which held up the right side brimme of his hat'. To this anonymous appraiser, Christian's stately appearance and diamond-encrusted beaver was part of his styling as a naval commander, an image that Christian would continue to pursue in the 1610s, when he commissioned voyages to the Arctic and Ceylon (Sri Lanka). Christian's dashing figure showed him to be 'a man of greate strength, activity, and indurance, such as are the markes of the best Conquerours'.[8]

Some of the finest surviving paintings that exhibit this style are portraits of ladies in beaver hats. In miniatures of prosperous gentry and aristocratic women, broad-brimmed hats stretch like bats across the composition. The whiteness of the faces glows against the starched ruffs and large black brims. One Jacobean portrait depicts an unknown lady in court dress, her cocked hat creating a disjuncture between her more masculine riding accessory and her otherwise formal attire. When paired with her black gown, white lace collar, and pearls dangling from ribbons, the beaver hat offers a pleasing deviance from expected decorum.

As with so many women in history who happened to sleep with famous men, Margaret Lemon is mostly remembered as a model and mistress. In the 1630s, she lived opulently with Anthony van Dyck in London. Yet Samuel Cooper's portrait miniature of Lemon from the mid-1630s conveys a confident, independent spirit. She wears her hair down, and curled, spilling over an intricate collar. In contrast to other portraits of her (coy gaze, various states of undress, adorned with flowers, and attended by cherubs), here she is almost completely covered, dressed in a masculine ensemble with a slashed black doublet and lace falling band. This painting wouldn't have quite the same panache without her distinctive black hat, likely a beaver: it is hard to imagine Lemon settling for less.

Beaver fur was fashionable, but functional, too. Consumers in the 1620s and 1630s had probably witnessed, or knew tales of, Londoners skating on a frozen Thames in 1607. Accounts of the Great Frost conjured a playful atmosphere where citizens swam on a cake of ice and glided on opalescent marble, snacking on spiced cakes, plums, and ale. But, practically speaking, people on both sides of the Atlantic were in the midst of a Little Ice Age: centuries of cooling conditions, and the expanding of glaciers in the Swiss Alps and those Arctic regions Frobisher sailed to, contributed to a significant dip in temperatures. The effects of these changes made survival harder for people, as erratic weather brought changing river flows and destroyed crops, triggering severe famine. Cold climates made a beaver's thick fur, designed to withstand frosty winters, particularly desirable.

A stone's throw from the frozen Thames, Jacobean felt-makers learned to work and manipulate North American pelts. They removed the undercoat of wool while preserving the longer guard hairs; compressed material; boiled the assembled pieces; and then stiffened, stretched, and brushed the hat after construction. Beaver hats could be exorbitantly expensive, depending on their cut, softness, and trimming, but the dense, insulating material found its way into cheaper alternatives. Demi-castors or 'felts', made from a mix of beaver and lower-grade furs such as rabbit, were an option for those with a smaller disposable income. Disputes arose when these objects were misleadingly marketed as beavers. It was not always possible for a buyer to see the difference between the materials, and they might only notice in the weeks and months that followed, as the cheaper materials collapsed the shape more quickly, and proved less resilient to the elements.[9]

Then as now, there's something depressing about unwittingly buying a knock-off. The anxiety over fake beavers, and the accompanying humiliation of being duped, was rife in early Stuart literature.

'Where did you buy your Felts?' one character asks another in John Cooke's popular comedy, *The City Gallant* (1614). 'Felts?' the gentleman asks, startled into defensiveness. 'By this light, mine is a good Beaver: / It cost mee three pound this morning.' In an anonymous satire, a young man named Rufus struts around in his hat until his companion strikes him and tells him it is a mere felt. Rufus strokes the material, gradually gaining a sense of its quality, until he realises he has been tricked into buying lower-grade wool. The pun on 'felt' in the final line – he would have never known, 'had he not *felt* it out' – highlights the tactility of the hat and its materials.[10] Understanding the quality of a thing involved handling and inspection.

The trajectory of a pelt from American wetland to English city involved many journeys and brokers, and there were multiple chances for buyers to be cheated along the way. Throughout the 1630s, petitioners complained to the Crown of the 'great abuses' and deceits that had been used in making beavers: 'corrupt mixtures, false workemanshipp, and vending of old for new'. Skins were sometimes sent in bulk from North America to Amsterdam and on to Russia for preparation before they were shipped to London to be fashioned into the final product, passing through various hands before they made it into artisans' workshops. Merchants were imprisoned in the Fleet for embezzling beaver furs from warehouses, and it was difficult for felt-makers to regulate production and ensure quality. Royal agents were commissioned to acquire the keys to warehouses and workshops to search out fakes that illegally entered the market, which were detrimental to guilds and trading companies but also to the king's taxable revenue.[11]

Meanwhile, in Wampanoag lands stretching from Wessagusset (Weymouth) to Pokanoket (in Rhode Island), Indigenous nations navigated the freshwater streams where beavers chewed down trees and made lodgings for their families. Travel accounts and private letters provide a link between the ecosystems of wetland and work-shop. Colonists knew that information about the rodents was relevant to those who made these furs into objects of human use. Beavers were wondrous creatures, wrote William Wood, with sharp teeth able to cut down thick trees. They meticulously built houses of wood and clay close to water's edge, 'three stories high, so that as landfloods are raised by great Raines, as the waters arise, they mount higher in their houses'. By art and industry, they created dams that drew human admiration. But the wisdom of the beaver made them wily, too, allowing them to escape 'the *English,* who seldome, or never kills any of them . . . so often deceived by their cunning evasions, so that all the Beaver which the *English* have, comes first from the *Indians*'.[12] Without Indigenous knowledge, there was no trade.

Indigenous inhabitants watched as English ships, those 'walking islands' that seemed to float across the horizon, began to dot the shore-lines. As beavers carried bark across streams and built their homes, the wooden ships and timber-frame houses of an invading new presence brought alterations to the land on a fast-growing scale. When the Puritan John Winthrop arrived in Massachusetts Bay on the *Arabella* in 1630, he warned his community in a sermon that they must be an example of godliness to all those who looked on them. But there could be no model society without economic survival. Colonists soon began trading for beaver skins with neighbouring Wampanoags. The colony served as a meeting place for traders and go-betweens. Merchants ben-efited from the arrival of the Puritans, those 'troopes of *Christs* Army, found as fit helpers to further their worke'.[13]

In Plymouth, the governor William Bradford carefully recorded the economic benefits of the beaver trade in his journal. Divine and eco-nomic matters jostled together in his entries, where notes on the plague and religious governance were interspersed with updates on the fate of pelts that colonists shipped across the Atlantic. One entry reported a large number of otter skins and *musquash* in addition to 494 pounds of beaver. Another recorded that God had enabled colonists to send home large quantities of beavers to pay off debts and encourage further overseas projects. Agents working for Bradford sent him updates of the safe delivery of his large parcels of beaver and otter skins.

As Bradford admitted, the colony's fledgling involvement in fur trading had started in 1620 with the *Mayflower*. No one 'ever saw a beaver skin till they came here and were informed by Squanto.'[14] Squanto, or Tisquantum, was a Pawtuxet man who served as a broker between settlers and local groups. There had also been 'a certain Indian' named Samoset who 'came boldly amongst them and spoke to them in broken English', having picked up the language from fishermen harvesting cod in Monchiggon (Monhegan Island).

Tisquantum had acquired his English in a harder way. Years earlier, an English merchant had trafficked him to Spain. Rescued by Jesuits after ostensibly converting to Catholicism, Tisquantum may have resided in England before finding a way back home. Bradford noted that Tisquantum lived with a merchant in Cornhill during his time in London. If so, he dwelled a few minutes' walk from the Royal Exchange, that entrepot of global trade that had opened during Elizabeth I's reign. There, he could have seen women and men like William Petre congregating in their customised beaver hats, smoking tobacco.

Tisquantum spent years working alongside the English in Massachusetts, teaching them to plant corn and source beaver, and saving their lives on multiple occasions. During this time, beaver financed the colony and kept it afloat, as Betty Booth Donohue writes. Read against the grain, English sources by Puritans in early colonial New England show 'Beaver as a hero . . . Beaver endures English warehouse captivity for the good of the Colony . . . Beaver is second only to corn as a Native nonhuman helpmeet for Plymouth.'[15]

In Passonagessit (Quincy), the London lawyer Thomas Morton established a settlement in opposition to the godly towns around him. We know little about his motivations for establishing a place he called Ma-re Mount, or Merrymount, where he encouraged English and Algonquian peoples to live together. They did not congregate around a chapel, but a maypole, that site of communal revelry at English folk festivals. Bradford described Morton's society as licentious and dissolute, drawing on pagan rituals and classical myths to express his horror at settlers dancing with 'Indian women . . . like so many fairies'.[16]

Morton was a settler, and his sympathy for Algonquians only extended so far. But he was also refreshingly impertinent, willing to critique colonists' double-dealing, often using the beaver to expose these tensions. To unveil the 'hypocrisy of puritans', he recounted how a minister had come to the settlement as a spy, preaching against the covetousness of fur traders while trying to acquire a beaver coat worn by one of the Indigenous inhabitants. At every turn, Puritans hoping 'for gaine in the Beaver trade' conspired against the denizens at Merrymount. To successfully trade for beaver, Morton stressed the significance of *wampum*, those white and purple shell beads current 'in all the parts of New England, from one end of the Coast to another'. While some had attempted to replicate *wampum*, none had 'attained to any composure of them, but that the Salvages [*sic*] have found a great difference to be in the one and the other; and have knowne the counterfett beads from those of their owne making'.[17] New England, Morton indicated, was full of dishonest traders and unholy acts, and had been long before traders in London could complain about demi-castors and counterfeits.

William Wood went further than Morton in condemning settlers' actions. In writing about the English who sought to 'uncloathe [Indigenous inhabitants] of their beaver coates', he exposed the dealings of merchants so desperate for pelts that they did anything to secure them. While Indigenous women wove coats of turkey feathers and lovingly wrapped their newborns in the softest beaver skins, scraping and rubbing the pelts and 'painting them with antique embroyderings in unchangeable colours', English merchants cozened and cheated their way to bundles of furs. Among the 'evill consequents' that the English had brought, with their rapaciousness and alcohol, was the 'unconscionable and forcive wresting of Beaver and Wampompeage [*wampum*]' – hardly the mutually beneficial free trade that propagandists praised back home.[18]

Wood admired the beaver, with its sharp incisors and its architectural know-how. Even as an outsider, he understood that animals were part of connected ecosystems that brought together humans and other animals in reciprocal relationships now disturbed by the arrival of fur traders. Large lobsters rested in long aquatic grasses, and every oyster bank, meadow, and marsh ground offered sustenance and pleasure. In trying to capitalise on the land, the English were continually getting lost, Wood admitted, but the Pequot, Narragansett, Abenaki, and other groups knew the 'swampie groves' and 'swift running rivers' perfectly – as perfectly as London citizens knew how to find the landmarks of Cheapside Cross or London Stone.

In the decades that followed, Indigenous collaboration, and resistance to English settlement, continued to shape trade and transatlantic policy-making. Wars on both sides of the Atlantic, including the Pequot War (1636–8), and the civil wars that ravaged the British Isles through the 1640s, severely disrupted the fur trade. Fierce competition raged between the English, French, and Dutch for territory on North American coastlines, often achieved through alliances with the powerful Haudenosaunee, a confederacy of Iroquois nations. Rivalries and negotiations emerging from European competition for the beaver trade had immense and long-lasting effects on Native lands and communities, dispersing nations and confederacies even as they assembled new ones.[19]

During the Restoration, several French traders sought an alliance with Charles II. They sought him out in Oxford, where the court had retired during a bout of plague, and then at Whitehall, where they pitched their proposal to reorient the fur trade further north, towards the Great Lakes via the St Lawrence River. Elite investors were beguiled. Turning towards the Canadian subarctic reignited their hopes, alive since Tudor times, of finding a north-west passage to China. The desire to find such a route had never really faded, even after the failures of Frobisher and Henry Hudson. In 1651, the 'Ferrar map', likely a collaboration between Virginia Ferrar and her father, John, offered a striking visual of English aspirations in North America. The map spanned from North Carolina, from the Algonquian settlement labelled 'Secotan' on the far left, to New England (a 'great trade of Furrs') and the Hudson River, and north towards Canada. As the region's waterways spread across the page, sea monsters and ships navigated a vast territory populated by animals including a porcupine, heron, and beaver. The 'Sea of China and the Indies' marked the route to the Pacific.

At the top, a portrait of Francis Drake stamped the whole thing with a fabricated legitimacy, harking back to Drake's stop-off in 'New Albion', or California, and his claims to various Indigenous lands during his circumnavigation of the globe. Over time, new conflicts and battles placed other names on such maps. In 1664, the Dutch surrendered New Amsterdam, built on Lenape homelands, to the English, where it was reincorporated as New York. In 1670, the joint-stock Hudson's Bay Company received its official charter. Its first transactions were conducted in bays, forts, and rivers renamed after those aristocrats who were lounging in their silks at court, dreaming of beaver hats and new streams of revenue to

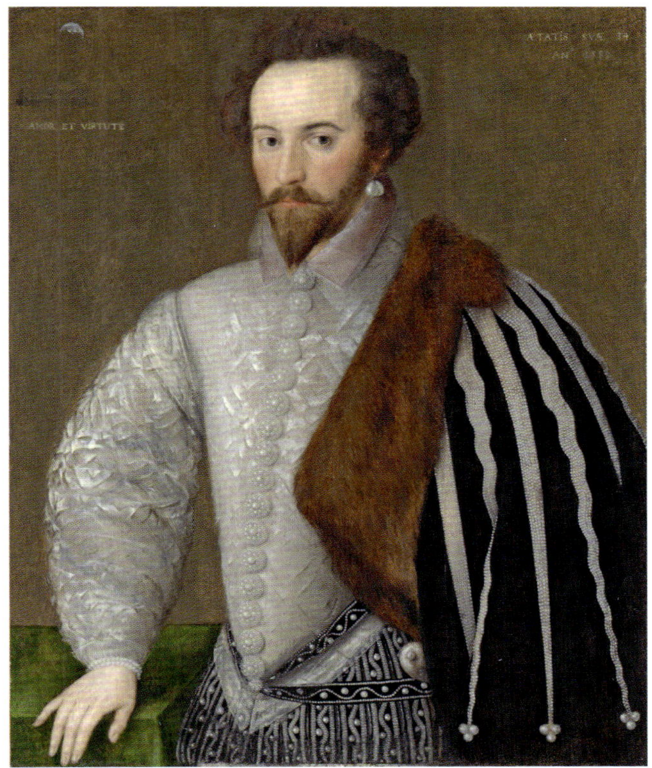

Despite the cascading pearls, Ralegh's double pearl earring takes centre stage here. Late Elizabethan portraits suggest a consistent link between the wealth of pearls and English aspirations in the Atlantic.

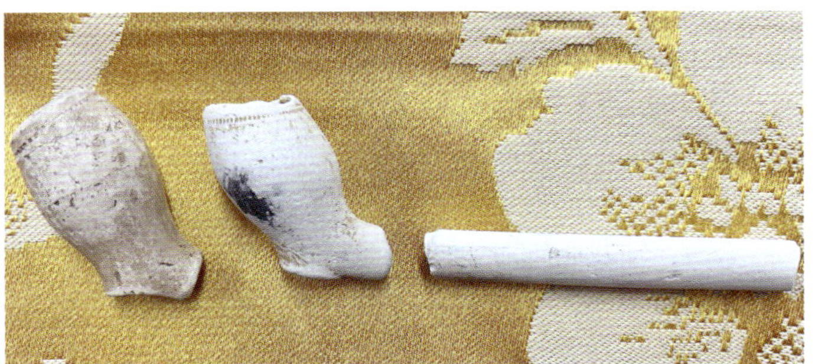

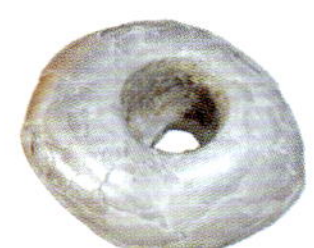

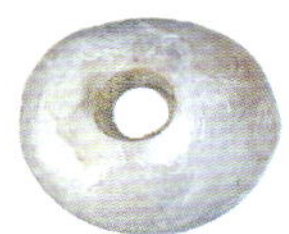

Above, left: These small pipe bowls reflect the high price of tobacco. John Donne poked fun at young gentlemen eager to 'excell / Th'Indians, in drinking [their] Tobacco well'.

Above, right: Drilled pearls from Jamestown testify to both English and Algonquian uses of pearls for adornment, including these Chesapeake freshwater varieties.

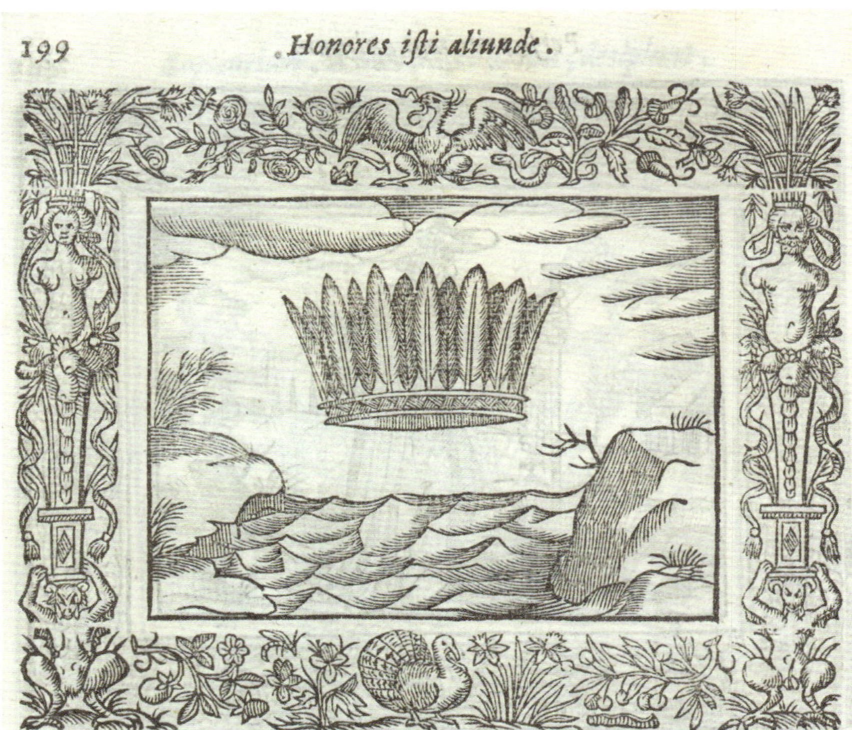

'Beautiful Indian plumes' appeared in Tudor and Stuart inventories, cabinets, and printed books. Indigenous adornments inspired fakes and imitations.

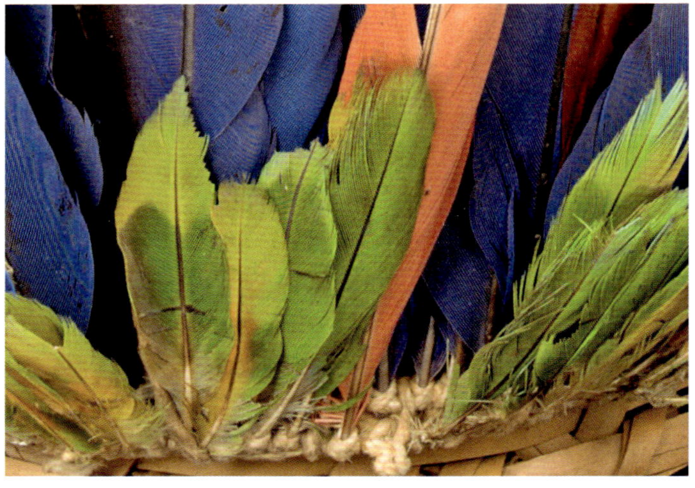

A feathered headdress, collected in the early nineteenth century in Brazil or Guyana, showing vivid macaw feathers and the use of cotton fibres to fasten feathers in place.

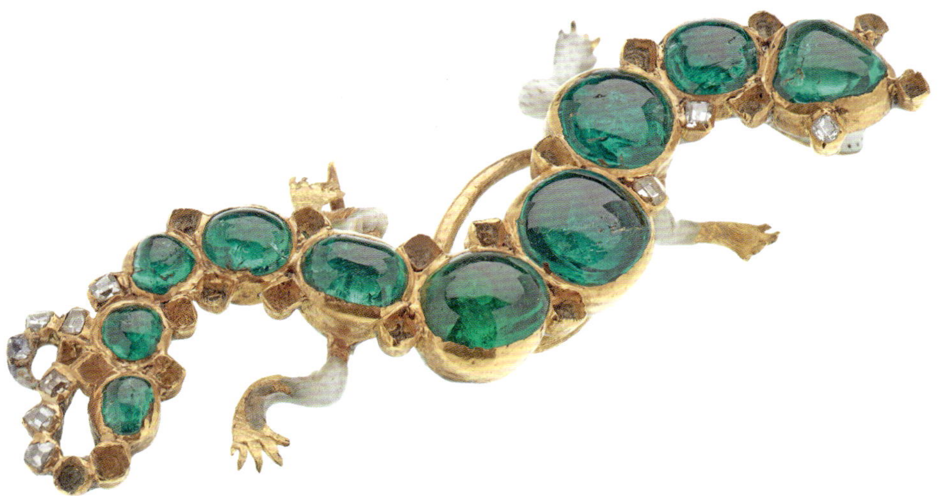

The emeralds in the Cheapside Hoard, including those in this salamander brooch, were formed in deposits in what is now Colombia, mined under perilous conditions.

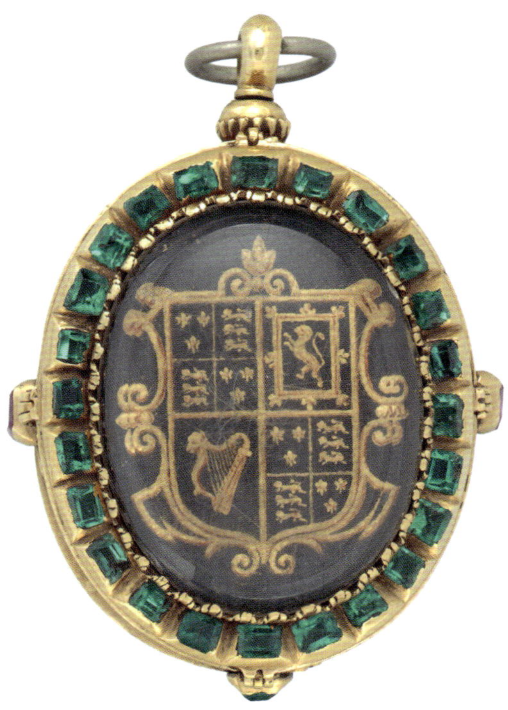

At the Jacobean court, emeralds studded everything from a turtle-shaped clock to this watch case. Nicholas Hilliard called emerald 'the most perfect green on earth'.

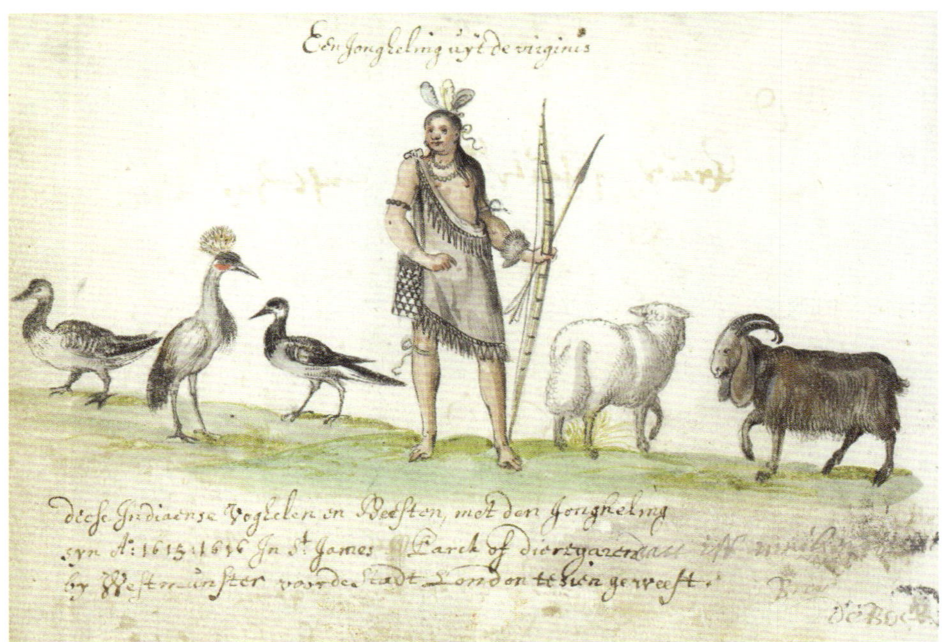

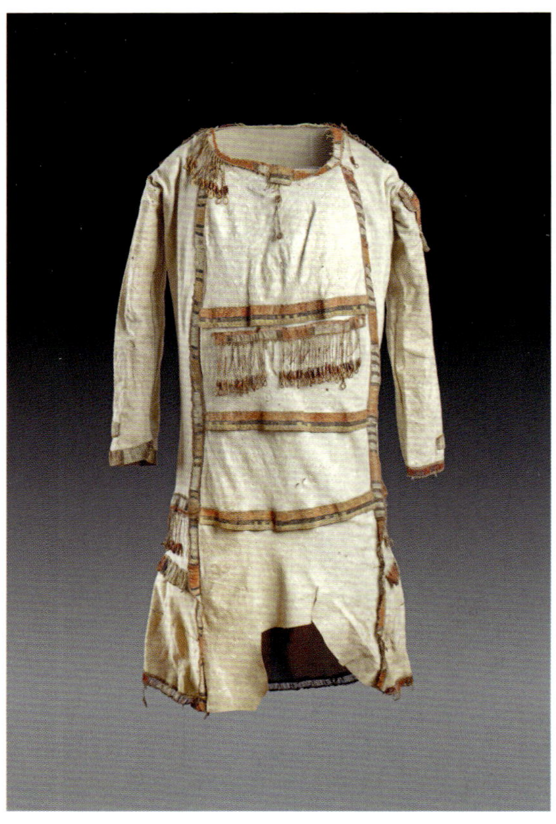

Above: In St James's Park, London, an Algonquian man – possibly the Powhatan Eiakintomino – wears fringed deerskin, his hair long over one shoulder, a woven bag tucked at his side.

Left: Thought to be the 'match-coat from Canada' listed in the Tradescant collection catalogue, made of fringed caribou skin and decorated with porcupine quills.

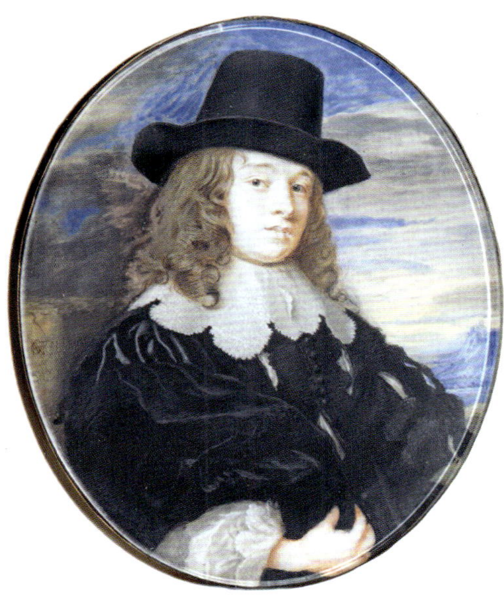

A beaver hat offers a pleasing deviance from expected decorum in this portrait of Margaret Lemon in more masculine attire. 'All the Beaver which the English have, comes first from the Indians', one New England colonist wrote in 1634.

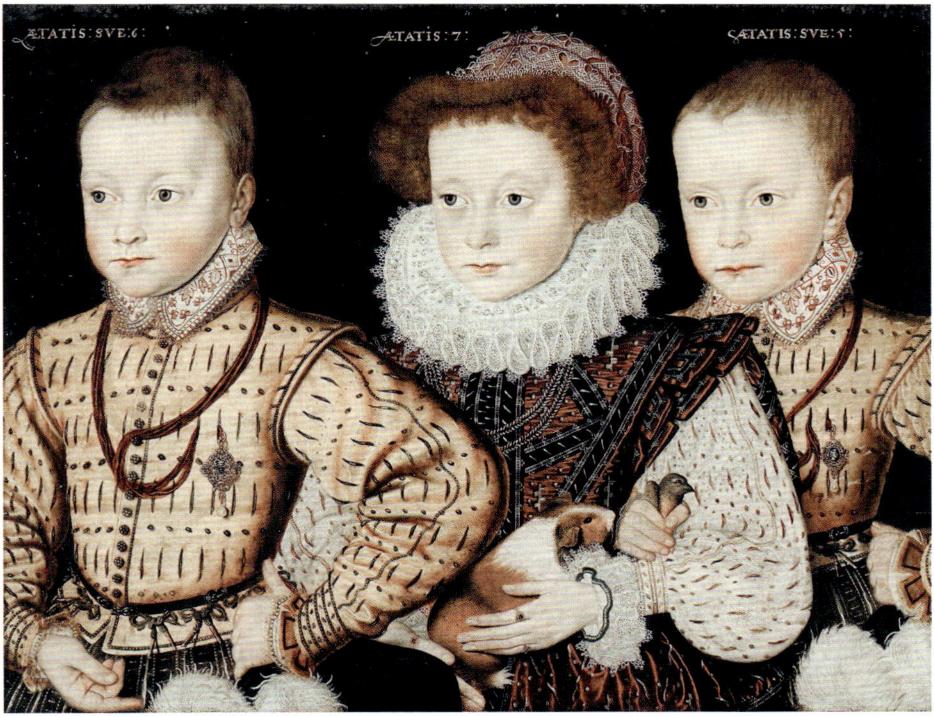

Three Elizabethan Children (*c.* 1580), the eldest cradling a guinea pig. Merchant and aristocratic households were inhabited by animals that had long held important places in Native communities.

Battata Virginiana ſiue Virginianorum, & Pappus.
Potatoes of Virginia.

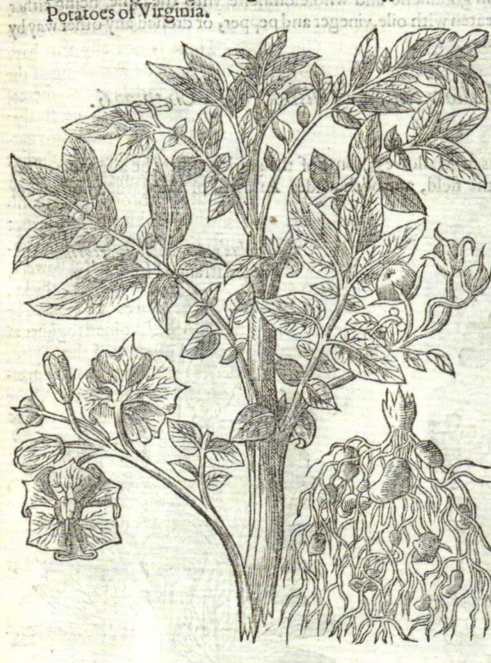

❧ *The deſcription.*

Virginia Potatoes hath many hollowe flexible branches, trailing vppon the grounde, three ſquare, vneuen, knotted or kneed in ſundry places at certaine diſtances; from the which knots commeth foorth one great leafe made of diuers leaues, ſome ſmaller, & others greater, ſet togither vpon a fat middle rib by couples; of a ſwart greene colour tending to rednes. The whole leafe reſembling thoſe of the Parſnep, in taſte at the firſt like graſſe, but afterward ſharp & nipping the toong: from the boſome of which leaues come foorth long rounde ſlender footſtalks, whereon do grow very faire and pleaſant flowers, made of one entire whole leafe, which is folded or plaited in ſuch ſtrange ſort, that it ſeemeth to be a flower made of ſixe ſundrie ſmall leaues, which cannot eaſily be perceiued, except the ſame be pulled open. The colour whereof it is hard to expreſſe. The whole flower is of a light purple color, ſtripped down the middle of euery folde or welt, with a light ſhew of yellownes, as though purple and yellow were mixed togither: in the middle of the flower thruſteth foorth a thicke fat pointell, yellow as golde, with a ſmall ſharpe greene pricke or point in the middeſt thereof. The fruite ſucceedeth the flowers, round as a ball, of the bignes of a little bulleſſe or wilde Plum, greene at the firſt, and blacke when it is ripe; wherein is contained ſmall white ſeede, leſſer than thoſe of Muſtarde. The roote is thicke, fat, and tuberous; not much differing either in ſhape, colour or taſte from the common Potatoes, ſauing that the rootes hereof are not ſo great nor long; ſome of them round as a ball, ſome ouall or egge faſhion, ſome longer, and others ſhorter: which knobbie rootes are faſtened vnto the ſtalkes with an infinite number of threddie ſtrings.

❧ *The place.*

It groweth naturally in America where it was firſt diſcouered, as reporteth *C. Cluſius*, ſince which time I haue receiued rootes hereof from Virginia, otherwiſe called Norembega, which growe and proſper in my garden, as in their owne natiue countrie.

❧ *The*

Above: John Gerard's *The Herball* (1597) celebrates the beauty of potato flowers and attests to the ubiquity of potatoes in England, as well as many other transatlantic flora.

Right: Sixteenth-century cucurbit (squash) seeds found at the Globe and Rose theatres suggest that audience members munched on a pumpkin snack while watching plays by Marlowe and Shakespeare.

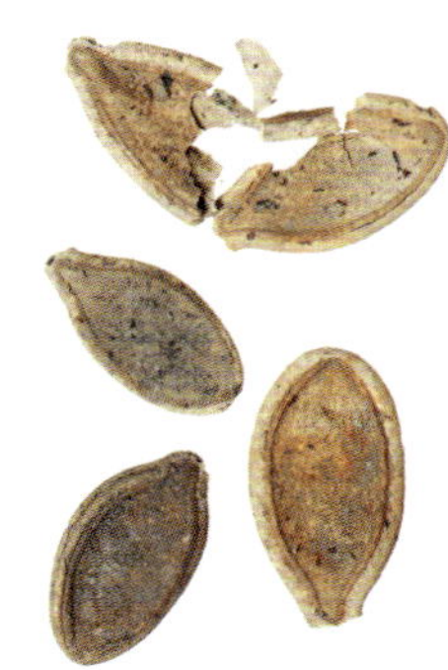

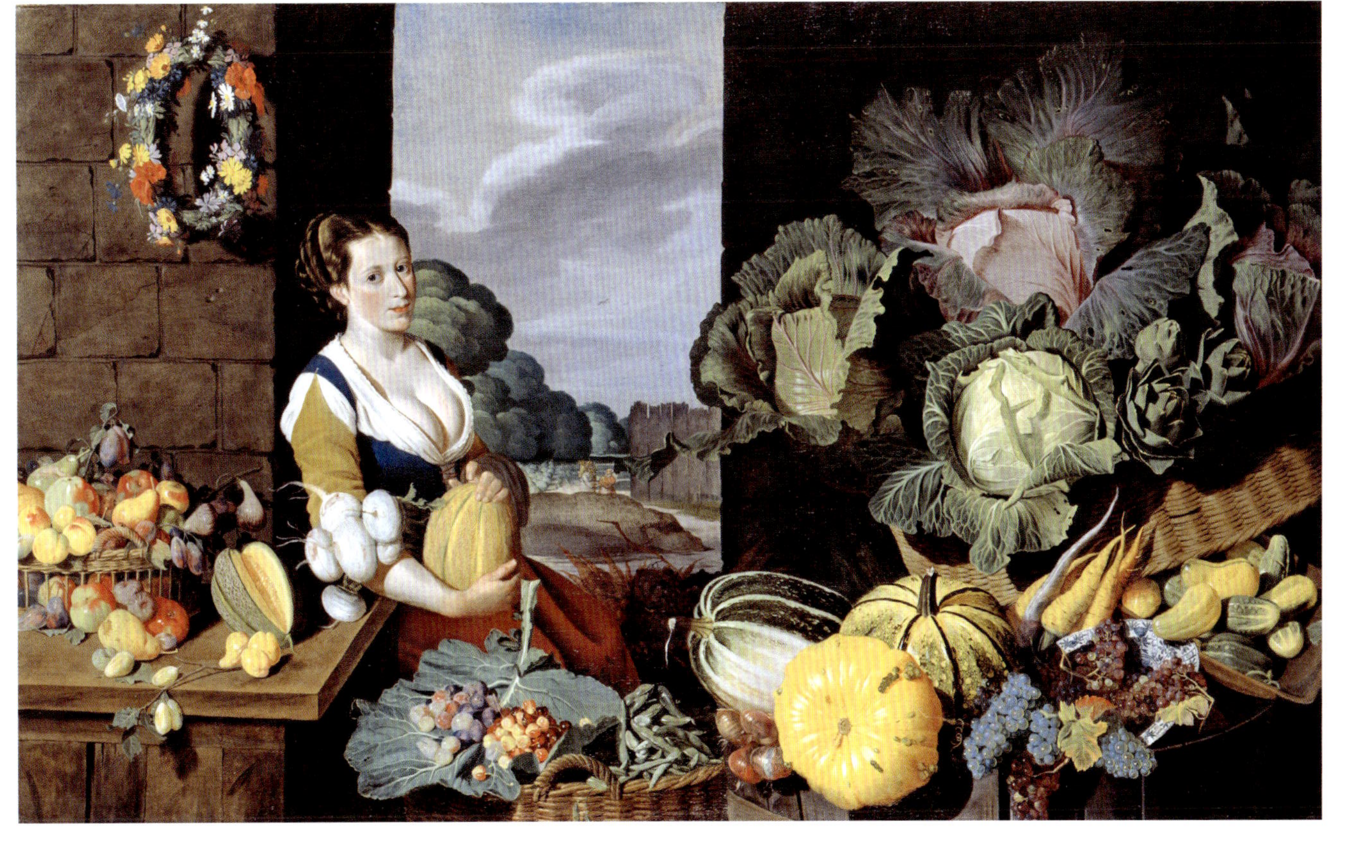

The Americas sneak into what may seem like an archetypally domestic still life in Nicholas Bacon's *Cookmaid with Still Life of Vegetables and Fruit* (c. 1620-25).

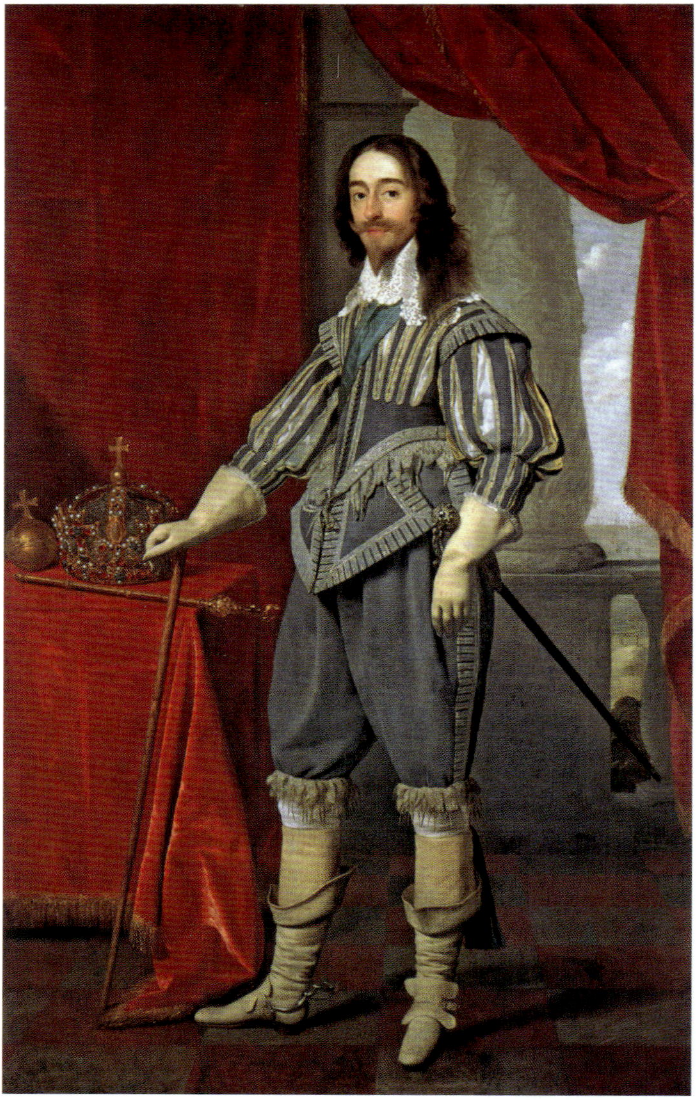

The crimson velvet of royal paintings and furnishings, like the rich fabric in Daniel Mytens's 1631 portrait of Charles I, is often cochineal – an American insect and dye.

Detail from Samuel Purchas's printed version of the Codex Mendoza,
which brought Mexica scripts into Renaissance libraries.

finance wars, or jewels for mistresses – Fort Charles, James Bay, Rupert River.[20]

Looking back on the events of the seventeenth century, the Narragansett elder Dawn Dove has written of how 'our ancestors who first met the Europeans, and those generations since' have lamented the Europeans' inability to see Mother Earth as anything but a commodity.[21] Beaver has become an important figure in Indigenous activism. Leanne Betasamosake Simpson (Michi Saagiig Nishnaabeg) uses stories of the beaver (*amik*) and their dams to think through the regenerative possibility of blockades and their role in resisting capitalist extraction. Beaver, she writes, are world-makers – they create sustaining habitats and also shift the landscape. They can point the way to a redeployment of resources creating different ways of living with each other, ways in which all members of the community, human or other-than-human, can benefit.[22]

Today, in the galleries and storage vaults of London's Victoria & Albert Museum, several seventeenth-century beaver hats are snugly locked away. The thickness and durability of the felt has served them well, helping them to survive these 400 years. To feel the bristly felt under one's fingertips is to touch the fragments of a beaver that lived in the same era as Tisquantum, Charles I, or the audacious Margaret Lemon.

Other hats survive only as mentions in texts. When the secretary John Pory wrote to his friend Dudley Carleton about life in 1610s Jamestown, he described a collier's wife walking through the settlement in flamboyant silk and a 'rough beaver hatt with a fair perle hatband'. The comment was a flippant one, gesturing to the pretensions of colonists whose fortunes had been made by tobacco. But the beaver hat in Jamestown is also a manifestation of the habits, tastes, and commodity chains that enabled colonial society to seem like a reflection of English life. A reworked, exported material serves to make the colony seem a suburb of the metropolis. In a small settlement built on swampy marshes, where resources were scarce, a beaver hat, likely manufactured in England from North American pelts, ends up back on its continent of origin, catching the eye of a richer man who wants to amuse his correspondent back home.[23] 'Rough', the well-connected, widely travelled Pory was keen to stress. He had been to Cambridge and Paris and Constantinople; he had seen plays on the Jacobean stage, where beaver hats mattered to the fashioning of the civil gentleman. It may be decorated with a pearl, but the hat is low-grade.

The hat worn by the woman in Jamestown was about more than self-expression or social aspiration. It owed its existence to many layers of labour and expertise. Like fashion supply chains today, the collier's wife's hat was part of a global system. As a beaver, it was bound to American landscapes, and to English access to a rodent that dwelled in the wetlands of Turtle Island. All that is left of the hat is Pory's glib remark. But, taken together, maps, travel books, diaries, petitions, inventories, poems, and portraits show that even a 'very pretty fashion' was never just that.

Lovelocked

In the Christmas season of 1597–8, seeking revenge for an insulting poem written by the law student Richard Martin, the young barrister John Davies armed himself with a dagger and cudgel and burst into Middle Temple Hall. Dressed in his cap and gown, Davies strode to where Martin sat dining with his friends and struck him violently over the head. Then he dashed out of the hall with his servant, rushing the short way to the River Thames, and escaped by boat to Oxford. The Middle Temple would have lost a serious advocate of Virginia plantation if Martin had been gravely injured in the attack; he would go on to serve on the council for the Virginia Company and to act on behalf of the colony in the House of Commons. But before those days of responsibility to come, gentlemen at the Inns of Court were lords of misrule, breakfasting on madeira wine and goading each other with barbs and quips that could land them in trouble.

Away from the confines of home – far from the eyes of watchful parents, pedantic tutors, entitled elder siblings – where did young Tudor and Stuart gentlemen spend their time? Where did they go when they had money in their pockets, and the pleasures of the city seemed endless? For those who were unsure where to start, perhaps intimidated by the capital after a bucolic adolescence spent hunting and attending local grammar school, one 1609 manual was there to help:

- Always sleep in. Nap a lot: mid-day slumbers are golden.
- Pace around your chambers in your tailor-made oversized shirt, or better yet, go completely naked.
- Wander the aisles of St Paul's Cathedral – not to pray, but to gossip about court scandals and disgraced playwrights.
- Spend the rest of your time in tobacco shops and browsing booksellers' stalls.
- Drink liberally, and cultivate eclectic and wide-range tastes.
- Whatever you do, don't cut your hair. Curse the puritanical pair of scissors that threatens to shorten your locks by even an inch.[1]

Thomas Dekker's counsel came in the form of a mock conduct manual, which poked fun at the rising genre of advice literature offering guidance on how respectable men and women should behave. But no matter how prescriptive such books tried to be, students were having none of it. At the Inns of Court, the young men seeking to enter fashionable London society were ready to shed the rules and counsel on which their elders had raised them. Maybe not forever; but they were young, often unmarried. This was their time. And it was in this boisterous, transgressive milieu that discussions about a flamboyant hairstyle became wrapped up in stories of shamans and warriors.

In 1628, vexed at the extravagant behaviour of his peers, the pious lawyer William Prynne waved his own, wholly unironic pair of puritanical scissors, and published a treatise dedicated entirely to condemning those long locks that Dekker had encouraged gentlemen to sport. His prime target was the 'lovelock' – a lock of hair worn longer than the rest, often styled to curl or braid over the left shoulder, by the heart. Calling his pamphlet *The Unloveliness of Lovelocks,* Prynne targeted the frizzled, cascading tresses that adorned London's youth. His argument was simple. These 'new-fangled Lockes', these 'Lascivious,

Exorbitant, and Fantastique *Haires*', were 'audacious' and 'sinister', serving as 'badges of our invirilitie'. Accusations of effeminacy came up a lot in Prynne's writing. Like many early Stuart moralists, he had a problem with gender fluidity. Prynne saw women behaving like men, and men like women, and envisioned the ruin of the entire civil Christian order. Crisping their hair made women insolent, and men 'womanish'. The barbershop had replaced the chapel. Young people spent more time studying their reflections than the Bible.[2]

In the time of Prynne's writing, wearing a lock of hair from a loved one signalled loyalty and attachment. Mothers wove their children's locks into bracelets and brooches. Cut locks were a marker of romantic love, too. They publicly declared private devotion, even obsession, harking back to the codes of chivalry and its favours and love tokens. In a miniature portrait of an unknown man from around 1600, possibly the first Earl of Northampton, a curly-haired courtier in a suit of armour and a multilayered ruff stands against a lush, velvety red curtain. Despite the intricate, burnished armour, our eye is drawn to something much more delicate: the enamelled pendant dangling from his ear. A strand of hair, incorporated into an embellished earring, trails across the ruff like a lover's tresses on a pillow in an erotic painting by Titian.

By the early seventeenth century, wearing one's own hair long on one side, often over the heart, was an extension of, or gesture to, this tradition. 'Will you bee Frenchefied with a love locke downe to your shoulders, wherein you may weare your mistresse favour?' one pamphleteer asked his upstart readers in 1592.[3] Prynne's argument tapped into religious concerns about declining standards in late Tudor and early Stuart England. The frontispiece to Samuel Ward's 1622 sermon, *Woe to Drunkards,* echoed Cicero's 'O tempora, O mores' to lament the decaying manners of the time. In the sermon's imagined chivalric past, knightly valour and Christian piety reigned supreme.

Underneath the symbols of masculine virtue at the top of the page, the frivolous new order came to life through its gaudy trappings: shoes decorated with ribbons and rosettes, cards and dice for gambling, expensive glassware for toasts, and tobacco pipes.

James I often asked his court preachers to deliver sermons against such vanities. Had not the fall of the Roman Empire been an abject lesson in the military weakness that accompanied too much luxury? My 'deare Feminine Masculine,' wrote the anonymous author of *Haec-vir* ('The womanish man') in 1620, 'why doe you curle, frizell and powder your hayres, bestowing more houres . . . in giving every thread his posture' than Caesar had in marshalling his armies? The bejewelled courtier with 'Indian Pearles' like two pears dangling from his ears, 'his Locks bedewed with waters of sweet savour', should be a target for ridicule, not imitation. To Prynne, lovelocks were voluptuous outward manifestations of a corrupt soul. We must '*reforme* our Heads, and Hearts, which distemper all our other members, with the Flux of sinne', he concluded, lest the English lose their military and mercantile power through distraction.[4]

In the midst of his diatribe about waning masculinity, Prynne does the unexpected. He offers a distinct origin story for lovelocks, one that brings Tsenacommacah and Algonquian sacred spaces to the heart of urban London. Although his tract made associations between lovelocks and societies from across the world, including Greek ancients, Nahua priests, and Japanese men, he specifically credited Indigenous Americans with the popularity of lovelocks in England. A certain Algonquian who had come into the realm encouraged this fashion by blaming the English for not wearing their hair longer, as Native 'priests' or shamans did.

Prynne referred to a 'reverend Historian', the geographical editor and Anglican churchman Samuel Purchas, 'who informes us in express tearmes: That our sinister, and unlovely Love-lockes, had their generation, birth, and pedigree [from] the Heathenish, and Idolatrous Virginians'. The Virginians, he wrote, 'doe weare a long Love-locke on the left side of their Heads (as our English Ruffians doe) in imitation of Ockeus their Devill-god'. Appearing to Algonquians in the form of a man with a long black lock on the left side of his head, Okeus was, in Prynne's imagination, the evil figure lurking behind Algonquian practices, so that 'if wee will resolve the generation of our Love-lockes, into their first and true originall; the *Virginia Devill Ockeus,* will prove to be the naturall Father'.[5]

Prynne had evidently been reading the 1617 edition of Purchas's popular *Purchas his Pilgrimage,* which mentioned lovelocks and the 'Virginian' in England by name. The book contained updated information about European travels to the Americas, including news from French and Spanish settlements in New France (Canada), Mexico, and Florida. Carrying on Hakluyt's legacy, Purchas had compiled this information using an assortment of printed books, unpublished manuscripts, correspondence, and in-person interviews with travellers.

At the time of his publication, numerous Algonquians lived in London as part of the Powhatan delegation that accompanied Matoaka across the Atlantic in 1616. Purchas was deeply committed to Virginian affairs, and he drew widely on intelligence from those who had newly returned from the Chesapeake, including a young interpreter named Henry Spelman; John Rolfe; the governor Thomas Dale; and '*Tomocomo,* at this present in London'. Tomocomo was the English name for Uttamatomakkin, a respected religious and political counsellor for Wahunsenaca (known by the English as 'Powhatan') and his brother, Opechancanough. He had been charged with gathering information about the English for the Powhatans back home.

According to Purchas, Uttamatomakkin had explained to colonists that Okeus, or Okee, was a deity the Powhatan associated with war, vengeance, and scarcity. In an attempt at cultural translation, the English began to equate this figure with the Christian idea of the devil. Since Okeus appeared to Algonquians in human form with a long lock of hair on one side, the lock served as a visual marker of this figure's shadowy association with paganism. And yet, even as the lock seemed to represent the darkest realms of spiritual evil, it migrated from Algonquian to English society. 'I have heard Sir *Thomas Dale,* and Mr *Rolph* of that opinion', Purchas wrote, that the wearing of a long lock on the left side 'was first by our Men in the first Plantation, little above thirtie yeeres since, borrowed from these Salvages'. Uttamatomakkin, 'so admiring this Rite . . . objected to our GOD this defect, that he had not taught us so to weare our haire'.[6]

In Purchas's retelling, the fashion for lovelocks went all the way back to Ralegh's Roanoke settlement in North Carolina in the mid-1580s. The Roanoke colonists, particularly Thomas Hariot, already had a reputation for making tobacco fashionable among wealthy Londoners after their return. But several Virginia colonists, from Governor Dale to the planter Rolfe, seemed to believe that 'our Men in the first Plantation' had introduced lovelocks to English society. In time, this style would spread as a result of increased encounters with the Powhatan after the establishment of Jamestown.

In 1609, John Smith placed the young Henry Spelman, Captain Argall's 'boy', in an Algonquian household to learn the language. Spelman had only been in Jamestown a few weeks. He was self-professedly headstrong, sent across the Atlantic by family members looking to reform his unruliness. In the end, Spelman found himself drawn to Algonquian life. In 1613, he wrote an account of the Powhatan. In his manuscript, which colonial promoters deemed unfit to disseminate too widely, Spelman wrote that he had been protected and well-treated among them. The women, he noted, worked hard to build houses, weave mats, and plant beans and maize.

He had learned the language and could now move freely between Algonquian villages and James Fort, quickly becoming, as Smith had hoped, a strategic asset in cross-cultural diplomacy and trade.

Spelman lived outside the Virginian political elite's circle of governors and council members. He was open about how his expectations of the Powhatan had been challenged, rather than confirmed, by living among them and seeing their laws and systems of justice at work. He, too, attributed distinctive hairstyles to Powhatan elites, both shamans and skilled hunters and fighters. The *quiakros* or 'priests are shaven on the right side of their head close to the skull [with] only a little lock left at the ear'. Warriors cut the hair on the right side of their head so that it would not hinder them when hunting with bows and arrows, but 'on the other side they let it grow and have a long lock hanging down their shoulder'.[7] In the highly fictionalised engraving printed in Smith's *The Generall Historie of Virginia* (1624), Smith was shown capturing the 'King of Pamaunkee' (Pamunkey) by wrapping his fist around Opechancanough's lock, his other hand gripping his pistol.

The Mattaponi oral history of Pocahontas's life recounts that many of the *quiakros* who voyaged to England in 1616 did so in disguise, hoping to gain intelligence for their leaders. The English had learned to identify them by their distinctive appearance. Uttamatomakkin's reputation, however, preceded him, and he openly operated as a Powhatan spiritual leader.[8] His hair may have served as a visual marker of his role as a powerful mediator, making the fashion among the English seem all the more subversive.

English Protestant associations between lovelocks and Indigenous fashions continued long after Uttamatomakkin returned home. Writing from Salem, Massachusetts, in 1630, the minister Francis Higginson wrote of how Algonquian hair 'is generally blacke, and cut before like our Gentlewomen, and one locke longer then the rest, much like to our Gentlemen which fashion I thinke came from hence into *England*'.[9]

In 1632, four years after publishing *The Unloveliness of Lovelocks*, Prynne produced an incendiary work against plays and actresses called *Histrio-mastix*. His indictment of women acting on stage was taken to be a targeted criticism of Henrietta Maria and, by extension, King Charles himself, leading to swift and severe punishment. Prynne was imprisoned and publicly punished, pilloried while his own book was burned before him. The pages that blazed and curled in the ash contained further denunciations of those 'frizled lockes', 'the very guise and fashion of the times'. Throughout *Histrio-mastix*, Prynne directed readers to his earlier work. 'See my *Unlovelinesse of Lovelockes*,' he wrote in the margins of multiple pages. Prynne cited '*Mr Purchas in his Pilgrim*' as evidence that men gravitated towards lovelocks because they preferred to imitate 'American Salvages'.[10]

As a lawyer, Prynne had addressed his book to a specific audience: the gentlemen of the four Inns of Court. Lincoln's Inn, Middle Temple, Inner Temple, and Gray's Inn were at the centre of fashionable London, institutions where up-and-coming gentlemen came to learn the workings of the law, and where members of the gentry might gain the required skills and training to become country clerks and justices of the peace. But the Inns were also known as England's 'third university', where aspiring writers and politicians went to polish their wits and gain connections that could be useful to their careers and social networks. Gentlemen who went there after Oxford and Cambridge were often in their mid- to late teens. Many studied at the Inns without the intention of actually passing the bar. Others took lodgings without even enrolling. They wanted to pace in their chambers in their long, embroidered shirts without their parents hovering over them, to read books about fencing and poetry, and go to plays that brought global travel to the stage. They wanted to find themselves.

Much of John Donne's early poetry is set in this environment of drama, prickly honour, and ruthless competition in and around London's four Inns of Court. In his 'Satire I', a student frets about abandoning the safety of his books to follow a companion into the bustling streets beyond his bedroom, with its posturing and elaborate honour codes. The speaker is convinced that his flighty friend, itching to be admired and see the world, will forsake him at the sight of more stylish or well-connected peers. Nonetheless, he gives in. He dresses, perhaps grabbing his wide-brim beaver hat on his way out. Once in the streets, the speaker's fears quickly transpire. The bustle of life in the narrow lanes and alleyways in and around the Inns of Court, with its booksellers and taverns and *flâneurs*, is too enthralling for any but those most virtuous or wary to resist.

The Inns connected ambitious gentlemen to political activities in Parliament and at the royal court, but they were also places of inventive, sometimes transgressive literary experimentation. Richard Martin's reputation as a wit, which helped him secure the role of Prince of Love in the 1597–8 festivities, also connected him to the poets and playwrights, including Donne, who were part of the Sirenical fraternity meeting at the Mermaid Tavern on Bread Street. Elizabethan tragedians experimented with blank verse, gentlemen wrote satires and saucy love poems, and barristers invited famous playwrights to contribute to those notorious Christmas revels. Shakespeare knew this milieu and wrote for it: his *Twelfth Night* was performed at the Middle Temple in 1602. The boisterous Sir Toby Belch first appears onstage after another raucous night out, and he is forever resisting the forces of authority that threaten his good spirits.

In 1613, the lawyer Matthew Carew complained to his friend that his son had entered the Middle Temple and had 'a chamber and studye, but I heare studieth the law very little.'[11] These were the anxieties of a father who knew what the Inns might do to an impressionable young man away from home. Sir Matthew had some reason to be concerned; this wayward student was Thomas Carew, who soon became associated with a coterie of daring and dissolute poets. In the 1620s, Thomas would pen 'The Rapture', one of the most erotic and oft-transcribed poems of his time. Pluck any few lines from it, and you get a taste of its primary, somewhat blasphemous, preoccupations:

> *Bathe me in juice of kisses, whose perfume*
> *Like a religious incense shall consume.*

In the years that followed, Carew inched his way into the exclusive inner circle of the court, eventually being sworn a Gentleman of the Privy Chamber and serving as 'sewer in ordinary' to Charles I, tasked with tasting the king's food before passing it to the monarch.

When Prynne railed against lovelocks, he was opposing these long-haired boys and their unholy dreams. It seems farfetched, but for him, the ostensible origins of the lovelock in Algonquian North America were intimately entangled with the lives of fashionable, disorderly young gentlemen in London. Purchas, Prynne, and New England ministers like Higginson were Protestants concerned with English piety following expansion into the 'pagan' Americas. They were also critical of the popularity of Catholicism at the English court. Queen Henrietta Maria, born at the Palais du Louvre in the same year as Henry Spelman had gone to live with the Powhatan, was a staunch Catholic, and Protestants feared she would seduce Charles – and the nation – away from the Protestant Church. To them, conformity to Protestantism had immense implications for the developing character of the English empire. Those gentlemen in and around the Inns who were inspired by Indigenous peoples, who succumbed to Algonquian practices like smoking or growing their hair long, and who, by extension, risked sympathising with Indigenous perspectives, seemed to revel in dissolving those boundaries that should remain between Christians and 'pagans', women and men.

During the 1610s and 1620s, the Chesapeake became the testing ground where the English sought to discover whether their entire model of colonisation was viable. Councillors and governors increasingly focused on occupying lands through plantation and long-term settlement. Though investors bitterly disagreed about how such settlements might be organised and governed – whether land should be parcelled out to individual landowners, or held in common by municipal corporations – both solutions required making claims to densely populated lands. The exportation of Protestantism and English ways of life served as justification. The English repeatedly excused their colonial efforts by professing their commitment to 'civilising' Algonquians, contrasting their plantation projects to the large-scale extraction and enslavement practices of Iberian colonial agents. The Catholic Church also sought converts, Protestants acknowledged, but was happy to accept merely the outward trappings of piety – the confessions and penance, the prayers to saints – whereas the English would gently guide and persuade Algonquians to search out the truth of the gospel deep in their hearts.

Increasingly, however, such a mission seemed perilous to the Protestant soul. It required sustained interaction with Indigenous peoples while refusing to accommodate their beliefs, ceremonies, and religious practices. The case of Henry Spelman appeared to prove the dangers of too much compromise. In the summer of 1619, Spelman came before the council at Jamestown's first General Assembly to answer charges that he had become too sympathetic to Algonquian causes. The council viewed this as unsettling evidence of the colonising project's fragility. Acting without remorse, Spelman 'had in him more of the Savage [than] of the Christian.'[12]

In the early 1620s, when the Virginia Company was at a crisis point and soon to be dissolved entirely, the Company council in London expressed consternation at the 'unwelcome newes, that had beene heard at large in publicke Court, that the *Indians* and [the colonists] lived as one Nation', with 'the Salvages as frequent in their houses as themselves'.[13] Authorities had vehemently advised against English cultural porousness, whether through Anglo-Indigenous marriages or friendship. 'We have sent boies amongst [the Powhatan] to learne their Language,' the minister Jonas Stockham reported, 'but they return worse than they went.' 'I am no States-man,' he concluded, but English ascendancy in Powhatan lands seemed impossible 'till their Priests . . . have their throat cut'.[14]

In associating lovelocks with Virginia, both Purchas and Prynne were picking up on English anxieties about the relationship between politics and cultural identity. What seems like an overblown reaction to a strand of hair became a flashpoint for deep-rooted fears of cultural transfer and extravagance, at a time when assimilation and sober-minded temperance were official policy. The denunciation of lovelocks flared at the same moment as tobacco emerged as Virginia's first cash crop. The 'faire unlovely generation of the Love-locke', from the Algonquian Chesapeake to metropolitan England, had infected the new wave of politically minded youth who were experimenting with who they wanted to be. Lovelocks adorned the heads of some of England's wealthiest imperial supporters, who busied themselves with financing, organising, and endorsing overseas voyages in those years before the civil wars, spearheaded by the young monarch who had taken the throne in 1625. Silver medals commemorating Charles I's dominion of the sea depicted the king in armour and his signature locks. On the reverse, a ship sailed underneath the words NEC META MIHI QUI TERMINUS ORBI ('Nor is that a limit to me, which is a boundary of the world'). For the younger generation, possible

Indigenous influences need not be a signifier of corruption, but rather of imperial ambition and cosmopolitanism.

As Prynne believed, lovelocks were the markers of those 'who make their will, and fancie, the onely rule by which they walke'.[15] Like a love-lock, fancy denoted a playful inventiveness of style, tottering on the verge of bad taste, tumbling headlong into its own golden spirals. In 1638, the poet and playwright William Davenant published *Madagascar* (1638), a lengthy poem that imagined a band of Cavalier lovers (as supporters of Charles I were known) conquering the island of Madagascar. He presented his conqueror-heroes as his friends might imagine themselves, honourably militant but also marvellously beauti-ful, landing on the island in a blaze of curly hair. These locks are important to their colonising mission. Conquest and the Cavalier aes-thetic go hand in hand: 'You may esteeme them lovers by their haire,' the speaker says.[16] Davenant wrote his poem in support of a project that had recently gripped the imagination of courtiers, including many of Henrietta Maria's favourites. The real-life poster boy for this project was Elizabeth of Bohemia's son Rupert, Charles I's nephew, whose portraits of the time depict him in those distinct tresses. Though Rupert never went to Madagascar, he eventually travelled to mainland Africa and the West Indies, seeking African and Indigenous allies and hunting ruthlessly for lucrative resources.[17]

As rich Englishmen boisterously defended their freedom to grow their hair long in defiance of their elders, they were enforcing a model of colonialism that deprived others of the freedom to choose their own ways of life. In Ireland, the English viewed Gaelic fashions and traditions as impediments to military success. Along with mantles, they targeted glibs, a style of hair worn longer in the front than at the back and sides. Colonists believed that glibs signalled the wearer's tendency towards subversion. Where necessary, English officers cut the glibs of captains and soldiers by force. Cutting them was 'the first token of obedyence'.[18] This was the context for a brutal little poem that found its way into an early Stuart commonplace book. Transcribed alongside various poems about love or Continental politics, the verses conveyed a fantasy of English conquest brought about by cutting hair. The peace-loving King James, the verses went, was 'too kind to cut', but Hugh O'Neill, Earl of Tyrone, and the other Gaelic lords needed to be subjugated, by the scissor as by the sword. They were 'barbarous boyes', due for a trim:

> *With Cizers to conforme ther lockes*
> *Unto the Soveraignes cutt.*[19]

The lovelock generation were the first to grow up at a time when the English had claimed territories in the Americas. Many were still toddling around country estates in their linens, or getting Latin beaten into them at grammar school, when Walter Ralegh sent colonists to Roanoke. When they were old enough to go to the Inns of Court and experience the excitement of metropolitan life, they were exposed to books and ideas that encouraged global travel and colonial participation. They could meet Uttamatomakkin, gain a glimpse of Matoaka at a court masque, or speak to one of the Algonquians residing in a merchant's house in the City. When Robert Hayman, who had studied at Lincoln's Inn, travelled to Newfoundland in the 1620s, he recalled being inspired to travel after Francis Drake himself had singled him out from a crowd in his childhood, offering him a fresh orange and blessing him with a kiss. This larger-than-life figure, the 'glory of this age', had deeply affected Hayman's 'little-little selfe'.[20] The Inns became the milieu where Hayman's fascination with crossing oceans finally moved from aspiration to real possibility.

Whether lovelocks were ever meant to reference a malign Chesapeake deity is, like many origin stories behind a trend, unverifiable – an act of fancy, one might say. But the golden curls that framed the ear, encircling those baroque pearls extracted from oysters in Venezuelan riverbeds, were nevertheless an aesthetic choice that promoted certain ideas and beliefs. In some ways, as Prynne believed, they were emblems of the times. Political ideas – about the control of resources, about who was entitled to wear what they wanted, or say what they wanted – were encapsulated in the freedoms and the extravagance that aristocrats flaunted.

For this generation, the baroque profligacy of 'womanish' curls ushered in a new sense of court style, captured in Van Dyck's vivid paintings of London's pretty young things. It signals how the aesthetic of the English Cavalier carried an imperial edge, and this can shape the way we think about the Stuart period as a whole. The English Empire didn't just erupt onto a world map from the later seventeenth century. Before Oliver Cromwell's military campaigns in the Caribbean, before the 1651 Navigation Acts and the rise of the English transatlantic slave trade during the Restoration (with help from Prince Rupert, incidentally), wealthy men and women were already at work revising their ideas of civility, privilege, and power, drawing on their interactions with specific peoples and lands in the Americas.

The Rich family is a case in point. Robert Rich, second Earl of Warwick, was a leading colonial councillor for Virginia and then New England, targeting Spanish power in the Atlantic through privateering and plunder. His brother, Henry Rich, first Earl of Holland, was Governor of the Providence Island Company, which set out to colonise parts of the Caribbean and Central America. Holland's own allegiances were rather slippery, wavering between support for Puritan factions in Parliament and sustaining a close personal relationship with members of the royal family, including Henrietta Maria. Both brothers used colonial affairs to style themselves as fashionable members of the landed elite. Both had passed through the Inner Temple. Both commissioned Van Dyck to paint their portraits. Even his enemies acknowledged that Holland was magnetic, with features that 'equalled the most beautiful Women'.[21]

In a full-length portrait from the 1630s, Holland's seafaring connections are visible in the soft blues and purples of sea and clouds painted prominently in the background. Several ships sail from the shoreline. They might allude to his military position as commander of Landguard Fort, Suffolk, or to his role as Governor to the Providence Island Company – minutes of the Providence Island court proceedings give an idea of the concerns about territorial expansion, trade, and acquisition that occupied Holland's time during these years. Holland looks like he has just stepped out of the preacher Samuel Ward's discourse about the sliding morality of the times, all heels and ribbons and lace. One imagines his servant is just out of the frame, ready to come in with some fortified wine in a crystal glass, or a pipe of tobacco sent directly from the Rich family's Bermuda plantations. His positioning expresses a belief in England's imperial possibilities and equally professes his dedication to the nation at home. With his heeled boots planted firmly on dry ground, Holland turns his gaze towards land, to the realm and England's wooded landscapes, even as his wealth blossoms from the transoceanic pursuits captured in the ships behind him. His wide-brim hat is in his hand, allowing us fully to take in the waves of his hair, rising and falling like the sea beyond.

Prickly Pears and
Danby's Gate

In 1634, a Miskitu man from the Caribbean coast could be spotted strolling under archways and painted ceilings at Charles I's court. The king befriended this Indigenous 'prince', though his name remains unrecorded in English archives. Charles financed his education, and invited him to private parties. Three years later, the man returned home, assuming leadership of his community after the death of his father.[1]

This Indigenous visitor came from a realm of tropical rainforests and freshwater swamps along the coast of present-day Nicaragua and Honduras, in environments alive with tapirs, macaws, and manatees. He could navigate gnarled mangrove forests and was probably skilled in hunting turtles. He came from the province that the Aztec/Mexica had called Taguzgalpa ('place of gold'), later known as the Mosquito Coast. The region spanned hundreds of miles from Cape Gracias a Dios, where the Wangki River (Río Coco) spilled into the Caribbean Sea, to the Río San Juan. The Miskitu were a dominant presence in these places. Spanish control did not extend to these lands; Franciscans attempted to establish missions there, but their efforts failed every time.[2]

The attendance of the Miskitu man at royal dinner parties was the result of a little-known Puritan project to establish a settlement on an island off the coast of Nicaragua in the 1630s. It was financed by some of England's wealthiest and most zealous Puritan elites, including the Earl of Warwick and his brother, the Earl of Holland. Its backers invested exorbitant amounts of capital into the scheme, designed to turn unruly paradises into plantations. Confident that the plantation would be an ideal source of commercially lucrative plants and animals, they named the island Providence, pitching it as a tropical alternative to the godly settlement in Massachusetts.

Cultivated green spaces in England had long offered places for spiritual devotion and reflection, experimentation and delight. In the sixteenth century, gardens became more extravagant, expanding into intricate landscapes that exhibited English encounters with the 'four parts of the world', and enhancing the status of those who could afford them. Mazes and fountains, French-style parterres and secret groves and grottoes modelled after classical villas offered a playground for the wealthy. Members of the public could pay to see John Tradescant's curiosities and gardens in Lambeth, which contained African and Persian flora, but also yellow wildflowers from New England and American beans. Apothecary shops and stalls in the fashionable Royal Exchange sold saps and leaves from around the world. The English fondness for gardens extended into embroidery work. Bright threads stitched glow-worms and butterflies, pomegranates and primroses onto bodices and nightcaps, creating wearable garden patches in linen and silk.

From Creation, God had instructed Adam and Eve to be cultivators and planters. To encourage colonialism, the clergyman Samuel Purchas cited Genesis 1:29: 'Behold, I have given you every herbe bearing seede, which is upon the face of all the earth.' Gardening was godly work, for the Creator had 'commissioned' humans to exert their dominion over nature.[3] Domestic projects to control fields and fenlands were discussed in terms of improvement and virtuous industry. While women were often bearers of plant knowledge in their role as household managers, gentlemen were also encouraged to play direct roles in overseeing their estates. In the early 1630s, the

MP and diarist John Oglander recorded that he had planted fruit trees at his estate 'with my owne handes', transforming the surroundings so that 'as of a rude Chaos I have now made it a fitt place for any Gentleman'.[4] In his essay 'Of Gardens', the statesman and natural philosopher Francis Bacon argued that well-maintained green spaces were at the heart of human identity. God had first planted a garden, not built a palace.[5] As an extension of one's house, gardens were reflections of their custodians, whether cultured or 'savage'.

In December 1606, a somewhat sickly George Percy, youngest son of a prominent aristocratic family from Northumberland, set off for the Chesapeake. After encounters with the Kalinago in the Caribbean, Percy recorded the relief he felt at finding a garden deep in the hurricane-ravaged forests of the Leeward Islands. After straying into thick woods on Nevis, he had stumbled on a garden, lush with cotton trees and guaiacum, the trees appearing artfully set by human hands. Weeks later, in Tsenacommacah, Percy again found comfort in what he saw as the almost miraculous presence of pleasure gardens in America. He followed a path of honeysuckles into a 'paradise' that looked like it belonged in a 'Garden or Orchard in England'.[6] In the weeks that followed, Percy was welcomed into an Algonquian village whose inhabitants offered him strawberries. Strawberries were important fruits for many Eastern Woodland groups, especially in the transition from spring to summer, which marked the seasonal arrival of these 'heart berries'.[7] Sharing in the strawberry harvest was a time of thanksgiving and reconciliation.

Percy's anxious attempts to navigate gardens and so-called wildernesses tell us a lot. Although his narrative contains multiple examples of Indigenous botanical knowledge and cultivation techniques, he could not help but view the gardens he encountered as marvels or miracles, as if they had sprung out of nowhere. When he found orchards that resembled those from home, he was quick to call them paradises, not places of Indigenous making. Biblical stories and travel books had primed colonists to look for a primordial landscape of fruitfulness and plenty on one hand, and a savage or alien terrain on the other. Francis Bacon had maintained that gardens were signs of the most advanced civilisations. When 'ages grow to Civility and Elegancie, Men come to *Build Stately,* sooner then to *Garden Finely*: As if *Gardening* were the greater perfection'.[8] If Algonquians were recognised as capable of cultivating the kind of luxuriant garden that appeared in estates like Percy's, then he might be forced to admit that they hardly needed 'civilising'.

Plenty of colonists knew that what they viewed as wildernesses were not wildernesses at all. Time and time again, Native inhabitants across the Americas saved settlers who had strayed too far from their settlements. They had 'oftentimes beene beholding to them for their guidance [through] the unbeaten Wildernesse', William Wood wrote from Massachusetts Bay. Many 'benighted coasters have been kindly entertained into [Wampanoag] habitations', resting and recovering much more comfortably than if they had been in some old countryside inn. Algonquians were entirely at home in 'the craggy mountaines, and the pleasant vales, the stately woods, and swampie groves, the spacious ponds, and swift running rivers, and can distinguish them as by their names as perfectly, and finde them as presently, as the experienced Citizen knows how to finde our Cheape-side crosse'.[9] Christina DeLucia has described these places as 'memoryscapes': 'geographies bearing layers upon thick layers of meanings, accessible to and transmitted by Indigenous past-keepers who learned to navigate particular terrain and routes'.[10] When William Bradford and the *Mayflower*'s other passengers settled in the lands of the Pawtuxet in 1620, and when English merchants and servants arrived in Central America, they entered into those storied places.[11]

In 1621, as colonists met with Native leaders in Pawtuxet, the 'place of little falls', England's first botanic garden was established in Oxford, near the Cherwell River. The Oxford Physic Garden, as it was known, was a place of study and experimentation. Its principal benefactor, the courtier and soldier Henry Danvers, first Earl of Danby, paid £5,000 to erect the walls and gates, offering an elaborate enclosure that proclaimed the university's prestige while protecting the area from trespassers. Vines and fruit trees were set against the walls, the air fragrant with blossoms.

By 1633, a large, rusticated stone arch completed the garden's building projects, inspired by the Renaissance mannerist architect Sebastiano Serlio. Its architect, Nicholas Stone, may also have designed the Duke of Buckingham's fanciful water gate near Embankment in London, where the king's favourite could leap off his boat and pass under an archway made of Portland stone into his adjacent gardens and residence after a night of revelries. Oxford's Danby Gate still stands today, a heavily ornamented structure with elongated niches, inscriptions, and a triangular pediment. It proclaims power and permanence.

Its Latin inscription can be translated, 'To the glory of God, in honour of King Charles, and for the use of the University and the public'. Those who passed into the garden from the gate were encouraged to frame their encounters through piety, kingly magnificence, and male-dominated scientific knowledge.[12]

The fashion for Italianate gates and arches in Stuart England was championed in no small part by the architect Inigo Jones. In his travels to Italy, Jones avidly studied his environs and jotted down notes in his copy of the great Renaissance architect Andrea Palladio's treatise on architecture. Back in England, alongside his larger-scale building projects, Jones designed arches for patrons keen to graft more fashionable entries onto old estates. In 1617, Anna of Denmark commissioned a painting of herself standing on the grounds of her residence at Oatlands, the white stone of Jones's new ornamental gateway gleaming against the piles of Tudor brick. Jones also incorporated arches into his set designs for masques, using them to convey civility and sophistication even in rustic scenes.

In 'Of Masques and Triumphs' (1625), Francis Bacon drew links between court entertainments and the classical processions staged to celebrate emperors' military victories in imperial Rome, highlighting their political function. Temporary triumphal arches were erected for city processions and festivals, including James's entry into London in 1604, where speeches and songs hailed the monarch as a descendant of Brutus, Prince of Troy and mythical founder of Britain. For a brief time, the streets of London were transformed into Rome, with towering painted arches of wood and plaster, flanked by statues and banners. Whether the newly columned doorway of a renovated hunting lodge or a massive triumphal arch, classical gateways were a declaration of power. They involved a kind of positioning or calibration, forcing those who walked through them to consider their own place in the world. In the glow of candlelight on the Banqueting House stage, arches served as a threshold, marking the moment when masquers stepped away from the stage and into the dancing space. This choreography mirrored the king's own movement from the fantasy realm of the masque to the realities of rule.[13]

Danby's arch, too, was a portal. It took the visitor from ignorance to knowledge, curiosity to dominion, theory to practice – even if Stone's architectural fancies were rather more ornate than a purist like Jones might approve. Within the botanical garden's walls, medicinal plants known in ancient Greece and Italy were cultivated alongside specimens from other continents for the purpose of study and pleasure. Over the course of the seventeenth century, through links to friends in Montpellier, Paris, Sicily, and Leiden, the garden's first Keeper, Jacob Bobart the Elder, amassed a large collection of foreign and domestic plants, from figs and local wildflowers to an evening primrose from North America. Eventually, the garden would contain avocados, sugarcane, and coffee, bringing into the university city specimens grown from Mexico to Barbados. Along with the collections that spiralled up walls and floated in ponds, Bobart and his son created a botanical library that included several *herbaria*, collections of dried plants pasted onto paper and kept in bound books. This process of gaining botanical knowledge reduced plants to specimens to be studied and catalogued. But the Bobarts' immense books, with maize and tobacco sent across oceans by friends and agents, survive today. Next to inky notes about their place of collection, 400-year-old sunflowers remain fixed to those pages, brittle but intact, their leaves faded but still green.

The year after the completion of Danby's Gate, the libertine poet Thomas Carew wrote a masque for Charles I and Henrietta Maria that brought fruitful gardens and classical pasts to the courtly stage. *Coelum Britanicum* (1634) began with a scene of decay, full of old arches and palaces, crumbling walls, and heaps of broken columns and statues, 'altogether resembling the ruines of some great City of the ancient Romans, or civiliz'd Brittaines'. An ageing Jupiter, resolved to reform the debauchery of his court, called on his fellow gods to help him expel corrupt matter and restore the celestial perfection of the Stuart reign. The performance ended with the stage transforming into a lush garden teeming with trees, fountains, and grottoes. Aristocrats descended from clouds to languish in the bountiful enclosure. Songs celebrated the royal couple's political power, upheld by the 'sacred seeds of Love' and their star-like brilliance.

Like the inscription to God, king, and science on Danby's Gate at the Oxford Physic Garden, Carew's masque captured the layered assumptions about civility, order, and political power that accompanied the governing elite's attraction to gardens. Avoid stagnation and moss at all costs, Bacon had advised in 'Of Gardens'. Barren seeds and withering buds must be expelled from the divine realms of the muses. It was no coincidence that one of the antimasques within the performance featured a band of wild, wood-dwelling Picts, 'the naturall Inhabitants of this Isle, ancient Scots and Irish'. Emerging from overgrowth and craggy mountains, these unruly, rustic forces submitted to the garlanded sovereign. The closing songs credited the Stuart dynasty with uniting the British Isles harmoniously together.[14]

As in the gardens beyond the Banqueting House, Indigenous plants and places entered into Carew's seemingly insular performance. Momus, trickster god of ridicule and satire, complained that corrupt and 'infectious persons' within the court should not be permitted to wander around imperilling the island's civil residents. They must embark on a ship for elsewhere, perhaps 'the plantation in *New-England,* which hath purg'd more virulent humors from the politique body, then *Guacum* and all the West-Indian druggs have from the naturall bodies of this kingdome'.[15] To Carew, whose allegiances lay with Charles and the Catholic Henrietta Maria, New England – that hotbed of radical Puritanism – had purged the realm of dissidents at home. To describe this purgation, Carew likened the state to a human body, subject to fluxes and change. The exodus of pestilential Puritans across the ocean had healed the state. Though he alluded to an assortment of drugs and medicines, Carew's mention of 'guacum' was intended as comic relief, since guaiacum was widely reputed to cure syphilis. The word derived from the Taíno word, *guayacán,* a wood that inhabitants of the Caribbean used to carve depictions of their *zemí,* or ancestor-spirits.[16] When Momus spoke the word under those decaying arches, he conjured English uses for the plant, but he also recalled the Taíno lifeways that lived in the language of tropical barks.

While Londoners sought out guaiacum from physicians to relieve a sexually transmitted disease, others learned about plants from books and their own horticultural experiments. With the rise of print, gardeners became household names. Alongside spiritual writings, romances, and cookbooks, literate women and men might keep at hand John Gerard's *The Herball, or Generall Historie of Plantes* (1597). Those who couldn't read could still enjoy the hundreds of illustrations that spanned its pages. Soon after it was published, Gerard received criticisms from fellow botanists for its errors and homely style, but the book was popular enough to be reprinted and revised numerous times. The new title page from a 1633 edition depicted Gerard as a distinguished practitioner, a formal ruff encircling his neck. In his left hand, he holds a flowering potato plant.

If nothing else, Gerard was an enthusiast. Nothing had 'provoked mens studies more, or satisfied their desires so much, as plants have done', he professed.[17] Flowers were nature's jewels, full of wonder while yielding their secrets to those who paid attention. But they also had odours and tastes that the most brilliant stones could not produce. Roses, palm trees, and orchids delighted the mind while ravishing the senses, connecting humans to God's wisdom and marvellous workmanship.

Gerard's book was one of the first Elizabethan herbals, or plant treatises, to include such an extensive array of plants from the Americas. It was an English guide to plants, but one that demonstrated how much Atlantic specimens had become part of Elizabethans' daily lives. Some had come to England from Mexico or Peru via European cities, others directly in the cargoes of English travellers returning from Puerto Rico or Virginia. This was no straightforward process of assimilation or absorption. He was conscious of plants inhabiting qualities and characteristics of their own. He wanted to allow them space to breathe, to spread themselves out in all their glory.

To grow something, one should understand, coax, cherish, and support each seed according to its needs. Specimens were never divorced from the places they came from, even if these origins could get muddled in their vast journeys. There was the 'Virginian Water-Melon' and the 'Virginia Potato'. Maize was, to 'the Virginians, *Pagatowr*'. Yellow henbane, or 'English tobacco', was dispersed across most parts of England, its pale yellow flowers dotting gardens in the summer months; but this, Gerard warned, was a 'doubtfull herbane', and not considered akin to the 'true' tobacco from islands such as Trinidad. The 'little Indian nut', the coconut, could be found in Africa and the East Indies, but also 'all the Islands of the West Indies'.[18]

Gerard described planting as a benign and virtuous process. While projectors were busy pursuing veins of gold and silver in faraway mountains, his labour was profitably directed to 'a harmlesse treasure of herbes, trees, and plants, as the earth frankely without violence offereth unto our most necessarie uses'.[19] For him, planting was a truly civil pursuit, fit for housewives and princes. Nourishing plants from the earth was not an act of violence, but care. While Pluto, god of riches, made 'forcible entry' into the earth to snatch wealth, subjecting metals to 'mysticall proofes, and chymicall trials', the pursuit of herbs brought health and vigour. In his masque, Carew had also contrasted the plenty of gardens to the hellish landscape of extraction. Gold was an 'excrescence', a poison, 'the true *Pandora's* box, whence issued all those mischiefes that now fill the Universe'.[20]

But although Gerard made a case for the gentility of planting, *trans*planting involved uprooting. Conflict and dispossession, too, lay behind the acquisition of plants. Ginger grew in Africa and the Canary Islands, as well as the Caribbean, gained after 'our men which sacked Domingo in the Indies [in 1586], digged it up there in sundry places wilde'. Gerard relied on the work of the Artois botanist Carolus Clusius, who travelled to London in 1581 specifically to purchase some of the flora, including roots and cacao pods, that Drake had gathered during his circumnavigation of the globe. During the 1580s and 1590s, George Clifford, third Earl of Cumberland, acquired cassava, maize, guavas, and cochineal in privateering voyages to Brazil and the West Indies. His access to these goods emerged from Anglo-Spanish warfare over territories and resources in the Atlantic. In June 1589, one Elizabethan councillor summarised these activities in a little scrawled note: 'Lord Cumberland, Frobisher, and others' went out to 'pilfer' and secure 'many rich Indian prizes'. When Cumberland besieged (and temporarily occupied) the Spanish city of San Juan, he navigated Puerto Rico with African go-betweens, and captured Spanish vessels filled with enslaved women and men.[21]

English backyards became little Caribbean spaces. 'The Indian Thistle groweth in Saint Johns Island in the West Indies, and prospereth very well in my garden,' Gerard informed his readers.[22] *The Herball* became an unexpected site for depicting Indigenous material culture. For an entry on various 'Indian fruits' from the West Indies, Gerard did not include an image of plants, but of kernels and seeds dangling from woven strings. These kernels were filled with stones and incorporated into adornments to be worn during ceremonial dances. To see examples of these (possibly Tupi) rattles, Gerard directed his readers to Tradescant's collection in Lambeth, where 'you may see these upon strings as they are here figured, among many other varieties'.[23]

When the botanist John Parkinson published *Paradisi in Sole* (1629), he aimed high, dedicating his herbal to the young queen, Henrietta Maria. The title page invited readers to draw a direct lineage between themselves and Adam and Eve as planters, but the image of paradise it depicted was a distinctly modern one, made possible through global traffic. Alongside biblical imagery, streaked tulips from Asia via the Ottoman Empire sprouted from the ground. Under the watchful gaze of cherubim, pineapples and prickly pears grew from the same soil as carnations and grapevines. Taller than humankind's first parents, these oversized plants proclaimed the nation's refined sensibilities. 'The Civill respects to be learned [from plants] are many,' Parkinson maintained, 'for the delight of the varieties both of formes, colours, and properties of Herbes and Flowers, have ever beene powerfull over dull, unnurtured, rusticke and savage people, led only by Natures instinct.'[24] How much more, then, should such knowledge preoccupy the minds of the English; to fail to cultivate nature, or to express an interest in the pleasures of botanical knowledge, was uncivil.

Like Gerard, Parkinson's sensitivity to the particularities of plants illuminated Atlantic specimens in estates and gardens. The red-flowered 'Indian Daffodill' came from the West Indies via Spain, 'and by the [Mexica] Indians in their tongue named AZCAL XOCHITL.' Gerard and Parkinson's books were gardening manuals, but also compilations, full of languages and places, bringing Nahua and Kalinago knowledge into English phrases. In some cases, singular plants were so rare that their journeys could be directly traced. The *Yuca sive Iucca,* 'the supposed Indian Iucca' (Parkinson was sceptical), was 'first brought into England (as Master Gerard saith) from the West Indies' by an apothecary's servant. Gerard cultivated the plant until his death, but it 'perished with him that got it from his widow, intending to send it to his Country house.'[25] Bananas and plantains might come from different global environments, but the bright green stalk that apothecary Thomas Johnson hung up in his London shop in 1633 had come from Bermuda. The bunch appeared on the frontispiece of the enlarged edition of *The Herball* that same year, artfully arranged atop an extravagant bouquet.

Other plants were more ubiquitous, including the crumple-leafed 'Indian Basil', sunflowers, potatoes, the 'Virginia *Pishamin*' or persimmon, the Virginia mulberry, pineapples, and the violet and white dogtooth flower, a type of orchid that 'the naturall people ... hold ... as a secret, loth to reveale it'. Two of the basils mentioned by Parkinson 'are greater strangers in our Country', coming from the West Indies and used to make sweet water. The sunflower, Parkinson wrote, was a 'stately plant, wherewith every one is now adayes familiar'. Even the humble parsley sprinkled on roasted and stewed meats had come to flavour domestic dishes as a result of transatlantic traffic. In addition to common and curled parsley, 'Virginia Parsley', though only 'of late knowne, yet is now almost growne common.'[26]

Perhaps more than any other Atlantic plant, the cactus – known as the prickly pear, hedge-hog thistle, prickly melon thistle, or Indian fig – bewildered herbalists. Melon, fig, or thistle? Aloe, or oversized cucumber? The hand of the divine was clearly at work: 'Who can but marvel at the rare and singular workmanship which the Lord God almighty hath shewed in this Thistle ... ?' The cactus contained many shapes and forms, becoming a sprawling mass of spikes and swelling stems, decorated with large flowers and vivid red fruits. It grew 'in many places of America ... The greater kinde in the more remote and hot Countries, as Mexico, Florida, &c. and in the Bermudas or Summer Islands'. The 'ribs on the outside are garnished or rather armed with many prickly stars ... so that without hurt to the fingers it cannot be touched'.[27]

Cactus plants, accustomed to the warmth of desert landscapes, stubbornly refused to thrive in England. The smaller, rounded cactus 'cannot endure the injurie of our cold clymate', Gerard wrote. Parkinson added that, although many cactuses were brought into England, and could be kept in the right conditions to grow, their flowers and fruits 'seldome or never commeth unto perfection with us ... for want of that heate and comfort of the Sunne it hath in his naturall place'.[28] By the time of Parkinson's writing, cactuses were known for their sprawling stems and their ability to regenerate. In a

1632 legal manual for women, a section on love and marriage declared that, to handle 'that matter [of wooing], *per genus & species,* would take up as much roome, as the Indian figge-tree, every third whereof, when it falleth to the ground, groweth to a body'.[29]

In the same year as Parkinson published his *Paradisi in Sole,* two ships belonging to Robert Rich, Earl of Warwick, navigated the coral reefs and volcanic islands some 150 miles from the Central American coast.[30] On Christmas Eve 1629, while people in England baked mince pies and decorated their chambers with sprigs of evergreen, colonists scrambled across cactus-dotted terrain. They soon established settlements on the islands of Santa Catalina and San Andreas, beginning the Anglo-Miskitu relations that led to the Miskitu man's presence at Charles I's court.

For the backers of the Providence Island project, profit and piety went hand in hand, though this created numerous tensions on the ground. The most prominent members of the Providence Island Company were aristocrats and leading members of the gentry, such as John Pym and Warwick, united by their commitment to reforming the commonwealth through intervention abroad. While Massachusetts Bay attracted many Puritans who came from merchant and yeoman backgrounds, the aristocrats behind the Providence Island ventures framed their project as a heroic national endeavour closely tied to high affairs of state, combining godly plantation with a strategic foothold in the Spanish Atlantic. The Earl of Holland was an enthusiast of the project, and close to the queen, using his proximity to Henrietta Maria to enlist her support for an Anglo-French alliance against the Spanish in the West Indies. Planting colonies would stabilise the English political economy while combatting Spanish power and asserting England's place in world affairs. The colony's governors thus wrote home with details about colonists' spiritual lives while also reporting on how lucrative crops would 'double or treble any mans estate in all England'.[31]

The English who arrived in Miskitu lands had been sent to cultivate a paradise in the Caribbean – a *paradisi in sole*, one could say. When he arrived on Providence Island in 1631, the governor Philip Bell quickly sent a report to investors to assure them that colonists were already experimenting with citrus fruits, sugarcane, ginger, and dyes. 'This your little Spot of Land will grow one of the gardens of the world,' he promised. Whether struck by the beauty of the lands they had encountered, or desperate to pander to those investors whose decisions influenced their very survival, those who wrote home emphasised the delicious fruits and fragrant airs that enriched their lives. The island's first minister, Lewis Morgan, called Providence 'the Eden of god'. In addition to cultivating the fruits that the island naturally produced, colonists had planted rhubarb, and were planning experiments with cloves and indigo: 'I doubt not but the Land will bear as well as any Land under heaven.'[32]

From the beginning, investors were preoccupied with how plantations in Caribbean soil might be coaxed and refined into producing a variety of crops for further export. The Company sent the Governor plants, roots, and seeds. Patrons promised future shipments of more slips and specimens, and demanded updates on which plants had been successfully transplanted. They were keen to prevent colonists from developing a tobacco-based economy akin to those of the Chesapeake and Bermuda. A society founded on a potent intoxicant was hardly a suitable model for a godly community, and a diverse agricultural economy, sustained by hard-working planters, would help prevent the colony from becoming too much like Virginia, with its reputation as a boisterous boomtown. In 1633, Providence Island councillors sent large quantities of cotton and instructed the men on the nearby Henrietta Island (San Andreas) to cultivate '*Mechoacan* [jalap] commonly called wild potatoes'.

In Company council meetings in London, Providence Island and Massachusetts affairs were often discussed at the same time, bundled together and containing intelligence about captains who sailed between the two colonies. Though investors encouraged white migrants to travel to the Caribbean coast, the population was always a diverse one. In 1634, Company members strictly admonished the colony's minister for viewing the conversions of Africans as ground for their manumission, showing both the presence of Africans on the island, and the Earl of Warwick's intention to keep them enslaved. The English war with the Pequot in New England led to colonists trafficking Indigenous women, men, and children to Bermuda and the Caribbean, including Providence.[33] The privateer Daniel Elfrith, in Warwick's employ, was a known slaver. Providence Island investors urged him to procure plants, such as annatto for dye, 'by negotiation and Traffique [with the Indians]', but they also accepted that enslaved Africans might be needed to search out the 'great quantities of silver ore' that were rumoured to exist. By the early 1640s, an eyewitness claimed that there were over 600 African and African-descended residents on the island.[34]

At the same time, the council warned Elfrith not to bring 'a [certain] Mulletto' and other mixed-heritage people into the colony for fear that competing loyalties might undermine the endeavour. This 'mulletto' was Diego al Mulato, a formerly enslaved man from Havana and an ally of the Dutch against the Spanish. In 1637, the English Dominican priest Thomas Gage would be unlucky enough to cross 'this Noble Captaine' on his way home from Central America. While Diego allowed him to keep his quilt, books, and clothes, he forced Gage to relinquish his precious stones and pieces of eight.

In 1644, an anonymous pamphlet, known as *Certaine Inducements to Well Minded People,* may have been assembled and distributed by members of the Providence Island Company to encourage subscribers to Caribbean projects. Its emphasis on tropical goods and the lament over the 'plundering and utter ruin of the Estates, by the cruelty of the Cavaliers' suggests Puritan leanings. Any who were strained with the burden of managing their estates, and 'willing out of Noble and Publique Principles, to transport themselves . . . into the *West Indies*', would find pearls, nourishing plantains, silky thread fashioned from pineapple leaves, and 'a barke of a Tree, which is white, that seemeth a compound of all Spices'.[35] In this pamphlet, Indigenous knowledge was woven into the language of Puritans and royalists. There is mention of the *tilboa* (from *tibla* in Miskitu), or tapir, whose whereabouts could be found 'by *Indian* and some *English* relations', and vanilla as 'dette' (*diti*).[36]

By then, Providence had already failed to become the tropical Eden that investors had hoped for. In 1641, Spanish and Portuguese forces took the island, ending an English colonial presence that had been over ten years in the making. The English lost Providence, however, just as other Caribbean colonies were taking off. On the eve of the civil wars, the English occupied parts of St Kitts, Antigua, Nevis, Montserrat, and Barbados. Planters began turning more concertedly to sugar production, soon causing a surge in enslaved labour as the plantation complex rapidly expanded.[37]

In 1631, the gentleman Henry Colt had admonished the unruly young men on Barbados for spending more time carousing and drinking than managing their lands. 'Your ground & plantations shewes what you are,' he had written. 'They lie like the ruins', disorderly and overgrown, when they should be nourished into pleasing landscapes of pleasure and industry.[38] Poor planting and garden management meant poor governance, an idea that had by now become fully embedded in English colonial ideologies. Ten years later, Barbados had become a large, multicultural colony. When the royalist planter Richard Ligon travelled there in the 1640s, he wrote of the thousands of indentured servants and enslaved Africans who produced the island's indigo, tobacco, sugar, and ginger. He expressed some sympathy for the fate of 'an Indian woman, a slave in the house' named Yarico, who had helped save an Englishman only to be betrayed and sold into slavery. But he also listed the enslaved as the 'commodities these Ships bring to this Iland'.[39]

On his way to Barbados, Ligon was enraptured by the African 'mistress' at the house of the Spanish Governor of St Jago (Santiago). He viewed the woman as a prized object, admiring the graceful way she wore striped linens, silks, and jewelled ribbons. In this moment of appraisal, he recalled the sugared parties at Whitehall's Banqueting House. This woman moved like Anna of Denmark, he wrote, when she would descend from her throne in a sea of green silks to dance in a masque. A long-dead Jacobean queen in masquing costume appears, like a mirage, in the colonial imaginary, far from home.

Time slips and circles on itself. Strawberry harvests give way to seasons marked by ice breaking on rivers and lakes, shimmering like beads. Centuries pass, but the past lingers.

Imagine a stately home. Carved cherubs and columns hark back to Italian Renaissance grandeur. There are stone gates, marble embellishments, and wide roads for the coaches. Fields and trees extend beyond the lawns, and nearby water sources keep these surroundings alive. This estate isn't in an English county, but a Caribbean island. At first view, this plantation is a pristine example of the classical style, with the same attention to order and proportion that characterised many Stuart mansions. But this is no healthy manor. The gardens have fallen to ruin. The idealised earthly paradise of this once heavily managed estate has turned to rot. The visitor who passes through feels queasy at the smell of decaying limes. Eucalyptus boughs creak under the weight of scavenging crows. It almost sounds like another scene from Carew's masque, but this is the scene the St Lucian poet Derek

Walcott paints in his poem, 'Ruins of a Great House' (1956).[40] By the time he wrote it, centuries of slavery and exploitation in the Caribbean, as elsewhere, had made the lush iconography of English estates inextricable from atrocity.

Why? Because, in some ways, these estates had started it all. Plantation in the Americas had happened when the kind of people who had been in the room to see Carew's masque – people with money and political power, people who had been taught that cultivating gardens and managing others were a measure of civility – decided that they wanted pineapples and plantains in their gardens, and that other islands and ecosystems were there to claim, and decorate with arches and urns. In Walcott's poem, time collapses for the narrator, who climbs over the ironwork and views the ruins of the old plantation, dwelling on the enslaved hands who contributed to its flourishing. Behind the crumbling facades, the ruined nature, are the Tudors and Stuarts: 'men like Hawkins, Walter Raleigh, Drake'. Those who first set out in search of gold and flowers; who imagined, like George Chapman in 1596, 'mansions [that] dance with neighbourhood' in the heart of tropical rainforests. The speaker struggles between rage and compassion, between fury at the pain of the imperial past and hope for a world where people care about the deaths of others.

If the English Renaissance has its sins, its literature, for Walcott, also offers a way through. John Donne is his ghostly interlocutor. Walcott cites several lines from Donne's 1624 reflection on death and compassion. No man is an island, disconnected from the rest, Donne insisted. 'Any Mans *death* diminishes *me*, because I am involved in *Mankinde*.' Send not to know for whom the bell tolls, marking the departed: 'it tolls for *thee*.'[41]

To the thousands of Indigenous and African women, men, and children who encountered the English, either in their homelands or across the Atlantic, the assertions about nature and control embodied by Danby's Gate stood at odds with their own ways of relating to land. What good was it to emblazon a name on imported stone, insisting on permanence and grandeur, at the expense of other life? Names of individuals are remembered, writes Susan M. Hill (Wolf Clan, Mohawk Nation), but the natural world, too, bears witness to the past, acts with its own agency, and carries history. Sweet potatoes and maize contained distinct properties and inner forms that connected them to the places they came from. Axomamma, the Incan Potato Mother. The Three Sisters – corn, beans, and squash. These stories were there in the thick rinds of tropical fruits, the sprawling petals of sunflowers, and the palo de Campeche from Yucatán, a wood coveted by artisans for the deep black dye that could be made from its bark. Land as Mother, not Land for Sale.[42]

In the short term, Providence Island loomed large in the English imperial imagination, bringing Caribbean flora, fauna, and people to the London of Henrietta Maria and Van Dyck. The Miskitu man had arrived at Whitehall at a key moment in English colonial development, as settlements from the Chesapeake to St Kitts became more stable in the reign of Charles I and the rate of colonial production escalated.[43] Several years before, the king had hosted the Mi'kmaq family of Segipt as a result of projectors' renewed interest in Canada. Tobacco and sugar, meanwhile, made the fortunes of a growing class of merchants who connected Puritan and Catholic patrons to Indigenous lands. These traders threw themselves into transatlantic commerce, becoming key agents in the diversification of colonial economies that accelerated the presence of fruits and vegetables in kitchens and herbals.

Had he wandered through the gardens in and around Whitehall or the City, London's Miskitu resident might have recognised some of the plants that grew around him, lingering at the places where cassavas and prickly pears asserted their stout presence in the damp climes of an island thousands of miles from home. If he was a healer, a *curandero* (herbal healer) or *sukia* (shaman), he would have listened and spoken to the plants, asking for their assistance, activating their properties through prayer.[44] As travellers, these plants were living records of other lands, holding other places in their seeds and blooms, as enduring as any classical arch. They kept other memories and places in their scents and vapours, so that, for a moment, tobacco smoke released the smell of volcanic earth or Chesapeake soil, and sassafras brought the aroma of the lands of the Nauset people, for a blade of sweetgrass 'puts you in touch with the spirit of sweetgrass everywhere'.[45] Near the classical facade of the Banqueting House, bells ring in the air. *Send not to know.* It is all connected.

Chilli Red in an
English Still Life

When was the last time you stopped to gaze at a still-life painting? Lost yourself in a fleck of paint capturing the gleam of light hitting a silver cup? Perhaps you are guilty of moving swiftly on, towards scenes of classical valour, or to the contour of a Renaissance nude. Admittedly, still lifes do not occupy a particularly elevated position in the history of art. It is easy to breeze past these paintings in a museum or in the creaky oak gallery of a country house. Can a tulip or a breakfast bun really compete with the vivid drama of a monarch on horseback, or the birth of Christ? History tends to be recalled through a full-length portrait, not a painting of a pumpkin. But alongside stately princes and heavenly scenes, images known as fruit or flower pictures edged their way into the seventeenth-century art market and English homes.

For millennia, artists had brought nature into art. Depictions of fruit and flower assemblages appear in the frescoes of Greek and Roman antiquity; in the Middle Ages, artists created a striking sense of realism through depictions of flora and fauna in books of hours, for example, the margins of these jewel-like devotional books crowded with plums, violets, and butterflies. But still life as we know it emerged as a new genre of painting in the sixteenth-century Netherlands. Beginning as relatively subdued depictions of 'still' or dead objects – a bundle of asparagus, a small bouquet – these tableaux quickly evolved into object-ridden subgenres: vegetable pieces; the still life in nature, where plants and vegetables remain rooted to the ground; breakfast pieces; banquet pieces; market scenes; shell pieces. *Vanitas* paintings, full of rotting figs, bubbles, skulls, and tobacco pipes, offer unsubtle reminders of our mortal existence.

Most sumptuous of all is the *pronk* still life: the showpiece, dripping in luxurious objects that mingled with the colourful variety of natural specimens. Perhaps the weirdest iteration of the still life painted in England is *The Paston Treasure* (*c.*1663), whose two figures, an African boy and a white English girl, are hardly able to escape the chaotic melange of stuff, much of which represented actual artefacts collected by the antiquarian William Paston during his travels to Europe, Palestine, and Egypt in the 1630s. Not a golden age, but a golden world, sparkling in a dark-edged composition overrun with beings and things, from a monkey to highly worked metals. As the tropical fruits and vegetables discussed elsewhere in this book appeared in the realm, they also came to be captured on canvas.

Little by little, these paintings were displayed in the kitchens, galleries, and cabinets of English merchants and aristocrats. A 1641 inventory of the Countess of Arundel's townhouse near St James's Palace shows that multiple still lifes provided the backdrop to an impressive array of nearly 500 pieces of Chinese porcelain, crystal flower vases, and silver-mounted cups. In her banqueting room, alongside marble statues and wicker baskets, the walls were decorated with paintings of artichokes and cherries, poultry, fish, and hares. Charles I's extravagant art collection included still lifes by Spanish, Italian, and Dutch artists. The Duke of Buckingham owned a floral still life by the Flemish painter Jan Brueghel. By the Restoration, a resident Dutch artist, Pieter Gerritsz van Roestraten, painted still lifes for aristocratic patrons including Charles II. The botanical illustrator Alexander Marshall, who painted sunflowers, blue and yellow macaws, porcupines, white-flowered bottle gourds, and sweet red peppers from the Americas, also became celebrated for his accomplished flower paintings.

From the beginning, still lifes have been highly symbolic compositions. The objects hold meanings, inviting spiritual contemplation. A butterfly can represent the soul, pomegranate seeds the blood of Christ, a candle the passing of time.[1] But they are also, inescapably, about things – about the presentness and elusiveness of objects, about the boundary between what we do and don't possess. Object becomes subject. We are encouraged to take in the presence and substance of a weighty lemon with a thick, curling rind, plopped before us to trick us into thinking we could reach out and grasp it. Such paintings are, by their very nature, about the gaze. In describing the atmosphere of still lifes, the American poet Mark Doty writes of 'the matrix in which we are held, the generous light binding together the fragrant and flavourful production of vineyard, marsh, and orchard'. In the still life, 'there is no end to our looking . . . we look in and in, to the world of things, in their ambiance of cool or warm light, in and in, as long as we can stand to look.'[2] The curtains that sometimes appear in a still life reinforce this notion of spectatorship and display.

Suspended in stillness, but not exactly tranquil. In more extravagant iterations of the genre, food rolls and sprawls across lavish but abandoned tables. It appears to be twilight. Have we woken up, collapsed under a banqueting table after a raucous bout of intoxication? Or are we suspended in a dream, next to a lobster and a ribbon? In addition to vineyard, marsh, and orchard, plantations creep in. The mystic calm is often made possible by a fracturing happening elsewhere – martial landings in the Chesapeake for tobacco or sassafras, the devastation of rainforest ecologies in the Maluku Islands of Indonesia for cloves and nutmeg. What is painted with such clarity, texture, and precision is also part of a botanical assemblage that is impossible to find in real life without human interference, brought together regardless of season or geographical consideration. Tulips with a husk of maize, peonies with pieces of eight. There is something unsettling about a seasonless flower, like supermarket roses that have been genetically engineered to grow year-round, their petals no longer fragrant.

Sometime towards the end of James I's reign, in the early 1620s, the gentleman artist Nathaniel Bacon produced the first known example of a still life by an English painter. A gushing enthusiasm for the vegetable world ran in Bacon's family. His uncle was the statesman Francis Bacon, whose scandalous fall from political power in 1621 following charges of corruption freed up time for scientific pursuits, and for writing essays, including 'Of Gardens' and 'Of Plantations'. Nathaniel Bacon brought his love of nature into painting, and he wanted posterity to know it. His marble funerary monument recorded how a lifetime of observation and experience had made him an expert in the history of plants, but had also taught him 'to conquer Nature by Art' with a brush.

Bacon's *Cookmaid with Still Life of Vegetables and Fruit*, now at Tate Britain, shows how the Americas sneak into what seems like an archetypally domestic still life. Bacon had travelled to the Netherlands and perhaps trained as an artist there. The large composition is clearly modelled on Dutch kitchen and market scenes. A milky white cookmaid sits in the midst of a large array of produce. Stark, clear light hits root vegetables and quinces, illuminating them like virtuous saints. Figs and plums, with their dusty coating of wax bloom, spill from a basket. The maid cradles a melon and tucks white turnips in the crook of her arm. The largest vegetables by far are the cabbages to the right of the painting, taking up a good proportion of the entire composition. The abundance of nature is bawdily equated to sex and a fertile landscape. The woman's plunging neckline invites comparisons between her own body and the fruit she holds. A voracious cabbage leaf reaches towards her like a roving hand.

In the painting, specimens from the Americas attest to the successful transplantation that gardeners such as John Gerard and John Parkinson wrote about in their herbals. Their presence is more subtle than what we see in *vanitas* still lifes, where dried tobacco leaves from the Americas spill from papers and silver boxes. Instead, the plant scientist Barrie Juniper has identified marrows, squashes, and pumpkins from North America. Additionally, the double-handed basket in the foreground may contain runner beans, which had come to Europe from Central America. Juniper also posits that the grapes sitting in the Chinese porcelain dish might be *Vitis labrusca,* the 'foxgrape' then recently brought from North America.[3] Certainly, vines and grape varieties were of prime interest for travellers to the Chesapeake. 'Vines here are in suche abundance, as where soever a man treads, they are ready to embrace his foote,' the secretary John Pory wrote from Jamestown in 1619. 'I have tasted here of a great black grape as big as a Damascin [damson], that hath a true Muscatell-taste; the vine whereof now spending itself to the topps of high trees, if it were reduced into a vineyard, and there domesticated, would yield incomparable fruit.'[4]

American insects made it into Bacon's composition, too, in the form of a pigment. Technical analysis has revealed that the red dye is cochineal, almost certainly from Central America, where the pigment was produced by Indigenous labourers who harvested and crushed the insects that grew on the *opuntia* prickly-pear cactus. Cochineal cultivation had existed long before Europeans invaded Indigenous homelands, and the skill of Native cultivators and craftspeople remained vital to the trade in subsequent centuries. Over the course of the 1500s, the cochineal trade in Europe boomed, radiating from Spanish port cities to other parts of Europe and Asia. 'The cheife

Merchandizes that come from *Mexicana* into *Europe*', wrote the Elizabethan humanist Thomas Blundevile, 'are these, Gold, Silver, Pearles, [and] Cochenilles, to d[y]e with.'[5] Thomas Hariot looked for cochineal in Roanoke in the 1580s, likening *metaquesúnnauk*, a pear-like fruit with a juicy red interior, to those in the West Indies that have 'a kind of red d[y]e of great price which is called Cochinile'. Unaware that cochineal was an insect rather than a plant, Hariot admitted he was unsure whether *metaquesúnnauk* 'be the true Cochinile or a bastard or wilde kinde'.[6]

Over centuries, Mesoamerican labourers and artisans refined the colour. They harvested the insects, dried or baked them, ground them to powder, and added a mordant such as alum to fix the colour. In Mexica/Aztec tomb paintings and dyed textiles, cochineal contained important sacred and political meanings, linked to blood and therefore to life itself. The Nahuatl word for cochineal is *nocheztli*, from *nochtli* (cactus) and *eztli* (blood). Only the female insect produced the high percentage of carminic acid that gave a vibrant red shade known as *chilichiltic*, chilli red.[7]

This brilliant red could be modified to create a range of rich hues from magenta to lilac. In Europe, where royal and religious vestments were often red or purple, the dye came to suffuse the garments worn by kings and cardinals in life and art. Cochineal was used to refer to both bug and colour, dye and paint. It appeared in everything from tapestries to the compositions of Van Dyck, Rembrandt, Caravaggio, and Velázquez.[8] Cochineal was steadfast, affixing itself readily to the fabrics European artisans worked with, such as wool and silk.

Where might Bacon have sourced the dye? Any number of gardeners, apothecaries, artists, cloth-workers, and merchants might have been able to help. In his herbal, John Parkinson discussed the 'bloody colour' of the grain or fruit of the cactus 'called by the Indians *Nocheztli Nopalli* ... so much sought after, and used by Dyers, for the excellency of the colour'.[9] Parkinson laid out the whole process of making the dye, from cultivating young *opuntia* to infesting them with the insects that were later gathered from the spiny segments. Eventually, cochineal appeared in English shops and dyers' workshops. When a lady admired the glow of a pearl against the vivid scarlet of a velvet cushion, the tiny female nymphs of the nopal cactus had helped produce that effect.

After silver, cochineal was the most lucrative substance to come from Central America. In 1591, Robert Cecil wrote to Elizabeth's Lord Chancellor about naval affairs, including significant shipments of cochineal and sugar. The merchant John Watts had brought three ships to Plymouth from Havana, laden with cochineal, gold, and silver: 'noe badd newse to my lord adm[i]rall when hee awoke this mornening'.[10] In 1597, the queen gave the Earl of Essex a gift of £7,000 gained from a cargo of cochineal that Essex may have captured from Spanish ships in his attack on Cádiz the summer before. Later that year, Cecil received an urgent dispatch about the importance of intercepting a cochineal shipment heading to London, whose cargo was so immense that it risked destabilising the commodity's value in the realm. At various points during James's reign, disgruntled dyers complained that corrupt mixtures were creating false dyes that depreciated the true red of 'pure' West Indies cochineal. This true dye continued to arrive with other lucrative American goods. A cargo from a wrecked Spanish vessel near the Isle of Wight in October 1635 yielded cochineal along with 16,000 pieces of eight, a wedge of silver, and animal furs.[11]

As English people knew when they raced to intercept cargoes and acquire the dye for textiles or paints, centuries of Indigenous experimentation and cultivation lay behind the absorbing red. Thomas Gage passed many cochineal farms and dye stalls in regional markets when he travelled across Central America in the 1630s. From 'no part of

America doth *Spaine* get more *Cochinil* then from one of the Provinces of *Chiapa*', he wrote. Perhaps these farms, maintained by various Mayan and Zoques communities, had supplied the cochineal that had been wrecked off the coast of England at the time of his travels.

The hub of cochineal production in Chiapas was also where Gage encountered a Spanish official he deeply disliked. Local colonial authorities liked to claim they were descended from Spanish dukes and conquistadors, he scoffed, but they were dim-witted company. When Don Melchor de Velasco asked Gage about life in England, Gage informed him that, for half the year, the sun appeared red like a patch of blood in the sky. As a result, the English were warlike and high-spirited, prone to wearing more scarlet than any other nation in the world. They 'delighted to goe [dressed] in red, and to bee like the Sun, so naturally they were brought to those Seas to single out such ships as from *America* carried the rich Commodity of *Cochinill*, whereof they make more use then *Spain* it selfe to d[y]e their cloaths and Coats withal'. The English would wear scarlet, Gage avowed, 'as long as any *Cochinill* is to be found in the *Indias*'.[12]

Gage's tale was not intended as a serious one. But plenty of Tudors and Stuarts, it turns out, were wearing and displaying cochineal. It appears in the portraits of Tudor queens, such as Catherine of Aragon. The flamboyant pinkish red of Francis Drake's cape, jerkin, breeches, and hose, in his showy full-length portrait from 1581 (now somewhat faded), is probably cochineal. The same with the orange cloak in Queen Elizabeth's surreal 'Rainbow Portrait' – which, recent technical analysis has revealed, was originally painted red, its inner lining once purple, not grey. The brilliant crimson velvet of royal paintings and furniture, like the swathes of rich fabric that surround Charles I in Daniel Mytens' 1631 portrait, is likewise cochineal. And it's tempting to suggest that, when Van Dyck painted himself in a loose-fitting, lustrous red jacket, reaching out to touch that resplendent sunflower, he did so with cochineal. *Chilichiltic.* Chilli red.

Back in the less flashy world of his rambunctious still life, Nathaniel Bacon was using cochineal to enhance the depth or lustre of cherries, poppies, and cabbage leaves. His use of the dye, and the North American squash varieties on display, indicate how plantation economies and trades were part of this early English example of the genre. And the giant lobster in *The Paston Treasure*? Cochineal, like the immense red curtain behind it that invites us to think of the painting, and global assemblages, as a kind of performance.

Not everyone thought the hybridisation of domestic gardens and transatlantic flora was a good thing. In 'The Mower against Gardens', the poet Andrew Marvell condemned the corruption caused by foreign species planted in English soil. He conjured the sinister image of a man who preens women in preparation for sex work:

> *With strange perfumes he did the roses taint,*
> *And flowers themselves were taught to paint.*

Covering the skin in cosmetics and 'strange' fragrances was an act conducted in the domain of the boudoir. In seeking rare specimens from around the world, wealthy English landholders became procurers, immoral agents of illicit desire, making flowers more seductive for their own sordid gain.

In the world of Marvell's mower, traffic and trade had forever altered the once-unadulterated landscape of the pastoral past:

> *Another world was searched, through oceans new,*
> *To find the* Marvel of Peru.
> *And yet these rarities might be allowed . . .*
> *Had* [man] *not dealt between the bark and tree,*

Forbidden mixtures there to see.
No plant now knew the stock from which it came;
He grafts upon the wild the tame.[13]

The 'Marvel of Peru', *Mirabilis jalapa,* had become popular in English gardens by the time of Marvell's writing. It was a flower that opened at dusk and emitted a sweet fragrance before closing again by morning, revealing itself only to partygoers, servants, and other wanderers of the night. Unusually, multicoloured flowers could grow on the same plant. Streaks of different colours blazed across a single petal. To find a flower that the Mexica had cultivated for centuries an ocean away created 'forbidden mixtures', encouraging a sensory gratification so baroque that it had become impossible to enjoy the fields and meadows in one's own backyard. For the mower – the reaper – a libertine garden was a perversion of nature.

These forbidden mixtures are precisely what the still-life genre captures. For the most part, these artworks do not show the fruits of an Edenic or Arcadian landscape, but rather collected and transported abundance. Not the pastoral nymph, wooed by a shepherd in an Elizabethan verse, but the nymph plucked from cactus fields by the hands of Nahua or Mayan cultivators. Still lifes show the effects of transplantation. Travel books, in turn, painted these hybrid compositions with words, enticing readers by turning colonial ecosystems into still lifes. A description of Bermuda written shortly after Bacon painted his *Cookmaid with Still Life* recorded the many varieties of colourful potatoes, tobacco, sugarcane, parsnips, 'exceeding large Radishes, the America bread, the Cassado root, the Indian Pumpi[o]n . . . also the English Artichoke', all of which satisfied a person's curiosity and delight, spread out like a tableau.[14] The land had become a hybrid garden, strange and familiar, where pineapples and English artichokes, pumpkins and radishes grew.

What would a Miskitu, Mi'kmaw, or African viewer have thought, seeing the tobacco leaves and pipes in a *vanitas*? Or a game still life, depicting wasteful piles of dead animals sprawled on tiled floors? When they hung in Stuart interiors, still lifes were placed in conversation with other objects. Depictions of fruits and vegetables might hang in long galleries, or in kitchens next to baskets full of foods gathered from the estate garden, where wealthy women experimented with transatlantic specimens to grow potatoes and Virginia parsley. A *vanitas* or *pronk* still life could appear in a dining room or gallery, next to torchères with African figures in feathered garments. When we add other layers of sociability to the scene – pinching tobacco out of a silver box engraved with the face of Charles I, gilt table globes, or banquet set pieces made of sugar – we gain a fuller idea of just how connected plantation and the civility of the English elite had already become. 'To dig for Wealth we weary not our limbs,' the poet Edmund Waller wrote in his panegyric to Oliver Cromwell. 'Gold (though the heaviest mettle) hither swims: / Ours is the Harvest where the Indians mow, / We plough the deep, and reap what others sow.'[15]

In the compositions themselves, however, uncertainty lingers. Bacon's *Cookmaid with Still Life of Vegetables and Fruit*, like wit poetry of the time, is a kind of *carpe diem,* a hearty invitation to succumb to sensual gratification before the season ends and the fruits sour. But even in their most exalted and ravishing iterations, something is amiss. Still-life paintings present a dissonant picture of appetites gone mad. If they entice with delectable fruits and gleaming chalices, they also provoke a consideration of the costs of desire. Though human figures rarely appear, they haunt these compositions. If there are vestiges of human bodies, they are probably skulls. These works lay out the results of our material longings. They invite us to consider a world that we have altered and embellished, and then abandoned, all for the seductive curve of a rare fruit. All is not right in the weird and opulent golden world. Unsettled objects come back to unsettle us.

In the end, these paintings offer us a dilemma. Forbidden fruit – that desire to obtain the rare or the unknown, to reach for new kinds of knowledge that might never have been for us – has always been a symbol of choice.[16] Can we find ways to pursue luxurious self-expression without the suffering of others? Will we continue to want things that usher destruction, somewhere out of the frame?

Epilogue

In 1620, the court clergyman John Williams preached a sermon before James I at his residence at Theobalds, condemning extravagant consumption and denouncing the absurdity of early Stuart tastes. Pride so possessed a man, Williams preached, that 'the *Indians* . . . must bee continually busied to tricke up and trimme him . . . in diving in their *seas* for pearles to adorne him', 'in digging to their Centre, for *golde* to lace him, in hunting their vermin for *smel[l]s* to fume him', all for the sake of admiration. If it was considered graceful and fashionable to collect feathers to plume an Englishman, the musk of rodents to bind scent, and 'the white excretions of *shel-fish* to decke him', then surely, Williams insisted, birds and beasts were more honourable than humans were.[1] An obsession with the sparkling, pearled body had set 'the remotest . . . Indians' an ocean away to labour endlessly for the sake of the English courtly aesthetic.

Williams's critique was, in essence, about how colonialism and outsourced labour had become written into the highest and most recognisable fashions of the era – styles that have equally come to embody what the Renaissance looks like to us. The bodies of the elite were wrought, moulded, and gilded, cast into figures that proclaimed England's budding colonial ambitions, achieved through piracy and plunder alongside plantation. The scale was unprecedented: piles of things, gathered and collected from Andean mountains, sacred burial sites, and Bermudian shipwrecks. The spoils from looted treasure ships made new fortunes, fuelling building projects and ventures to other parts of the world. An 'Indian mine in a Lambs skinne', one Elizabethan character gleefully calls the wealth in his leather purse.[2] Lustrous, flat-tailed denizens of Chesapeake wetlands supplied the fur that merchants and artisans turned into hats, accessories that have become so ubiquitous in portraits of royals, merchant women, Puritans, and Catholic Gunpowder Plotters that it's hard to imagine the seventeenth century without them. As they wrote treatises endorsing Native dispossession, grew potatoes and pumpkins in their gardens, and brawled over Virginia Company affairs under the arcades of the Royal Exchange, Londoners' skins touched and carried evidence of Atlantic economies and ecosystems.

Two years before Williams preached his sermon, at the same royal residence, James had ordered two newly erected brick houses to be demolished after the owners turned them into tobacco shops. This information survives as a hasty postscript in a letter, a reminder of how much James abhorred tobacco. We can hear the groans of his courtiers who forgot their supply at home but wanted a puff of something punchy between banqueting courses. The tobacco houses at Theobalds also signal the prevalence of this Indigenous plant across England. It was right there, in a letter about state offices and the Duke of Buckingham's sympathy for the imprisoned Ralegh after his return from the Orinoco – a note about the tobacco dried and stocked in country estates, in buildings and shops, creating new rural and urban spaces of sociability and conversation, decades before the establishment of coffeehouses.

In the early eighteenth century, the writer Joseph Addison wrote a story from the perspective of a shilling. The history of Tudor Atlantic crossings provided the foundation for this speaking coin's tale of circulation and fiery alteration. The silver had been forged in a village in Peru and transported as an ingot in one of Francis Drake's ships, before being minted into a coin in London. The coin is 'taken out of my Indian habit, refined, naturalised, and put into the British mode, with the face of Queen Elizabeth on one side'. He passes through many hands, changing the fates of others even as they change his own fortunes. Eventually, he triggers literary innovation by inspiring a poet to pen a new work.[3]

It is telling that Addison traces the silver to the sixteenth-century Viceroyalty of Peru. He is aware that transatlantic metals, both real and longed for, were a catalyst for the prosperity and refinement that would follow in the century to come. Throughout its misadventures, the shilling's alchemical transformation into the 'British mode' does not erase the story of its origins and migrations. These stories jostle within him as he becomes an eyewitness to the upheavals of a society soon torn from within by civil war; a society whose wealth, from the time of the Tudors, became entangled with transatlantic economies, war, and dispossession. 'From the new world, her silver and her gold, / Came, like a tempest, to confound the old,' one poet wrote in the 1650s.[4]

Not all were optimistic about this moment of colonial opportunity. In criticisms – short verses here and there, satires, plays, sermons against luxury – Tudor and Stuart writers lamented and ridiculed the avarice of fellow citizens. One of Ben Jonson's most biting satires about humankind's endless capacity for greed was *Volpone* (1607), performed the same year as the establishment of Jamestown. 'Good morning to the Day; and next, my Gold,' the duplicitous Volpone rhapsodises in his opening monologue. Around 1609, just as the Virginia Company launched a campaign that idealised North America as an endlessly yielding Eden, the court poet Samuel Daniel warned Prince Henry of what imperial indulgence could lead to. Conquest was a series of 'ill events', bringing destruction and downfall to the coloniser. Powerful states had been weakened by claiming sovereignty over wide dominions.[5]

The Age of Gold, one merchant wrote, had pushed the English into voluntary exile from their homes, imprisoning God's creatures in putrid ships and exposing bodies to discomfort and pain through a thousand perils.[6] For the poet John Beaumont, the pursuit of a golden world hindered the possibility of ever recovering the Golden Age. The precious metals carried in the ribs of ships brought feuds and boundless avarice. For him, tobacco was the herb that might assuage the world's wounds and sorrows. There was no need for alchemists to labour vainly with 'distillations of the quintessence'.[7]

In many ways, Jacobean criticisms came too late. Beaumont viewed tobacco as a remedy for discord, but by then Europeans had already turned the plant into a colonial commodity, disrupting long-standing connections between Indigenous peoples and their homelands. Several years later, when James I asked his subjects why they could not welcome a friend but by lighting a pipe, the answer was that society had already begun to change drastically. Members of the gentry and aristocracy staked their fortunes and their lives on expansionist projects that turned them into colonial landlords. Everyday sociability and plantation affairs were developing hand in hand. 'Most younger *Brothers* sell their Lands to buy *Gu[i]anian Plumes*: like *Icarus* to fly,' one satire quipped in 1618, ever searching for those 'rarer *Rarities* . . . [j]ust now to be discovered', never leaving without 'his *Looking-glasse*, / In a *Tobacco* box'.[8] The mirror in the tobacco box presents the gentleman with his portrait in miniature, shifting and blinking, encased in a container that emits the heady smell of a plantation-sourced intoxicant.

'No age hath ever wit refined so far,' the oracle proclaimed, in that entertainment about an Amazonian prince performed for Queen Elizabeth in 1595. 'Seated between the old world and the new, / A land there is no other land may touch.' But of course, the prophecy was wrong.

Today, all that remains of Whitehall Palace, that centre of Tudor and Stuart state power and intrigue, is its Banqueting House. A fire destroyed the labyrinth of council chambers, cloisters, galleries, and royal bedrooms in the late seventeenth century, reducing its buildings to rubble and ash. Only Inigo Jones's neoclassical masterpiece survives, designed by the same hand that sketched the costumes for those feathered Virginian princes in *The Memorable Masque.* It seems fitting somehow. In the Banqueting House, state power met pure luxury and high fantasy. It was the crucible where ideas of Englishness and global power could be projected as benign, magnificent, harmonious. A place where imperial aspirations and diplomatic negotiations, fuelled by sugared confections and dances under triumphal arches, were carried out in surroundings that consciously harked back to the civilisation of Rome. The vision of English imperial identity that came down through the centuries was reliant on the fictions that a place like the Banqueting House allowed for, with its columns and jewels and stories of sea goddesses. James I was so proud of its construction that he included it in one of his most regal state portraits. A Latin inscription was drafted, perhaps to appear in the hall:

> James, first king of Great Britain built from the ground up this hall, which strikes the eye of its majesty ... equal of any marble buildings throughout Europe, intended for festive occasions ... to the eternal glory of his name and of his most peaceful empire, he left it for posterity.[9]

The building, and the Jacobean past, looms in the Anishinaabe writer Gerald Vizenor's *The Heirs of Columbus* (1991). It is an exuberant, irreverent rescripting of the colonial story, one that signals the important place that early Stuart England can hold in Indigenous historical memory. Felipa Flowers is a trickster-poacher character who has devoted her life to retrieving sacred Native belongings from private collections and museums. When she receives a mysterious letter from a London antiquarian bookseller named Pellegrine Treves, informing her that he has recently found the whereabouts of Pocahontas's bones (long believed to have been buried at Gravesend, following her death in 1617), she crosses the Atlantic in search of the Algonquian woman whose life had become so entangled in early Stuart political desire. In London, Treves invites Felipa to a recreation of a masque at the Banqueting House, where the revelries of old have been revived. The masque is the same one that Matoaka attended in 1617, staged on the day that the louche George Villiers became Earl of Buckingham.

Music and laughter can be heard down the corridors as Felipa enters the building, her deerskin moccasins treading softly against the polished floor. Through the doors of the Banqueting House, time seems to collapse. If Felipa looks up, she'll see James I ascending into heaven, painted by the baroque master Peter Paul Rubens. In the crowd, amidst sweets and intoxicating liquors glowing like rubies, she sees panthers purring on tables and flashes of the hand talkers – the Native healers and tricksters who communicate through touch. Felipa is haunted by the thought of Matoaka twisting her body into the restrictive silhouettes of court attire.[10]

After the masque, she walks through London in her moccasins. They are blue, linked to the blue light of survivance, that radiating throughline of Native presence and Native stories. Blue is the colour of the Atlantic, appearing in the old chime that 'in 1492, Columbus sailed the ocean blue', but it is also the colour of creation and story-telling, of rocks that reveal ancient memories, and the rivers that spread them. Blue is the colour of Arnaq's tattoos and the cotinga feathers in Mesoamerican codices, of Arctic ice and flying fish. 'Blue is imagination,' one character says. It is healing and possibility. Felipa finds London lonely, full of statues and lofty stone, permeated by an inescapable cold. She views the monuments around her as vestiges of the golden world: 'banners of blood and gold decorate a pallid facade that honoured the glories of the Crown'. They celebrate an empire whose seeds were sown in the time of Drake and Queen Elizabeth, James I and those duchesses with their cabinets and travel books. 'Too much romance,' she tells the bookseller Treves, 'subdues our humour and miseries.'[11]

For a long time, the Americas of the English Renaissance have been viewed only as commodities and curiosities. They have been seen as colourful references to English seafaring and transatlantic adventuring, or evidence of the quirky habits of collectors and their ostentatious cabinets. Romance has had a lot to do with it, both in the Tudor sense of 'an extravagant fabrication, a wild falsehood, a fantasy', and in a more contemporary one, a 'feeling or sense of wonder, mystery, remoteness from everyday life . . . [often through] association with adventure, heroism, chivalry'.[12] Too much romance leads to histories of Frobisher and Ralegh that aren't also about Inuit makers and Arawakan interpreters. Too much romance is an account of Elizabethan pearl mania that isn't also about African divers, canoes, and Cumanagoto lands. As Williams preached in 1620, the story of colonial consumption involves a whole community of other creatures – parrots and oysters, or, for that matter, muskrats and prickly pears.

Too much romance disconnects these environments, and the labour and expertise of Native peoples, from Renaissance art and politics. It's easier to imagine a picture of the past where intrepid knights and sea captains crossed oceans on quasi-mythical quests, and where ordinary subjects knew little about the distant lands that seemed magically to engender the potatoes, sugar, or silver that ended up on their dining tables. In chronicling a two-way influence through migrations and travelling things – through *un*settlement – the story becomes infinitely more variable. The people, plants, animals, and cultural belongings presented in this book offer proof of vast, multilingual processes and exchanges whose influences on the Tudors and Stuarts have only begun to be investigated and confronted. Different material remains help to tell different stories, requiring various forms of collaboration and expertise. Many cultural belongings that were present in early modern England no longer survive, but some do – an obsidian mirror, a jaguar-skin codex, *wampum* belts, feathered pouches, claw necklaces, embroidered deerskin garments. Others might yet come to light, lying packed away in an attic next to some damaged Tudor portraits, or newly attributed after remaining uncatalogued or mislabelled for so long. Perhaps some of the Algonquian-made arrows sent yearly to Charles I from Maryland will be found at Windsor Castle.

These pieces of the past call attention to Indigenous perspectives and knowledge, in histories that have often disregarded or obfuscated what was always present. They are tangible evidence of how Native peoples have long been, and remain, 'actors on a world stage'. They demonstrate how, as Glicéria Tupinambá put it, 'we also occupied, reclaimed the Old World', through a flow of objects and influences that '[subvert] the very direction of colonialism'.[13] They show that, even as lawyers drafted charters and MPs justified settlements with the stated intention of 'civilising' others and altering their ways of life, Indigenous presences were always coming in – not only from Virginia or Massachusetts, but from Mexico, Providence Island, and Brazil. Leanne Betasamosake Simpson (Michi Saagiig Nishnaabeg) has spoken about how making canoes, dyeing and weaving threads, and observing the seasonal arrival of strawberries are all 'tiny bits of poetry doing the work of the otherwise', opening up spaces that can live 'outside of colonialism'.[14] By searching for copper-and-gold figures or Caribbean roots and gums in early modern England, and even within Renaissance texts and performances, we afford them little spaces of their own.

As secret Catholics hid rosaries under floorboards to avoid persecution, powerful women staked a claim in national politics, and corrupt favourites rose and fell, Tudor and Stuart England housed Indigenous and African knowledge-holders, dusk-blooming Peruvian flowers, and Muzo emeralds. Plants from invaded lands sprouted in English plots, and there were Hispaniola crocodiles in St James's Park. Patronesses engaged in transatlantic affairs, while the bodies of female insects gave the world chilli red. A gold mine appeared on a stage in Whitehall, a blazing emblem of the ruling elite's imperial fancies, at the same time as Epanow, with trickster flair, found a way home. Broken tobacco pipes were strewn across theatres, taverns, gardens, riversides, and country estates. These fragments can still be unearthed today, their insides charred from use. They connect us to a time when an accomplished artist painted himself with a sunflower, and when hopes for another golden age, free of greed and cruel extraction, still lingered like summer light.

Acknowledgements

This book is the result of many years of research and conversation, beginning with my own travels from the Pacific coast of North America to a tiny medieval university in coastal Scotland. Since then, the work of many scholars – friends, acquaintances, strangers – has helped guide my way, and I have tried to indicate my indebtedness to them in my citations.

I would like to thank Stephanie Pratt (Dakota) for her generosity and insights over the years. Having first admired from afar her expertise on representations of Indigenous Americans in British art, and her dedication to changing British perceptions of Native peoples, I feel fortunate to now consider her a friend as well as a collaborator. I am grateful to Stephanie as well as Hugh Foley, Misha Ewen, Olivia Carpenter, and Ana de Oliveira Dias for reading drafts of this book; to Kerry Apps and Emily Stevenson for casting their eyes over details relating to privateering earls and merchant networks; and to colleagues and friends at the University of York, and the University of Oxford before that, for their perceptive questions and observations on everything from Cavalier poetry to featherwork. My thanks to Nandini Das for her counsel throughout the book-writing process, and for her wholehearted support of my research since my postdoc.

I am delighted that the book features two new graphics by the Cherokee artist Rebecca Lee Kunz, and I greatly appreciate her willingness to collaborate on this project. In the UK, Caroline Dodds Pennock and David Stirrup's long-standing efforts to foster meaningful dialogue and partnerships between Indigenous and non-Indigenous writers, artists, and activists have been invaluable. I have learned much from their research, and from Indigenous scholars and artists on both sides of the Atlantic, including Robbie Richardson (Mi'kmaq), whose conversations and work have helped shape my approaches.

Thank you to my agent, Emma Bal at Madeleine Milburn Agency, for her support and sage advice through the years, and to Phoebe Fawcett for seamlessly stepping in during Emma's leave. My editor at Faber, Fiona Crosby, has been there at every step, and her guidance and discernment have helped me find a voice for this project. Jessica Case, my US editor at Pegasus Books, and the wider Faber and Pegasus teams (including Joanna Harwood, Jo Stimfield, Lara Weisweiller-Wu, Amanda Russell, Raminta Uselytė, and Nicole Maher) have provided endless assistance and enthusiasm throughout this process. The producers at BBC Radio kindly granted permission to print some of the reworked material from 'Boy with a Pearl Earring', my essay that first aired on BBC Radio 3 in March 2022, and from my 'postcard' on still lifes for 'The Botanical Past', an episode of *Free Thinking* that aired on 1 June 2021.

The sources consulted for this book would have remained beyond my reach without the help of archivists, librarians, and institutions in the UK and US. Fellowships and grants have financially supported this research over the years, including from the Folger Shakespeare Library in Washington, DC; Huntington Library in Pasadena, California; Yale Center for British Art in New Haven, Connecticut; Omohundro Institute of Early American History and Culture in Williamsburg, Virginia; Eccles Institute for the Americas at the British Library; Pasold Research Fund; Leavis Fund at the University of York (Department of English and Related Literature); and Paul Mellon Centre for Studies in British Art in London. I am further indebted to curators at the Ashmolean, Oxford University Herbaria, Oxford Botanic Garden, Pitt Rivers Museum, British Museum, London National Portrait Gallery, National Trust, and Victoria and Albert Museum for granting me access to objects in their collections, and to the archaeologists and historians at Historic Jamestowne, especially Jim Horn and Merry Outlaw. Having freelanced for the National Portrait Gallery for many years now, I am grateful to the curators and education team for inviting me to imagine what new stories and possibilities might come of asking different questions of Tudor and Stuart paintings.

Like the Elizabethan poets, dreamers, and degenerates who share the traveller's road in *The Pilgrimage to Parnassus*, friends old and new have met me along the course of my studies to offer motivation and healthy doses of distraction. I am beholden to all of them for their wit, care, and good humour, and to my parents for always kindling my love of the past. Though I spend a lot of time in the sixteenth century, I am best in the twenty-first: it is here that Inès came into the world, a now-three-year-old whose inexhaustible curiosity and freewheeling wordplay serve as continual inspiration. Finally, I thank H for his love and encouragement, and for his serious engagement with my work. His sensitivity to the value of poetry and a well-turned line has always charmed me, but it has also helped me become a better writer. *Let sea-discoverers to new worlds have gone.* We carve out something else.

Notes

INTRODUCTION

1 'A device by the Earl of Essex for the Queen's entertainment', 17 November 1595, National Archives, SP 12/254, f. 139.

2 George Chapman, 'De Guiana, carmen Epicum', in Lawrence Kemys, *A relation of the second voyage to Guiana* (1596; STC 14947), sig. A4v.

3 John Donne, 'Upon Mr Thomas Coryat's *Crudities*' and 'The Sun Rising' in *The Complete Poems of John Donne*, ed. Robin Robbins (London: Routledge, 2013), pp. 106–7, 243.

4 Fulke Greville, *The life of the renowned Sir Philip Sidney*, 1651, in D. G. Wing, *Short-title catalogue of books printed in England, Scotland, Ireland, Wales, and British America . . . 1641–1700*, 2nd edn (1994) (hereafter 'Wing'), B4899, p. 133.

5 Quoted in Roger Kuin, 'Querre-Muhau: Sir Philip Sidney and the New World', *Renaissance Quarterly*, 51:2 (1998), pp. 549–85, at p. 562.

6 Kuin, 'Querre-Muhau', p. 564.

7 Kuin, 'Querre-Muhau', p. 563.

8 *The Tempest*, Act II, sc. i, 137–46.

9 Quoted in Mordechai, 'Projectors and Learned Projects in Early Modern England', *The Seventeenth Century*, 32:1 (2017), pp. 63–79, at p. 64.

10 Walter Hamond, *A paradox* (1640; STC 12735), sig. Ev.

11 Samuel Daniel, *Tobacco battered; & the pipes shattered* (1617; STC 23582a), p. 85.

12 William Heath, 'The Goulden Arte, or, The Jewell House of Gemes', early 17th century, British Library, ff. 2r, 41r–48v.

13 Ned Blackhawk, *The Rediscovery of America: Native Peoples and the Unmaking of US History* (New Haven, CT: Yale University Press, 2023), p. 3.

14 *The Tempest*, Act V, sc. i, 181–4.

15 Greville, *The life of the renowned Sir Philip Sidney*, p. 126.

16 Jerry Brotton, *This Orient Isle: Elizabethan England and the Islamic World* (London: Allen Lane, 2016); Nandini Das, *Courting India: England, Mughal India, and the Origins of Empire* (London: Bloomsbury, 2023);

Matthew Dimmock, *Elizabethan Globalism: England, China, and the Rainbow Portrait* (New Haven, CT: Yale University Press, 2019); Anna Whitelock, *The Sun Rising: James I and the Dawn of a Global Britain* (London: Bloomsbury, 2025).

17 See Imtiaz Habib, *Black Lives in the English Archives, 1500–1677: Imprints of the Invisible* (Aldershot: Ashgate, 2008); Kim Hall, *Things of Darkness: Economies of Race and Gender in Early Modern England* (Cornell, NY: Cornell University Press, 1995); Noémie Ndiaye, *Scripts of Blackness: Early Modern Performance Culture and the Making of Race* (Philadelphia, PA: University of Pennsylvania Press, 2022).

18 *Gesta Grayorum, or, The history of the high and mighty prince, Henry Prince of Purpoole* (1688; Wing C444), p. 33.

19 William Wood, *New Englands prospect* (1634; STC 25957), p. 62.

20 *King Lear*, Act III, sc. ii, 1–3.

21 Richard Brathwaite, *A solemne joviall disputation* (1617; STC 3585), p. 155; *The Noble Gentleman*, in *Comedies and tragedies written by Francis Beaumont and John Fletcher* (1647; Wing B1581), p. 27.

22 *An Experimentall discoverie of Spanish practises* (1623; STC 22077), pp. 36, 39, 47.

23 Vincent T. Harlow (ed.), *Colonizing Expeditions to the West Indies and Guiana, 1623–1667* (London: Hakluyt Society, 1925), p. 102; Susan Dwyer Amussen, *Caribbean Exchanges: Slavery and the Transformation of English Society, 1640–1700* (Chapel Hill, NC: University of North Carolina Press, 2007).

24 Luke Taylor, 'Bolivian Indigenous groups assert claim to treasure of "holy grail of shipwrecks"', *Guardian*, 29 March 2024, www.theguardian.com/environment/2024/mar/29/bolivia-shipwreck-colombia-treasure [accessed 13 August 2025]; Ruth Lopez, 'International Scrap Over Treasure', *Art Newspaper*, 10 January 2024, www.theartnewspaper.com/2024/01/10/international-scrap-over-treasure-laden-spanish-galleon-that-sunk-off-the-colombian-coast-in-1708 [accessed 17 April 2024].

25 Kathryn N. Gray and Amy M. E. Morris (eds), *Matoaka, Pocahontas, Rebecca: Her Atlantic Identities and Afterlives* (Charlottesville, VA: University of Virginia Press, 2024), p. 1 [discussing the work of Jean O'Brian and Patrick Wolfe].

26 Jelena Porsanger, 'An Essay about Indigenous Methodology', *Nordlit*, 15 (2004), pp. 105–20; 'A Toolkit for Respectful Collaboration with Indigenous Peoples', IPCA Knowledge Basket, www.ipcaknowledgebasket.ca [accessed 25 August 2025]; Daniel Heath Justice, *Why Indigenous Literatures Matter* (Ontario: WLU Press, 2018).

27 On how to recover Indigenous perspectives in European texts, see also Caroline Dodds Pennock, *On Savage Shores: How Indigenous Americans Discovered Europe* (London: Weidenfeld & Nicolson, 2022).

28 John Nicholl, *An houre glasse of Indian newes* (1607; STC 18532), sigs. B3r–Cv; Walter Ralegh, *The discoverie of the large, rich, and beautiful empire of Guiana* (1596; STC 20634), p. 48.

29 Saidiya Hartman, 'Venus in Two Acts', *Small Axe*, 25 (2008), pp. 1–14, at p. 12; Tiya Miles, *All That She Carried: The Journey of Ashley's Sack, a Black Family Keepsake* (London: Profile, 2023) [proof copy], pp. 300–1; Marisa Fuentes, *Dispossessed Lives: Enslaved Women, Violence, and the Archive* (Philadelphia, PA: University of Pennsylvania Press, 2016).

30 Quoted in Gray and Morris (eds), *Matoaka, Pocahontas, Rebecca*, p. 8.

31 Gerald Vizenor, *Manifest Manners: Narratives on Postindian Survivance* (Lincoln, NE: University of Nebraska Press, 1999), p. vii.

32 John Jacob Berlu, *The treasury of drugs unlock't* (1690; Wing B1980), pp. 16, 27; Megan Peiser, 'Citing Seeds, Citing People: Bibliography and Indigenous Memory, Relations, and Living Knowledge-Keepers', *Criticism*, 64:3 (2022), pp. 521–31, at pp. 524, 527.

33 Nicaise Le Fèvre, *A discourse upon Sr Walter Rawleigh's great cordial* (1664; Wing L928), p. 25.

34 John Donne, *A sermon . . . Preached to the Honourable Company of the Virginian Plantation* (1624; STC 7052), p. 13.

35 Robbie Richardson, 'Decolonizing Eighteenth-Century Studies: An Indigenous Perspective', *Studies in Eighteenth-Century Culture*, 52 (2023), pp. 35–9, at p. 35.

SEALSKIN PARKAS AND A YELLOW JERKIN

1 Louis-Jacques Dorais, *Words of the Inuit: A Semantic Stroll through a Northern Culture* (Winnipeg: University of Manitoba Press, 2020), p. 21; George Best, *A true discourse of the late voyages of discoverie, for the finding of a passage to Cathaya* (1578; STC 1972), p. 67.

2 Betty Issenman, *Sinews of Survival: The Living Legacy of Inuit Clothing* (Vancouver: University of British Columbia Press, 1998), pp. 43, 65–76.

3 Coll Thrush, *Indigenous London: Native Travellers to the Heart of Empire* (New Haven, CT: Yale University Press, 2016), p. 2.

4 Quoted in Roger Kuin, 'Querre-Muhau: Sir Philip Sidney and the New World', *Renaissance Quarterly*, 51 (1998), pp. 549–85, at p. 562.

5 Best, *A true discourse*, sig. A3r.

6 Best, *A true discourse*, sig. A3v.

7 Thomas Wood to Richard Bagot, 10 October 1576, Folger Shakespeare Library, MS L.a.987.

8 Nicole Blackwood, 'Meta Incognita: Some Hypotheses on Cornelis Ketel's Lost English and Inuit Portraits', *Netherlands Kunsthistorisch Jaarboek*, 66:1 (2016), pp. 28–53, at p. 36.

9 Blackwood, 'Meta Incognita', p. 34.

10 Best, *A true discourse*, p. 25.

11 Best, *A true discourse*, p. 68.

12 *Thomas Platter's Travels in England, 1599*, tr. and ed. Clare Williams (London: Jonathan Cape, 1937), p. 201.

13 John Tradescant, *Musaeum Tradescantianum, or, A collection of rarities* (1656; Wing T2005), pp. 7, 33, 48.

14 Dionyse Settle, *A true reporte* (1577; STC 22265), sigs. C6r–v.

15 Exodus 31:1–5.

16 'An Abstract of the Journall of Master *Henry Hudson*, for the Discoverie of the North-west Passage, begunne the seventeenth of April, 1610' in Samuel Purchas, *Purchas his pilgrimes* (1625; STC 20509), p. 597; 'James Hall his Voyage forth of *Denmarke* for the discovery of *Greeneland*, in the years 1605' in ibid.,Purchas, *Purchas his pilgrimes*, p. 817.

17 Settle, *A true reporte*, sig. B7r; Aaju Peter et al., 'The Seal: An Integral Part of Our Culture', *Etudes/Inuit/Studies*, 26:1 (2002), pp. 167–74, at p. 167.

18 Issenman, *Sinews of Survival*, pp. 44, 53; Sylvie Pharand, *Caribou Skin Clothing of the Igloolik Inuit* (Iqaluit: Inhabit Media, 2012).

19 William C. Sturtevant and David Quinn, 'This New Prey: Eskimos in Europe in 1567, 1576, and 1577', in Christian F. Feest (ed.), *Indians in Europe: An Interdisciplinary Collection of Essays* (Lincoln, NE: University of Nebraska Press, 1989), pp. 61–140, at p. 130; 'Skin: Stitching the Surface', *Inuit Art Quarterly*, 31 (summer 2018); '25+ Ways Inuit Artists Have Historically Used Pantone's Colour of the Year', *Inuit Art Quarterly* blog, 3 January 2020, www.inuitartfoundation.org/iaq-online/pantone's-classic-blue-in-inuit-art [accessed 30 March 2024].

20 On the significance of traditional tattooing as a process of recovering histories ruptured by colonialism, see the work of tattoo artists such as Maya Sialuk Jacobsen and Angela Hovak Johnston (Inuit Tattoo Revitalization Project). Angela Hovak Johnston, *Reawakening our Ancestors' Lines: Revitalizing Inuit Traditional Tattooing* (Toronto: Inhabit Media, 2017); *Ancestral Threads*, dir. Sean Stiller (2023); Maya Sialuk Jacobsen (Greenlandic Inuk), 'Ancestral Threads', *Canadian Art*, Spring 2019 issue, www.canadianart.ca/essays/ancestral-threads/ [accessed 1 March 2024].

21 Settle, *A true reporte*, sig. B8r.

FLORIDA AND ROANOKE IN WATERCOLOUR

1 Katherine Coombs, '"A Kind of Gentle Painting": Limning in 16th-Century England', in Kim Sloan (ed.), *European Visions: American Voices* (London: British Museum, 2009), pp. 77–84; Timea Tallian, 'John White's Materials and Techniques', in Sloan (ed.), *European Visions, American Voices*, pp. 72–6.

2 Henry Peacham, *The compleat gentleman* (1622; STC 19502), p. 105.

3 Coombs, '"A Kind of Gentle Painting"', pp. 77–8.

4 Kim Sloan, 'Introduction', in Sloan (ed.), *European Visions, American Voices*, p. 1.

5 Richard Hakluyt to Francis Walsingham, 7 January 1584, in Richard Hakluyt, *A particuler discourse concerning the greate necessity and manifolde commodities*, ed. David B. Quinn and Alison M. Quinn (London: Hakluyt Society, 1993), pp. 197–8.

6 John Donne, 'The Storm', in *The Complete Poems of John Donne*, ed. Robin Robbins (London: Routledge, 2013), p. 66.

7 Coombs, '"A Kind of Gentle Painting"', p. 77.

8 Helen C. Rountree and Wesley D. Taukchiray, *Manteo's World: Native American Life in Carolina's Sound Country Before and After the Lost Colony* (Chapel Hill, NC: University of North Carolina Press, 2021), pp. 87–8, 93.

9 Rountree and Taukchiray, *Manteo's World*, Ch. 1.

10 Rountree and Taukchiray, *Manteo's World*, p. 75.

11 Kim F. Hall, Scott Manning Stevens, and L. Lehua Yim, 'On Critical Indigenous Studies and Early Modern Critical Race Studies: A Tri-Interview', in Noemie Ndiaye and Lia Markey (eds), *Seeing Race Before Race: Visual Culture and the Racial Matrix in the Premodern World* (Tempe, AZ: Arizona State University Press, 2023), pp. 217–28, at p. 221.

12 Rountree and Taukchiray, *Manteo's World*, p. 88.

13 'The fifth voyage of Master John White', in Richard Hakluyt, *The principal navigations, voyages, traffiques and discoveries of the English nation* (1599–1600; STC 12626a), p. 293.

14 Stephanie Pratt, 'Truth and Artifice in the Visualization of Native Peoples: From the Time of John White to the Beginnings of the 18th Century', in Sloan (ed.), *European Visions, American Voices*, pp. 33–40, at p. 34.

15 Pratt, 'Truth and Artifice', p. 35.

16 Christina J. Faraday, 'Lively Limning: Presence in Portrait Miniatures and John White's Images of the New World', *British Art Studies*, 17 (2020) [online].

17 Theodor de Bry, *The King and Queen taking a Walk for their Amusement*, 1591, State Archives of Florida, www.floridamemory.com/items/show/294805 [accessed 13 May 2024].

18 Jerald T. Milanich, *Florida Indians and the Invasion from Europe* (Gainesville, FL: Library Press at University of Florida, 2018), p. 2; Alejandra Dubcovsky and George Aaron Broadwell, 'Writing Timucua', *Early American Studies*, 15:3 (2017), pp. 409–41, at p. 413.

19 René Goulaine de Laudonnière [tr. Richard Hakluyt], *A notable historie containing foure voyages* (1587; STC 15316), sig. Q4v.

20 Jacques le Moyne's narrative, translated and printed in Theodor de Bry, *Grand Voyages* (1591), in *Narrative of Le Moyne* (Boston, MA: James R. Osgood, 1875), p. 17.

21 Deborah E. Harkness, 'Elizabethan London's Naturalists and the Work of John White', in Sloan (ed.), *European Visions, American Voices*, pp. 44–50, at pp. 44–7.

22 Verlyn Klinkenborg, 'Introduction', in *The Drake Manuscript* (London: André Deutsch, 1996), p. xvi.

23 *The Drake Manuscript*, p. 266.

24 *The Drake Manuscript*, pp. 265–7.

RAKÍOCK CANOES

1 Thomas Hariot, *A briefe and true report of the new found land of Virginia* (1590; STC 12786), 'To the gentle Reader'.

2 Hariot, *A briefe and true report*, p. 6.

3 Richard Hakluyt to Francis Walsingham, 7 January 1584, in Richard Hakluyt, *A particuler discourse concerninge the greate necessity and manifolde commodities*, ed. David B. Quinn and Alison M. Quinn (London: Hakluyt Society, 1993), pp. 197–8; Coll Thrush, *Indigenous London: Native Travellers to the Heart of Empire* (New Haven, CT: Yale University Press, 2016), pp. 33–5.

4 Thrush, *Indigenous London*; Michael Leroy Oberg, *The Head in Edward Nugent's Hand: Roanoke's Forgotten Indians* (Pennsylvania, PA: University of Pennsylvania Press, 2010), p. 58.

5 Oberg, *The Head in Edward Nugent's Hand*, p. 98; Meredith Hanmer, *The baptizing of a Turke* (1586; STC 12744).

6 Alden Vaughan, 'American Indians in England', *Oxford Dictionary of National Biography*, www.doi.org/10.1093/ref:odnb/71116 [accessed 3 July 2025].

7 Hariot, *A briefe and true report*, p. 30.

8 Samuel Purchas, *Purchas his pilgrimes* (1625; STC 20509), p. 1813.

9 Hariot, *A briefe and true report*, pp. 24, 27.

10 Hariot, *A briefe and true report*, 'On the chief Ladyes of Secota'.

11 Hariot, *A briefe and true report*, pp. 13, 15, 18–19.

12 Hariot, *A briefe and true report*, pp. 7–9, 11; Dawn Dove, 'In Order to Understand Thanksgiving, One Must Understand the Sacredness of the Gift', in Siobhan Senier (ed.), *Dawnland Voices: An Anthology of Indigenous Writing from New England* (Lincoln, NE: University of Nebraska Press, 2014), p. 527.

13 Arthur Barlowe, 'The first voyage made to the Coasts of America', 1584, in Henry S. Burrage (ed.), *Early English and French Voyages* (New York. NY: Charles Scribner, 1906), p. 229.

14 Barlowe, 'The first voyage made to the Coasts of America', p. 233.

15 Hariot, *A briefe and true report*, p. 23, and 'Their manner of fishynge in Virginia'.

16 John Smith, *The generall historie of Virginia, New England, and the Summer Isles* (1624; STC 22790), p. 10.

17 Smith, *The generall historie*, pp. 141–2.

18 Smith, *The generall historie*, p. 215.

19 Smith, *The generall historie*, p. 39.

20 Hariot, *A briefe and true report*, p. 23.

21 Hariot, *A briefe and true report*, pp. 16, 20, 25, 28, 31.

22 Peter Mancall, *Hakluyt's Promise: An Elizabethan's Obsession for an English America* (New Haven, CT: Yale University Press, 2007), p. 157; Thrush, *Indigenous London*, p. 58; Vaughan, 'American Indians in England'.

23 Sir John Davies to the Earl of Salisbury, 24 August 1609, Hatfield House, CP 127/133r.

AN AZTEC CODEX IN OXFORD

1 Daniela Bleichmar, 'History in Pictures: Translating the *Codex Mendoza*', *Art History*, 38:4 (2015), pp. 682–701; Samuel Purchas, *Purchas his pilgrimes* (1625; STC 20509), p. 1066. On the terms 'Aztec' and 'Mexica', including their overlaps and distinctions, see Caroline Dodds Pennock, *On Savage Shores: How Indigenous Americans Discovered Europe* (London: Weidenfeld & Nicolson, 2022), pp. xvi, 3–4. The use of 'Mexica' here partly raises attention to the linguistic world of Hakluyt's and Purchas's own works, which talk about 'Mexican' histories, at a time when 'Aztec' was not yet used to refer to Nahua peoples.

2 Stephen Parmenius, *De Navigatione* (1582), in Robert J. Barnett, 'New World Colonization and the *De Navigatione* of Stephen Parmenius', *Intertexts*, 1:2 (1997), pp. 159–68, at p. 160.

3 Purchas, *Purchas his pilgrimes*, p. 1066; Peter Mancall, *Hakluyt's Promise: An Elizabethan's Obsession for an English America* (New Haven, CT: Yale University Press, 2007). On the technique and artistry of Mesoamerican codices and the value of the Codex Mendoza, see also the work of Joanne Harwood.

4 On Aztec/Mexica warfare, see Caroline Dodds Pennock, 'A Warlike Culture? Religion and War in the Aztec World', *History and Anthropology*, 34:1 (2023), pp. 99–122.

5 Frances F. Berdan and Patricia Reiff Anawalt, *The Codex Mendoza, Vol. II* (Berkeley, CA: University of California Press, 1992), pp. 112–14; 'Codex Mendoza', *c.* early 1540s, Bodleian Library, Oxford, MS Arch. Selden. A.1, f. 46.

6 Florentine Codex, *c.*1577, book 8, f. 25. Translated in the *Digital Florentine Codex*, Getty Research Institute, www.florentinecodex.getty.edu/ [accessed 21 November 2025].

7 *Cantares Mexicanos: Songs of the Aztecs*, tr. John Bierhorst (Stanford, CA: Stanford University Press, 1985), songs 24, 40, 44.

8 Michel de Montaigne, 'Of Cannibals' and 'Of Coaches', in *Essays written in French by Michael Lord of Montaigne*, tr. John Florio (1613; STC 18042), pp. 104, 512–14.

9 Purchas, *Purchas his pilgrimes*, p. 30.

10 Pennock, *On Savage Shores*.

11 *Cantares Mexicanos*, Song 20; Caroline Dodds Pennock and Amanda Power, 'Globalizing Cosmologies', *Past & Present*, 238, Issue suppl_13 (2018), pp. 88–115.

12 Caroline Dodds Pennock, 'Aztecs Abroad? Uncovering the Early Indigenous Atlantic', *American Historical Association*, 125:3 (2020), pp. 787–814, at p. 793.

SILVER VESSELS AND PIECES OF EIGHT

1 'The Pilgrimage to Parnassus', in *Three Parnassus Plays (1598–1601)*, ed. J. B. Leishman (London: Ivor Nicholson & Watson, 1949), p. 124.

2 John Donne, 'On Love's Progress', in *The Complete Poems of John Donne*, ed. Robin Robbins (London: Routledge, 2013), p. 349.

3 'Notes of the West Indies' in Samuel Purchas, *Purchas his pilgrimes* (1625; STC 20509), p. 1420; Kris Lane, *Potosí: The Silver City That Changed the World* (Oakland, CA: University of California Press, 2019), pp. 1–2, 18.

4 Lane, *Potosí*; Allison Margaret Bigelow, *Mining Language: Racial Thinking, Indigenous Knowledge, and Colonial Metallurgy in the Early Modern Iberian World* (Durham, NC: University of North Carolina Press, 2020), pp. 242–3; Nicholas A. Robins and Nicole A. Hagan, 'Mercury Production and Use in Colonial Andean Silver Production: Emissions and Health Implications', *Environmental Health Perspectives*, 120:5 (2012), pp. 627–31; Danila Sokolov, 'Vulcan's Gold: Poetic Metallurgy in the English Renaissance', *Modern Philology*, 121:3 (2024), pp. 272–95, quoted at p. 283.

5 Glyn Redworth, 'Philip I of England, Embezzlement, and the Quantity Theory of Money', *Economic History Review*, 55:2 (2002), pp. 248–61; Christopher Heaney, 'Marrying Utopia: Mary and Philip, Richard Eden, and the English Alchemy of Spanish Peru', in Jorge Cañizares-Esguerra (ed.), *Entangled Empires: The Anglo-Iberian Atlantic, 1500–1800* (Philadelphia, PA: University of Pennsylvania Press, 2018), pp. 85–104, at p. 94.

6 Lane, *Potosí*; Raphael Holinshed, *The first volume of the chronicles of England, Scotlande, and Irelande* (1577; STC 13568b), p. 117; 'Account of Spanish monies', 23 May 1572, National Archives, SP 70/123, f. 154.

7 'Account of Spanish monies', f. 154.

8 Peter Bakewell, 'Technological Change in Potosí: The Silver Boom of the 1570s', in Peter Bakewell (ed.), *Mines of Silver and Gold in the Americas* (London: Routledge, 1997), pp. 79–95, at p. 75; Petition of George Barkworth to Secretary [Robert] Cecil, 1598, The National Archives, SP 12/269, f. 52.

9 Philip Nichols, *Sir Francis Drake revived* (1626; STC 18544); Robert C. Schwaller (ed.), *African Maroons in Sixteenth-Century Panama: A History in Documents* (Norman, OK: University of Oklahoma Press, 2021).

10 'The Cabildo of Panama to the Crown, February 24, 1573', and 'Cristóbal Monte's Report on Drake's April Raid (1573)', in *African Maroons in Sixteenth-Century Panama*, pp. 112–13, 117.

11 'Robos y daños que hacían los corsarios ingleses en Indias', 1575, General Archive of the Indies, Seville, PATRONATO,265,R.25; 'Disposiciones que tomaban los ingleses para ir a América', 1573, General Archive of the Indies, PATRONATO,265,R.21; 'Devolución de bienes robados por los ingleses: Tierra Firme', 1570, PATRONATO,265,R.14.

12 Nicholas Quemerforde, Alderman of Waterford, to Secretary Fenton, 7 November 1586, National Archives, SP 63/126, f. 202.

13 Purchas, *Purchas his pilgrimes*, p. 603; 'Memorandum of the weight and value of bullion in silver and gold brought from the Indies', 7 June 1596, National Archives, SP 12/259, f. 28.

14 'The Queen to the Officers of the Exchequer', October 1602, National Archives, SP 12/285, f. 81.

15 Addenda 1591, 23 Dec 1591, 'A Discourse of the Indies', in W. Noel Sainsbury (ed.), *Calendar of State Papers: Colonial, America, and West Indies: Vol. 9, 1675–1676 and Addenda 1574–1674* (London: Her Majesty's Stationery Office, 1893), pp. 28–40; Peter Bakewell, 'Notes on the Mexican Silver Mining Industry in the 1590s', in Bakewell (ed.), *Mines of Silver and Gold*, pp. 171–97, at pp. 171–2.

16 'A discourse written by one *Miles Philips* Englishman', in Richard Hakluyt, *The principal navigations, voyages, traffiques and discoveries of the English nation* (1599–1600; STC 12626a), p. 479.

17 'A discourse written by one *Miles Philips*', pp. 470, 481.

18 'A discourse written by one *Miles Philips*', pp. 481–4.

19 *By the King a proclamation against the uttering of light Spanish silver coine* (1613; STC 8485).

20 Francis Fletcher, *The world encompassed by Sir Francis Drake* (1628; STC 7161), p. 3; Jemma Field, *Anna of Denmark: The Visual and Material Culture of the Stuart Courts, 1589–1619* (Manchester: Manchester University Press, 2020), p. 92.

21 Robert Lewes, *The merchants mappe of commerce* (1638; STC 21094), p. 63.

22 Pippa Shirley, 'Mannerism', in Philippa Glanville (ed.), *Silver* (London: V&A, 1996), pp. 24–7.

23 'Rare 16th Century Ewer and Basin Acquired for the Nation', National Museums Scotland, 1 November 2023, https://media.nms.ac.uk/news/rare-16th-century-ewer-and-basin-acquired-for-the-nation [accessed 16 April 2024].

24 Annie-Marie Desaulty and Francis Albarede, 'Copper, Lead, and Silver Isotopes Solve a Major Economic Conundrum of Tudor and Early Stuart Europe', *Geology*, 41:2 (2013), pp. 135–8.

25 William Heath, 'The Goulden Arte, or, The Jewell House of Gemes', *c.*1603, British Library, Stowe 1071, f. 2r.ff., 44r–v.

26 Heath, 'The Goulden Arte', f. 48r.

27 Heath, 'The Goulden Arte', f. 2r.

28 Quoted in Sokolov, 'Vulcan's Gold', p. 283.

29 Jonathan Barth, *The Currency of Empire: Money and Power in Seventeenth-Century English America* (Ithaca, NY: Cornell University Press, 2021), p. 13.

30 John Beaumont, *The metamorphosis of tabacco* (1602; STC 1695), sig. Dv.

31 John Battie, *The merchants remonstrance* (1648; Wing B1158), p. 21.

32 William Vaughan, *The golden fleece* (1626; STC 24609), p. 9.

33 Battie, *The merchants remonstrance*, p. 23; Ben Jonson, *The staple of newes* (1631; STC 14753.5), p. 58; Charles Cotton, *The confinement a poem* (1679; Wing C6385), p. 56. On the effects of colonial extraction on Indigenous communities in the twenty-first century, see Joseph Zárate, *Wars of the Interior*, tr. Annie McDermott (London: Granta, 2021), pp. 61–72.

34 Beaumont, *The metamorphosis of tabacco*, sig. A3r; Vaughan, *The golden fleece*; Nathaniel Baxter, *Sir Philip Sydneys ouránia* (1606; STC 1598), sig. E3v.

35 Thomas Gage, *The English-American* (1648; Wing G109), p. 124.

'A GUIANA IDOLL OF GOLD & COPPER'

1 Nicholas J. Saunders, *The Peoples of the Caribbean: An Encyclopaedia of Caribbean Archaeology and Traditional Culture* (Santa Barbara, CA: ABC-CLIO, 2005), pp. xiv, 115.

2 Robert Blust, 'Tumbaga in Southeast Asia and South America', *Anthropos*, 87, no 4/6 (1992), pp. 443–57, at p. 443; Scott Fulton and Sylvia Keochakian, 'The Conservation of Tumbaga Metals from Panama at the Peabody Museum, Harvard University', *Objects Specialty Group Postprints*, 12 (2005), pp. 76–90, at p. 76.

3 Bartholomé de las Casas, *The Spanish colonies* (1583; STC 4739), sig. E4r.

4 Richard Hakluyt (tr.), *Divers voyages touching the discoverie of America* (1582; STC 12624), sigs. F3v–F4r.

5 'Inventory of ores, plans, MSS, jewels, &c found on the body of Sir Walter Ralegh, with note of their disposition, as delivered to the Lieutenant of the Tower, Sir Lew[is] Stukeley, or Sir Geo[rge] Calvert', 10 August 1618, National Archives, SP 14/98, f. 116r.

6 Richard Hakluyt, *A Discourse of Western Planting*, ed. Leonard Woods (Cambridge: Wilson, 1877), p. 67.

7 Joyce Lorimer, 'Introduction', in Joyce Lorimer (ed.), *English and Irish Settlement on the River Amazon* (London: Hakluyt Society, 1989).

8 Lorimer (ed.), *English and Irish Settlement on the River Amazon*, pp. 30–1.

9 William Davies, *A true relation of the travailes and most miserable captivitie of William Davies* (1614; STC 6365), sig. C3r.

10 Walter Ralegh, *The discoverie of the large, rich, and beautiful empire of Guiana* (1596; STC 20634), pp. 15–16.

11 Ralegh, *The discoverie*, p. 4.

12 Neil Whitehead, 'The Historical Anthropology of Text: The Interpretation of Ralegh's *Discoverie of Guiana*', *Current Anthropology*, 36:1 (1995), pp. 53–74, at p. 61.

13 Ralegh, *The discoverie*, pp. 93, 15–16.

14 Ralegh, *The discoverie*, p. 43.

15 Ralegh, *The discoverie*, pp. 7, 40, 46, 53, 48; on the interpreters in Guiana who assisted the English, see also Caroline Dodds Pennock, *On Savage Shores: How Indigenous Americans Discovered Europe* (London: Weidenfeld & Nicolson, 2022), pp. 108–11.

16 Ralegh, *The discoverie*, p. 56.

17 Ralegh, *The discoverie*, pp. 70, 80.

18 Ralegh, *The discoverie*, p. 80.

19 Peter Martyr, *The decades of the newe worlde of west India*, tr. Richard Eden (1555; STC 647), pp. 177, 204.

20 Ralegh, *The discoverie*, p. 80.

21 Manari Ushigua, 'Of the Forest', *Granta*, 153 (2020), p. 133.

22 Ralegh, *The discoverie*, pp. 81, 7.

23 Ralegh, *The discoverie*, p. 7.

24 *Triumphalia de victorri Elizabethae* (1589), quoted in Winfried Schleiner, '"Divina Virago": Queen Elizabeth as an Amazon', *Studies in Philology*, 75:2 (1978), pp. 163–80, at p. 171.

25 Ralegh, *The discoverie*, pp. 23–4.

26 Robert Harcourt, *A relation of a voyage to Guiana* (1613; STC 12754), p. 14; Alden T. Vaughan, *Transatlantic Encounters: American Indians in Britain, 1500–1776* (Cambridge: Cambridge University Press, 2006), p. 36.

27 [Francis Bacon], *A Declaration of the Demeanor and Cariage of Sir Walter Raleigh* (1618; STC 20652.5), p. 4.

28 Quoted in Vaughan, *Transatlantic Encounters*, p. 37.

29 Lorimer (ed.), *English and Irish Settlement on the River Amazon*, pp. 181, 192–8.

30 V. S. Naipaul, *The Loss of El Dorado: A Colonial History* (London: Picador, 2001), p. 91.

31 Harcourt, *A relation of a voyage to Guiana*, 'Preface'; Michael Drayton, *The second part, or a continuance of Poly-Olbion* (1622; STC 7229), p. 9.

32 Harcourt, *A relation of a voyage to Guiana*, p. 38 and 'Preface'.

33 Ralegh, *The discoverie*, 'To the Reader'.

34 Harcourt, *A relation of a voyage to Guiana*, p. 39.

BOY WITH A PEARL EARRING

1 John Donne, 'The Sun Rising', 'To his Mistress Going to Bed', and 'A Funeral Elegy', in *The Complete Poems of John Donne*, ed. Robin Robbins (London: Routledge, 2013), pp. 247, 328, 861.

2 Francis Lenton, *The young gallants whirligigg* (1629; STC 15467), p. 12.

3 Pliny the Elder, *The historie of the world* [tr. Philemon Holland] (1634; STC 20030), pp. 256–7.

4 Pliny, *The historie of the world*, pp. 254, 256.

5 José de Acosta, *The naturall and morall historie of the East and West Indies*, tr. E. G. (1604; STC 94), p. 252.

6 Molly A. Warsh, *American Baroque: Pearls and the Nature of Empire, 1492–1700* (Chapel Hill, NC: University of North Carolina Press, 2018), pp. 1, 7–8, 11.

7 Warsh, *American Baroque*, p. 55.

8 Imtiaz Habib, *Black Lives in the English Archives, 1500–1677: Imprints of the Invisible* (Aldershot: Ashgate, 2008), pp. 23–4.

9 'The Observations of Sir Richard Hawkins', in Samuel Purchas, *Purchas his pilgrimes* (1625; STC 20509), p. 1411.

10 'Account of pearls delivered to the Queen', 1586, National Archives, SP 46/17, f. 189.

11 Karen Raber, 'Chains of Pearls: Gender, Property, Identity' in Bella Mirabella (ed.), *Ornamentalism: The Art of Renaissance Accessories* (Ann Arbor, MI: University of Michigan Press, 2011), pp. 159–81, at p. 169.

12 Pierre de Bourdeille, quoted in Ana Howie, 'Materializing the Global: Textiles, Color, and Race in a Genoese Portrait by Anthony van Dyck', *Renaissance Quarterly*, 76:2 (2023), pp. 589–644, at p. 612.

13 'Spanish money brought to the Tower', May 1572, National Archives, SP 70/123, f. 185; 'Spoils on Spanish vessels', 25 April 1573, National Archives, SP 70/127, f. 53.

14 Thomas Hariot, *A briefe and true report of the new found land of Virginia* (1590; STC 12786), pp. 11–12.

15 Janet Ambers, Duncan Hook, and Antony Simpson, 'John White's Watercolours: Analysis of the Pigments', in Kim Sloan (ed.), *European Visions: American Voices* (London: British Museum, 2009), pp. 67–71, at p. 68.

16 Hariot, *A briefe and true report*, p. 30; Mark Nicholls (ed.), 'George Percy's "Trewe Relacyon": A Primary Source for the Jamestown Settlement', *The Virginia Magazine of History and Biography*, 113:3 (2005), pp. 212–75, at p. 245.

17 Florentine Codex, *c*.1577, book 8, f. 17r; book 11, f. 64v.

18 John Smith, *The generall historie of Virginia, New England, and the Summer Isles* (1624; STC 22790), pp. 3, 77; *Virginia richly valued*, tr. Richard Hakluyt (1609; STC 22938), sig. A3v.

19 John Bulwer, *Anthropometamorphosis* (1653; Wing B5461), p. 539.

20 Gerard Malynes, *Consuetudo, vel lex mercatoria* (1622; STC 17222), p. 78; 'The several sorts of Pearl with their names and prices, in Margarita, as also

what they are sold for in St Domingo', May 1585, National Archives, SP 12/178, f. 194; 'Spanish money brought to the Tower', May 1572, National Archives, SP 70/123, f. 185; 'Spoils on Spanish vessels', 25 April 1573, National Archives, SP 70/127, f. 53; 'Commission to Rich. Hawkins to attempt some enterprise with a ship, bark, and pinnace against the King of Spain', October 1593, National Archives, SP 12/245, f. 205; [Unknown] to Lord [Unknown], May 1596, National Archives, SP 12/257, f. 172.

21 Lewis Stucley [Stukley], *To the Kings most excellent Majestie* (1618; STC 23401), p. 8.

22 John Chamberlain to Sir Dudley Carleton, 1 August 1613, in W. Noel Sainsbury (ed.), *Calendar of State Papers: Colonial, Vol. I* (London: Her Majesty's Stationery Office, 1860), pp. 14–15.

23 Heather Miyano Kopelson, '"One Indian and a Negroe, the first thes Ilands ever had": Imagining the Archive in Early Bermuda', *Early American Studies*, 11:2 (2013), pp. 272–313.

24 *The Rich Papers: Letters from Bermuda, 1615–1646*, ed. Vernon A. Ives (Toronto: University of Toronto Press, 1984), p. 229; Kerry Apps, 'Enslavement in the English Atlantic World, 1616–1641' (unpublished MA thesis, Cambridge University, 2022), p. 85; Michael J. Jarvis, *In the Eye of All Trade: Bermuda, Bermudians, and the Maritime Atlantic World, 1680–1783* (Chapel Hill, NC: University of North Carolina Press, 2012), p. 27; Henry Earl of Northampton to the King, August 1612, in *Calendar of State Papers: Colonial, Vol. I*, p. 14.

25 Smith, *The generall historie*, p. 199; Apps, 'Enslavement in the English Atlantic World', p. 55.

26 Warsh, *American Baroque*, p. 251.

27 Quoted in Diana de Marly, *Fashion for Men: An Illustrated History* (New York, NY: Holmes & Meier, 1985), p. 46.

28 Molly Warsh, 'A Political Ecology in the Early Spanish Caribbean', *The William and Mary Quarterly*, 71:4 (2014), pp. 517–48, at p. 545.

29 Kevin Dawson, 'A Sea of Caribbean Islands: Maritime Maroons in the Greater Caribbean', *Slavery & Abolition*, 42:3 (2021), pp. 428–48, at pp. 431–2.

30 Walter Ralegh, *The discoverie of the large, rich, and beautiful empire of Guiana* (1596; STC 20634), p. 52.

FEATHERS AND FAKES

1 Nicholas Saunders to Robert Cecil, 30 June 1596, Hatfield House, CP 41/97.

2 Amy Buono, 'Crafts of Colour: Tupi Tapirage in Early Colonial Brazil', in Andrea Feeser, Maureen Daly Goggin, and Beth Fowkes Tobin (eds), *The*

Materiality of Colour: The Production, Circulation, and Application of Dyes and Pigments, 1400–1800* (Abingdon: Routledge, 2012), pp. 235–49, at p. 238.

3 Jessica O'Leary, 'The Uprooting of Indigenous Women's Horticultural Practices in Brazil, 1500–1650', *Past & Present*, 262:1 (2024), pp. 45–83, at pp. 53 (fn. 23), 46.

4 Amy J. Buono, 'Tupi Featherwork and the Dynamics of Intercultural Exchange in Early Modern Brazil', in Jaynie Anderson (ed.), *Crossing Cultures: Conflict, Migration, Convergence* (Melbourne: Melbourne University Press, 2009), pp. 349–55, at pp. 349–50; Carlos Fausto, 'Of Enemies and Pets: Warfare and Shamanism in Amazonia', *American Ethnologist*, 26:4 (2008), pp. 933–56; Nicholas J. Saunders, *The Peoples of the Caribbean: An Encyclopaedia of Caribbean Archaeology and Traditional Culture* (Santa Barbara, CA: ABC-CLIO, 2005), p. 2.

5 Quoted in Susanna Burghartz *et al.*, 'Introduction: Materializing Identities', in Susanna Burghartz *et al.* (eds), *Materialized Identities in Early Modern Culture, 1450–1750: Objects, Affects, Effects* (Amsterdam: Amsterdam University Press, 2021), p. 36.

6 Stefan Hanß, 'Material Encounters: Knotting Cultures in Early Modern Peru and Spain', *The Historical Journal*, 62:3 (2019), pp. 583–615.

7 Mary Wroth, *The Countesse of Mountgomeries Urania* (1621; STC 26051), pp. 461, 417, 497; Hanß, 'Material Encounters'; Stefan Hanß, 'The Material Creativity of Affective Artefacts in the Dutch Colonial World: Imaging and Imagining Early Modern Feather Fans', *Current Anthropology*, 65:2 (2024), pp. 196–234.

8 Thomas More, *Utopia*, ed. George M. Logan and Robert M. Adams (Cambridge: Cambridge University Press, 1989), p. 105.

9 Roger Barlow, *A brief summe of geography* (London: Hakluyt Society, 1932), pp. 151, 158, 161, 172.

10 Clements R. Markham (ed.), *The Hawkins' Voyages during the Reigns of Henry VIII, Queen Elizabeth, and James I* (London: Hakluyt Society, 1878), pp. 3–4.

11 Stuart Piggott, 'Brazilian Indians on an Elizabethan Monument', *Antiquity*, 38:150 (1964), pp. 134–6.

12 André Thevet, *The new found worlde, or Antarctike* [tr. Thomas Hacket?] (1568; STC 23950), pp. 39, 94.

13 Thevet, *The new found worlde*, pp. 116–17.

14 Buono, 'Crafts of Colour', p. 235.

15 Buono, 'Crafts of Colour', p. 238.

16 *Thomas Platter's Travels in England, 1599*, tr. and ed. Clare Williams (London: Jonathan Cape, 1937), pp. 171–3.

17 [Nehemiah Grew], *Musaeum regalis societatis* (1685; Wing G1952A), pp. 62, 373.

18 George Percy, 'Observations', p. 13; John Brereton, *A briefe and true relation of the discoverie of the north part of Virginia* (1602; STC 3611), p. 11; John Smith, *The generall historie of Virginia, New England, and the Summer Isles* (1624; STC 22790), p. 30; Buck W. Woodard, 'Degrees of Relatedness: The Social Politics of Algonquian Kinship in the Contact Era Chesapeake' (unpublished MA thesis, William & Mary, 2008), p. 69; William Wood, *New Englands prospect* (1634; STC 25957), p. 90.

19 Henry Peacham, *Minerva Britanna* (1612; STC 19511), p. 199.

20 Robert Greene, *Greenes, groats-worth of witte* (1592; STC 12245), sig. Fv.

21 Theodore de Bry, *America* (Cologne: Taschen, 2019), p. 311.

22 *The world encompassed by Sir Francis Drake* (1628; STC 7161), pp. 73–4.

23 J. Frederick Fausz, 'An "Abundance of Blood Shed on Both Sides": England's First Indian War, 1609–1614', *The Virginia Magazine of History and Biography*, 98:1 (1990), pp. 3–56, at p. 42.

24 Smith, *The generall historie*, p. 144; James I, *A counterblaste to tobacco* (1604; STC 14363), sigs. B2r, Cr.

25 'The Governor and Council of Virginia to the Earl of Southampton, and the rest of the Council', 3 April 1623, in W. Noel Sainsbury (ed.), *Calendar of State Papers: Colonial, Vol. I* (London: Her Majesty's Stationery Office, 1860), pp. 41–2.

26 Betty Booth Donohue, *Bradford's Indian Book: Being the True Roote & Rise of American Letters as Revealed by the Native Text Embedded in 'Of Plimoth Plantation'* (Gainesville, FL: University of Florida Press, 2011), pp. 17–18.

27 Donohue, *Bradford's Indian Book*, pp. 77–9.

28 Glicéria Tupinambá, 'An Indigenous Woman Troubling the Museum's Colonialist Legacy: Conversation with Glicéria Tupinambá' [interviewed by Bruno Brulon Soares], *Museum International*, 74:3–4 (2022), pp. 10–23, at p. 16.

29 George Chapman, *The memorable maske* (1613; STC 4981), sig. D4v.

30 [Nathaniel Butler], *The historye of the Bermudaes or Summer Islands*, ed. J. Henry Lefroy (Farnham: Ashgate, 2010), p. 196.

31 William Davenant, *The Cruelty of the Spaniards in Peru* (1658; Wing D321), pp. 1–2, 27.

32 George Abbot, *A briefe description of the whole world* (1664; Wing A62), p. 279; Aphra Behn, *Oroonoko and Other Writings*, ed. Paul Salzman (Oxford: Oxford University Press, 1994), p. 7; John Tradescant, *Musaeum Tradescantianum, or, A collection of rarities* (1656; Wing T2005), p. 51.

33 Thomas Baskerville to Robert Cecil, 8 May 1596, in *Calendar of the Manuscripts of the Most Honourable the Marquess of Salisbury, Part VI* (London: Her Majesty's Stationery Office, 1895), p. 173; also George Trenchard and Ralph Horsey to Robert Cecil, 31 July 1596, in *Calendar of the Manuscripts*, p. 300; Thomas West to Robert Cecil, 31 August 1595, in *Calendar of the Manuscripts*, p. 357.

34 Edmund Spenser, *The Faerie Queene*, ed. Thomas R. Roche (London: Penguin, 1987), p. 552.

35 Nicholas Saunders to Robert Cecil, 13 July 1596, Hatfield House, CP 42/40.

36 'The Letters of Lord Burghley, William Cecil, to his Son Robert Cecil, 1593–1598', *Camden Fifth Series*, 53 (2017), p. 234.

37 Jamille Pinheiro Dias, 'Environmental Thinking and Indigenous Arts in Brazil Today', *Journal of Latin American Cultural Studies*, 31:1 (2022), pp. 141–57, at p. 142.

38 Tupinambá, 'An Indigenous Woman Troubling the Museum's Colonialist Legacy', pp. 21–2.

COLOMBIAN EMERALDS IN THE CHEAPSIDE HOARD

1 Hazel Forsyth, *London's Lost Jewels: The Cheapside Hoard* (London: Museum of London, 2013), p. 136.

2 'The Cheapside Hoard', Museum of London, www.museumoflondon.org. uk/discover/cheapside-hoard-collection-focus [accessed 10 April 2024]; James Howell, *Londinopolis* (1657; Wing H3090), title page.

3 'Relación de Santa Marta', in J. Michael Francis (ed.), *Invading Colombia: Spanish Accounts of the Gonzalo Jiménez de Quesada Expedition of Conquest* (University Park, PA: Pennsylvania State University Press, 2007), p. 67.

4 Kris Lane, *Colour of Paradise: The Emerald in the Age of Gunpowder Empires* (New Haven, CT: Yale University Press, 2010), p. 28; Forsyth, *London's Lost Jewels*, p. 134; Brian Brazeal, 'The History of Emerald Mining in Colombia: An Examination of Spanish-Language Sources', *The Extractive Industries and Society*, 1:2 (2014), pp. 273–83, at p. 275.

5 Lane, *Colour of Paradise*, pp. 48–50; Ron Ringsrud, 'The Coscuez Mine: A Major Source of Colombian Emeralds', *Gems & Gemology*, 22 (summer 1986), pp. 67–79; Luis Duque Gómez et al., *Sweat of the Sun, Tears of the Moon: Gold and Emerald Treasures of Colombia* (Los Angeles, CA: Natural History Museum Alliance of Los Angeles County, 1981).

6 'Epítome de la conquista del Nuevo Reino de Granada', in Francis (ed.), *Invading Colombia*, p. 74.

7 Lane, *Colour of Paradise*, p. 52; 'Epítome de la conquista del Nuevo Reino de Granada', pp. 79–80.

8 Walter Ralegh, *The discoverie of the large, rich, and beautiful empire of Guiana* (1596; STC 20634), sig. A4v.

9 Lane, *Colour of Paradise*, pp. 53–62. On the revitalisation of historically invaded communities in Colombia, see Paola Andrea Sánchez-Castañeda, 'Memory in Sacred Places: The Revitalisation Process of the Muisca Community', *Urban Planning*, 5:3 (2020), pp. 263–73.

10 'Stuff delivered to the Lady Jane, usurper, at the Tower', [July] 1553, *Calendar of the Cecil Papers in Hatfield House, Vol. 1: 1306–1571* (London: Her Majesty's Stationery Office, 1883), pp. 120–34.

11 'Jewelry', 1530, National Archives, SP 1/58, f. 212; 'Royal Jewels', 6 October 1519, National Archives, SP 1/19, f. 42; 'Account of Jewels', 1527, National Archives, SP 1/46, f. 40; 'French news from Italy', 12 May 1540, National Archives, SP 1/160, f. 31.

12 Thomas Nichols, *A lapidary* (1652; Wing N1145), pp. 30, 99; George Frederick Kunz, *The Curious Lore of Precious Stones* (London: Dover, 1972), p. 28; Tom Blaen, '"Not used to be worn as a Jewel": The Wearing of Precious Stones in Early Modern England – Ornaments or Medicine?', *Geological Society*, 452 (2017), pp. 261–5, at pp. 261–3.

13 Pliny the Elder, *The historie of the world* [tr. Philemon Holland] (1634; STC 20030), pp. 611–12; Bruce R. Smith, *The Key of Green: Passion and Perception in Renaissance Culture* (Chicago, IL: University of Chicago Press, 2010), p. 64.

14 Francisco López de Gómara, *The pleasant historie of the conquest of the Weast India*, tr. Thomas Nicholas (1578; STC 16807), dedicatory epistle.

15 López de Gómara, *The pleasant historie of the conquest of the Weast India*, pp. 205, 363, 384.

16 'A discourse how Hir Majesty may annoy the King of Spayne', 6 November 1577, National Archives, SP 12/118, f. 30.

17 José de Acosta, *The naturall and morall historie of the East and West Indies*, tr. E. G. (1604; STC 94), 'To the Reader' and pp. 248–50.

18 Gerard Malynes, *Consuetudo, vel lex mercatoria* (1622; STC 17222), pp. 266–7; Samuel Chappuzeau, *The history of jewels* (1671; Wing C1959).

19 Bernardino de Mendoza to the King, 8 January 1581, *Calendar of State Papers, Spain, Vol. 3, 1580–1596*, ed. Martin A. S. Hume (London: Her Majesty's Stationery Office, 1896), pp. 71–82.

20 Lane, *Colour of Paradise*, pp. 66, 87–8.

21 'Observations of things most remarkable, collected out of the first part of the Commentaries Royall', in Samuel Purchas, *Purchas his pilgrimes* (1625; STC 20509), p. 1481.

22 Bartolomé de las Casas, 'A briefe Narration of the destruction of the *Indies* by the *Spaniards*', in Purchas, *Purchas his pilgrimes*, pp. 1591–2.

23 Daniel Packer, 'Jewels of "Blacknesse" at the Jacobean Court', *Journal of the Warburg and Courtauld Institutes*, 75:1 (2012), pp. 201–22, at p. 203; 'The value of a great looking glasse', January 1604, National Archives, SP 14/6, f. 21r; 'An Inventory of the Effects of Henry Howard', ed. Evelyn Philip Shirley, *Archaeologia*, 42 (1870), pp. 347–78, at p. 349; Memorial for Sec[retary] Windebank, January 1640, National Archives, SP 16/439, f. 28.

24 Francis Bacon, *Sylva sylvarum, or, A naturall historie* (1627; STC 1168), pp. 67, 258.

25 Packer, 'Jewels of "Blacknesse" at the Jacobean Court', pp. 2–3.

26 Quoted in Forsyth, *London's Lost Jewels*, p. 100; Lane, *Colour of Paradise*, pp. 11–12.

27 'List, by Sir Tho[ma]s Roe, of goods', March 1618, in W. Noel Sainsbury (ed.), *Calendar of State Papers: Colonial, East Indies, China and Japan, Vol. 3, 1617–1621* (London: Longman, 1870), pp. 145–6.

28 Lane, *Colour of Paradise*, p. 7.

29 Chappuzeau, *The history of jewels*, sigs. A2r–v, A6r; Forsyth, *London's Lost Jewels*, p. 156.

30 Forsyth, *London's Lost Jewels*, pp. 105–27; Lane, *Colour of Paradise*, p. 121.

31 Lane, *Colour of Paradise*, pp. 121–2; 'Court Minutes: 16 January 1633', in W. Noel Sainsbury (ed.), *Calendar of State Papers: Colonial, East Indies and Persia, Vol. 8, 1630–1634* (London: Her Majesty's Stationery Office, 1892), pp. 339–50.

32 Warwick Bray, 'The Lost Emerald Mines of Ecuador: Contrasting Patterns of Emerald Use in Native South America', *Andean Past*, 13 (2022), pp. 75–107, at p. 91.

33 Carlie Porterfield, 'Ring with Emerald Recovered from 400-Year-Old Shipwreck Raises $1.2 Million for Ukraine at Auction', *Forbes*, 8 December 2022, www.forbes.com/sites/carlieporterfield/2022/12/08/ring-with-emerald-recovered-from-400-year-old-shipwreck-raises-12-million-for-ukraine-at-auction/ [accessed 18 April 2024].

34 Luke Taylor, 'Bolivian Indigenous groups assert claim to treasure of "holy grail of shipwrecks"', *Guardian*, 29 March 2024, www.theguardian.com/environment/2024/mar/29/bolivia-shipwreck-colombia-treasure [accessed 13 August 2025]; Ruth Lopez, 'International Scrap Over Treasure', *Art Newspaper*, 10 January 2024, www.theartnewspaper.com/2024/01/10/international-scrap-over-treasure-laden-spanish-galleon-that-sunk-off-the-colombian-coast-in-1708 [accessed 17 April 2024].

35 Barten Holyday, *A survey of the world in ten books* (Oxford, 1661; Wing H2533), p. 9.

A GOLD MINE AT WHITEHALL PALACE

1 George Chapman, *The memorable maske* (1613; STC 4981), sig. A4r.

2 George Chapman, 'De Guiana, carmen Epicum', in Lawrence Kemys, *A relation of the second voyage to Guiana* (1596; STC 14947), sig. A4v.

3 Daniel Price, *Prince Henry his first anniversary* (1613; STC 20299), p. 4.

4 Thomas Campion, *Songs of mourning bewailing the untimely death of Prince Henry* (1613; STC 4546), sig. Av.

5 *The last terrible tempestious windes and weather* (1613; STC 25840), sig. C3r.

6 *The wonders of this windie winter* (1613; STC 25949), sig. A3r.

7 W. R. Streitberger, *The Master of the Revels and Elizabeth I's Court Theatre* (Oxford: Oxford University Press, 2016), p. 29.

8 Patricia Crouch, 'Patronage and Competing Visions of Virginia in George Chapman's *The Memorable Masque* (1613)', *English Literary Renaissance*, 40:3 (2010), pp. 393–426, at p. 398; 'Virginia Company of London', *Encyclopedia Virginia*, www.encyclopediavirginia.org/entries/virginia-company-of-london/ [accessed 7 August 2025].

9 Chapman, *The memorable maske*, sigs. Ar–A2r.

10 Chapman, *The memorable maske*, sig. Av.

11 Thomas Middleton, *The triumphs of truth* (1613; STC 17903), sig. B4v.

12 Antonio Foscarini to the Doge and Senate, 10 May 1613, in H. F. Brown (ed.), *Calendar of State Papers Relating to English Affairs in the Archives of Venice, Vol. 12, 1610–1613* (London: His Majesty's Stationery Office, 1905), pp. 529–45.

13 Imtiaz Habib, *Black Lives in the English Archives, 1500–1677: Imprints of the Invisible* (Aldershot: Ashgate, 2008), pp. 333, 336–7.

14 *Thomas Platter's Travels in England, 1599*, tr. and ed. Clare Williams (London: Jonathan Cape, 1937), pp. 163–4.

15 Album amicorum of Michael van Meer, 1614–1617, Edinburgh University Library, La.III.283, f. 254v; Stephanie Pratt, 'Truth and Artifice in the Visualization of Native Peoples: From the Time of John White to the Beginnings of the 18th Century', in Kim Sloan (ed.), *European Visions: American Voices* (London: British Museum, 2009), p. 6.

16 Foscarini to the Doge and Senate, 10 May 1613, p. 532.

17 Chapman, *The memorable maske*, sigs. B3r–Dr.

18 Chapman, *The memorable maske*, sigs. A2r, D2r.

19 Chapman, *The memorable maske*, sig. D4v.

20 Chapman, *The memorable maske*, sigs. E2r, E4r–Fr.

21 *The order and solemnitie of the creation of the High and mightie Prince Henry* (1610; STC 13161), sig. F3v.

22 Alden T. Vaughan, *Transatlantic Encounters: American Indians in Britain, 1500–1776* (Cambridge: Cambridge University Press, 2006), pp. 60–1; James Rosier, *A true relation of the most prosperous voyage* (1605; STC 21322), sig. C3r.

23 Vaughan, *Transatlantic Encounters*, pp. 65–6.

24 See stories by John Bear Mitchell (Penobscot Nation), including 'Tribes and their Interactions with the Ship Builders', *Maine's First Ship*, 7 July 2022, www.mfship.org/wabanaki-center/ [accessed 21 November 2025], and 'Rediscovering the Story in Ourselves', *Metcalfe Institute of Rhode Island*, 21 October 2023, www.youtube.com/watch?v=W2TL5Y3LkLc [accessed 23 October 2024]; Harald E. L. Prins and Bunny McBride, *Asticou's Island Domain: Wabanaki Peoples at Mount Desert Island, 1500–2000* (National Parks Service, 2007).

25 *Collections of the Massachusetts Historical Society, Vol. VI* (Boston, MA: American Stationers' Company, 1837), pp. 59–60.

26 John Smith, *The generall historie of Virginia, New England, and the Summer Isles* (1624; STC 22790), p. 204.

27 'Device, n.', *Oxford English Dictionary*; Anthony Munday, *Chrusothriambos: The triumphes of gold* (1611; STC 18267), sig. A3v.

28 Walter Hamond, *A paradox* (1640; STC 12735), sigs. D2v–D3r.

TOBACCO LEAVES AND LAUREL CROWNS

1 Edmund Gardiner, *The trial of tabacco* (1610; STC 11564), p. 5.

2 Thomas Hariot, *A briefe and true report of the new found land of Virginia* (1590; STC 12786), p. 16.

3 Quoted in Dane T. Magoon, 'Chesapeake Pipes and Uncritical Assumptions: A View from Northeastern North Carolina', *North Carolina Archaeology*, 48 (1999), pp. 107–26, at pp. 120–1; Hariot, *A briefe and true report*, p. 16.

4 William Strachey, 'The historie of travaile into Virginia Britannia', *c.*1612, British Library, Sloane MS 1622, ff. 102r–105r; Kevin P. Groark, 'The Angel in the Gourd: Ritual, Therapeutic, and Protective Uses of Tobacco (*Nicotiana tabacum*) among the Tzeltal and Tzotzil Maya of Chiapas, Mexico', *Journal of Ethnobiology*, 30:1 (2010), pp. 5–30; Marcy Norton, *Sacred Gifts, Profane Pleasures: A History of Tobacco and Chocolate in the Atlantic World* (Ithaca, NY: Cornell University Press, 2008).

5 Nicolás Monardes, *Joyfull newes out of the newfound world* [tr. John Frampton] (1577; STC 18006), sigs. Jv, J3v; John Cotta, *A short discoverie of the unobserved dangers of several sorts of ignorant and inconsiderate*

practisers of physicke (1612; STC 5833), p. 5; Anthony Chute, [*Tabacco*] (1595; STC 5262.5), pp. 46–9; John Bonoeil, *His Majesties gracious letter to the Earle of South-Hampton* (1622; STC 14378), p. 61.

6 *Poems, by J[ohn]. D[onne]* (1633; STC 7045), sigs. Tt3r, Tt4v; *Thomas Platter's Travels in England, 1599*, tr. and ed. Clare Williams (London: Jonathan Cape, 1937), pp. 170–1.

7 Barten Holyday, *Technogamia* (1618; STC 13617), sig. D3r.

8 Thomas Middleton and Thomas Dekker, *The roaring girle* (1611; STC 17908), sig. C3r.

9 *Thomas Platter's Travels*, p. 171; Thomas Dekker, *The guls horne-booke* (1609; STC 6500), sig. Er.

10 C. T., *An advice how to plant tobacco in England* (London, 1615; STC 23612), sig. A4v.

11 John Beaumont, *The metamorphosis of tabacco* (1602; STC 1695), sig. Bv.

12 *The poeticall essayes of Sam. Danyel* (1599; STC 6261), sig. F2v.

13 James I, *A counterblaste to tobacco* (1604; STC 14363), sig. B2r.

14 James I, *A counterblaste to tobacco*, sigs. C4v, Cr.

15 John Deacon, *Tobacco tortured* (1616; STC 6436), sigs. Cc2r–v.

16 Linwood 'Little Bear' Custalow and Angela 'Silver Star' Daniel, *The True Story of Pocahontas: The Other Side of History* (Golden, CO: Fulcrum, 2007), pp. 73–5; 'Tobacco trade', 18 April 1621, quoted in Lauren Working, *The Making of an Imperial Polity: Civility and America in the Jacobean Metropolis* (Cambridge: Cambridge University Press, 2020), p. 152.

17 'A report of S[i]r George Yeardleys going Governor to Virginia', 5 December 1618, Ferrar Papers, FP 93.

18 Raphael Thorius, *Hymnus tabaci*, tr. Peter Hausted (London, 1651; Wing T1040), sig. A7r.

19 Richard Brathwaite, *A solemne joviall disputation* (1617; STC 3585), p. 179; Josuah [Joshua] Sylvester, *Tobacco battered, & the pipes shattered* (1616; STC 23582a), pp. 86, 90.

20 Megan Peiser, 'Citing Seeds, Citing People: Bibliography and Indigenous Memory, Relations, and Living Knowledge-Keepers', *Criticism*, 64 (2022), pp. 521–31, at p. 526; Raglan Maddox *et al.*, 'Reflections on Indigenous Commercial Tobacco Control: "The dolphins will always take us home"', *Tobacco Control*, 31:2 (2022), pp. 348–51, at p. 348.

DUCHESSES AND PRETTY PAMPHLETS

1 Peter Mason, 'André Thevet, Pierre Belon and *Americana* in the Embroideries of Mary Queen of Scots', *Journal of the Warburg and*

Courtauld Institutes, 78:1 (2015), pp. 207–21; Peter Mason, 'Mary's Armadillo', in Mark Thurner and Juan Pimentel (eds), *New World Objects of Knowledge* (London: University of London Press, 2021) [online edition].

2 Richard Eden and Richard Willes, *The history of travayle in the West and East Indies* (1577; STC 649), 'The Epistle Dedicatory'.

3 Eden and Willes, *The history of travayle*, p. 236.

4 Eden and Willes, *The history of travayle*, sigs. A4r, T3r.

5 Eden and Willes, *The history of travayle*, sig. V2r.

6 Sylvester Jourdain, *A discovery of the Barmudas* (1610; STC 14816), p. 8; *The Tempest*, Act I, sc. ii, 229.

7 William Strachey, 'True repertory', in Louis B. Wright (ed.), *A Voyage to Virginia in 1609: Two Narratives* (Charlottesville, VA: University of Virginia Press, 2013), pp. 3, 14, 16, 37.

8 Strachey, 'True repertory', pp. 65–6.

9 George Best, *A true discourse of the late voyages of discoverie* (1578; STC 1972), p. 51.

10 *The Earl of Stirling's Register of Royal Letters Relative to the Affairs of Scotland and Nova Scotia from 1615 to 1635,* Vol. I (Edinburgh: Printed for Private Circulation, 1885), p. xxxii.

11 *The Earl of Stirling's Register*, p. xxxii.

12 Nathaniel Brent to [Dudley] Carleton, 7 February 1618, National Archives, SP 14/96, f. 25.

13 Walter Ralegh to the queen, [1611], National Archives, SP 14/67, f. 196.

14 '[Unknown] to the queen, 1610', in G. Dyfnallt Owen (ed.), *Calendar of the Manuscripts of the Most Honourable the Marquis of Salisbury, Vol. 21: 1609–1612* (London: His Majesty's Stationery Office, 1970), p. 276.

15 John Gilbert to Robert Cecil, 27 April 1596, in Owen (ed.), *Calendar of the Cecil Papers: Vol. 6*, pp. 155–64.

16 Misha Ewen, *The Virginia Venture: American Colonization and English Society, 1580–1660* (Philadelphia, PA: University of Pennsylvania Press, 2022), pp. 45–7.

17 John Smith, *The generall historie of Virginia, New England, and the Summer Isles* (1624; STC 22790), 'To the Illustrious and Most Noble Princesse'.

18 *Henry VIII*, Act V, sc. iv, 31–3.

19 Smith, *The generall historie*, p. 122.

20 Karenne Wood, 'Amonute, 1617', in Kathryn N. Gray and Amy M. E. Morris (eds), *Matoaka, Pocahontas, Rebecca: Her Atlantic Identities and Afterlives* (Charlottesville, VA: University of Virginia Press, 2024), p. xv.

21 [Nathaniel Butler], *The historye of the Bermudaes or Summer Islands*, ed. J. Henry Lefroy (Farnham: Ashgate, 2010), p. 282; Alden T. Vaughan, *Transatlantic Encounters: American Indians in Britain, 1500–1776* (Cambridge: Cambridge University Press, 2006), p. 93.

22 William Camden, *Annales* (1625; STC 4497), p. 426.

23 Walter Ralegh, *The discoverie of the large, rich, and beautiful empire of Guiana* (1596; STC 20634), p. 52.

24 Saidiya Hartman, 'Venus in Two Acts', *Small Axe*, 12:2 (2008), pp. 13–14.

25 Robin Wall Kimmerer, *Braiding Sweetgrass: Indigenous Wisdom, Scientific Knowledge, and the Teachings of Plants* (Minneapolis, MN: Milkweed Editions, 2013), pp. 6–7, 50; Isabel Altamirano-Jiménez and Nathalie Kermoal, 'Introduction', in Nathalie Kermoal and Isabel Altamirano-Jiménez (eds), *Living on the Land: Indigenous Women's Understanding of Place* (Alberta: Athabasca University Press, 2016), pp. 10–12.

26 Robert Wilkinson, *The merchant royal* (1607; STC 25657).

27 Margaret Cavendish, *Poems and Fancies* (1653; Wing N869), p. 164.

28 Margaret Cavendish, *The Blazing World and Other Writings*, ed. Kate Lilley (London: Penguin, 1994), p. 47.

29 Cavendish, *The Blazing World and Other Writings*, p. 223.

30 Cavendish, *The Blazing World and Other Writings*, p. 124.

31 Anne Bradstreet, *Tenth muse lately sprung up in America* (1678; Wing B4166), p. 16; Lucy Munro, 'Frances and Judith: Parallel Lives', *Engendering the Stage*, https://engenderingthestage.humanities.mcmaster.ca/2022/06/07/frances-and-judith-parallel-lives-2/ [accessed 5 December 2024].

32 Aphra Behn, *Oroonoko* (1688; Wing B1749), p. 5.

33 John Tradescant, *Musaeum Tradescantianum, or, A collection of rarities* (1656; Wing T2005), pp. 47–51; Tara Prindle, 'Porcupine quillwork and hair', *Native Tech: Native American Technology and Art*, www.nativetech.org/quill/index.php [accessed 10 May 2025].

34 William Morrell, *New-England, Or, A briefe enarration* (1625; STC 18169), p. 21.

35 William Wood, *New Englands prospect* (1634; STC 25957), p. 96.

36 Cristina L. Azocar and Ivana Markova, 'Pocahontas Chic', in Gray and Morris (eds), *Matoaka, Pocahontas, Rebecca*, pp. 204–23, at p. 213; Chloe Wigston Smith, *Needlework and Empire: Material Entanglements in the Eighteenth-Century Atlantic World* (New Haven, CT: Yale University Press, 2024), p. 108.

37 Margaret Cavendish, *The worlds olio* (1655; Wing N873), 'The Preface to the Reader'.

38 Kimmerer, *Braiding Sweetgrass*, p. 256.

FROM THE ARK

1 Caroline Grigson, *Menagerie: The History of Exotic Animals in England* (Oxford: Oxford University Press, 2016), pp. 8–9.

2 Grigson, *Menagerie*, p. 10.

3 *The Jew of Malta*, Act I, sc. i, 37.

4 Grigson, *Menagerie*, pp. 18, 23.

5 John Gilbert to Robert Cecil, 16 March 1596, in R. A. Roberts (ed.), *Calendar of the Cecil Papers in Hatfield House: Vol. 6, 1595* (London: Her Majesty's Stationery Office, 1895), p. 99.

6 Marcy Norton, 'Going to the Birds: Animals as Things and Beings in Early Modernity' in Paula Findlen (ed.), *Early Modern Things: Objects and their Histories, 1500–1800* (London: Routledge, 2021), pp. 51–81, at pp. 64, 69–70; José Barreiro, *Taíno: A Novel*, 3rd edn (Wheat Ridge, CO: Fulcrum, 2023), p. 127.

7 Richard Flecknoe, *A relation of ten years in Europe, Asia, Affrique, and America* (1656; Wing F1232), p. 73.

8 Norton, 'Going to the Birds', p. 70; Bruce Thomas Boehrer, *Animal Characters: Nonhuman Beings in Early Modern Literature* (Philadelphia, PA: University of Pennsylvania Press, 2010).

9 Grigson, *Menagerie*, p. 24; Boehrer, *Animal Characters*, pp. 81–2.

10 Henry, Earl of Southampton, to Earl of Salisbury, 15 December 1609, National Archives, SP 14/50, f. 130.

11 Fabienne Pigière *et al.*, 'New Archaeozoological Evidence for the Introduction of the Guinea Pig to Europe', *Journal of Archaeological Science*, 39:4 (2012), pp. 1020–24, at p. 1021.

12 Susan D. deFrance, 'Guinea Pigs in the Spanish Colonial Andes: Culinary and Ritual Transformations', *International Journal of Historical Archaeology*, 25:1 (2021), pp. 116–43.

13 John Crouch, *Flowers strowed by the muses* (1662; Wing C7298), p. 11.

14 Grigson, *Menagerie*, p. 10; Susan E. James and Katlijne van der Stighelen, 'New Discoveries Concerning the Portrait of the Family of William Brooke, 10th Lord Cobham', *Dutch Crossing*, 23:1 (1999), pp. 66–101, at pp. 85–6.

15 William Harrison, *The Description of England*, ed. Georges Edelen (Ithaca, NY: Cornell University Press, 1968), p. 129; Fynes Moryson, *An itinerary* (1617; STC 18205), p. 150.

16 John Parkinson, *Paradisi in sole paradisus terrestris* (1629; STC 19300), pp. 518, 296.

17 Boehrer, *Animal Characters*, pp. 141–4. On the turkey's possible religious symbolism, as in the Puritan William Strickland's choice to put a turkey

on his family's coat of arms in 1550, see Adrian Green, *Boynton Hall Simply Told* (Richard Marriott Trust: n.p., 2025), pp. 23, 80.

18 Jemma Field, *Anna of Denmark: The Visual and Material Culture of the Stuart Courts, 1589–1619* (Manchester: Manchester University Press, 2020), pp. 93, 104; John Fletcher, *The night-walker* (1640; STC 11072), sig. B2v.

19 Marjorie Swann, *Curiosities and Texts: The Culture of Collecting in Early Modern England* (Philadelphia, PA: University of Pennsylvania Press, 2001), p. 2.

20 'Account of payments made by Endymion Porter at command of his Lord [the Marquis of Buckingham]', 1620, National Archives, SP 15/42, ff. 73v–74r.

21 Quoted in Grigson, *Menagerie*, p. 22.

22 Quoted in Graham Perry, *The Golden Age Restor'd: The Culture of the Stuart Court, 1603–42* (Manchester: Manchester University Press, 1981), p. 137.

23 John Tradescant to Edward Nicholas, 31 July 1625, National Archives, SP 16/4, f. 226.

24 15 May 1626, *Journal of the House of Lords, Vol. 3, 1620–1628* (London: His Majesty's Stationery Office, 1802), pp. 618–27.

25 Vera Keller, 'The "framing of a new world": Sir Balthazar Gerbier's "Project for Establishing a New State in America", c.1649', *The William and Mary Quarterly*, 70:1 (2013), pp. 147–76, at p. 154; John C. Appleby, 'An Association for the West Indies? English Plans for a West India Company, 1621–29', *The Journal of Imperial and Commonwealth History*, 15:3 (1987), pp. 213–41, at pp. 219–22.

26 Examination of Elizabeth Done, 11 October 1628, National Archives, SP 16/118, f. 54v.

27 John Wesley Murray Lee (ed.), *The Calvert Papers, Vol. I* (Baltimore, MD: Murphy, 1889), pp. 11–12.

28 Leonard Calvert to Cecil Calvert, 25 April 1638, in Lee (ed.), *The Calvert Papers, Vol. I*, p. 193; John Lewger to Lord Baltimore, 5 January 1639, in Lee (ed.), *The Calvert Papers, Vol. I*, p. 198.

29 *A relation of the successefull beginnings of the Lord Baltemore's plantation in Mary-land* (1634; STC 4371), pp. 2–5.

30 'The Haudenosaunee Creation Story', *Oneida Indian Nation*, www.oneidaindiannation.com/the-haudenosaunee-creation-story/ [accessed 14 August 2025].

31 Norton, 'Going to the Birds', pp. 62–3, 67; Melissa Marie Legge and Margaret Robinson, 'Animals in Indigenous Spiritualities: Implications for Critical Social Work', *Journal of Indigenous Social Development*, 6:1 (2017), pp. 1–20, at p. 9.

32 Manari Ushigua, 'Of the Forest', *Granta*, 153 (2020), p. 129.

33 Norton, 'Going to the Birds', pp. 72–3.

34 Legge and Robinson, 'Animals in Indigenous Spiritualities', p. 8.

35 *A relation of the successefull beginnings*, p. 4.

36 George Chapman, 'In Sejanum Ben Jonson', in Ben Jonson, *Sejanus his fall* (1605; STC 14782), sig. A4; William Bullock, *Virginia impartially examined* (1649; Wing B5428), p. 56.

37 A. M. Williams (ed.), *Conversations at Little Gidding: 'On the Retirement of Charles V' and 'On the Austere Life'* (Cambridge: Cambridge University Press, 1970), pp. 71–2.

38 Quoted in Beverly A. Straube, 'Incorporating the Other: A Seventeenth-Century Virginia Indian Basket Rendered in Clay', *Chipstone*, 2011, www.chipstone.org/article.php/488/Ceramics-in-America-2011/Incorporating-the-Other:-A-Seventeenth-Century-Virginia-Indian-Basket-Rendered-in-Clay [accessed 2 August 2024].

PORTRAIT OF A LADY IN A BEAVER HAT

1 Ben Jonson, *The fountaine of selfe-love, Or, Cynthias revels* (1601; STC 14773), sig. C3v.

2 Heidi Bohaker, '"Nindoodemag": The Significance of Algonquian Kinship Networks in the Eastern Great Lakes Region, 1600–1701', *The William and Mary Quarterly*, 63:1 (2006), pp. 23–52, at pp. 32–9; Megan Bang *et al.*, 'Muskrat Theories, Tobacco in the Streets, and Living in Chicago as Indigenous Land', *Environmental Education Research*, 20:1 (2014), pp. 37–55; Leanne Betasamosake Simpson, *A Short History of the Blockade: Giant Beavers, Diplomacy, and Regeneration in Nishnaabewin* (Edmonton: University of Alberta Press, 2021).

3 Walter Cary, *The present state of England expressed in this paradox* (1626; STC 4734), pp. 10–12.

4 Quoted in John C. Appleby, *Fur, Fashion and Transatlantic Trade During the Seventeenth Century: Chesapeake Bay Native Hunters, Colonial Rivalries and London Merchants* (Woodbridge: Boydell and Brewer, 2021); Ann M. Carlos and Frank D. Lewis, *Commerce by a Frozen Sea: Native Americans and the European Fur Trade* (Philadelphia, PA: University of Pennsylvania Press, 2010).

5 Henry Fleet, 'A Brief Journal of a Voyage', in Edward D. Neill (ed.), *The Founders of Maryland as Portrayed in Manuscripts, Provincial Records and Early Documents* (Albany, NJ: Munsell, 1876), pp. 16, 28–37; Appleby, *Fur, Fashion and Transatlantic Trade*, pp. 86–7.

6 *A treatise of New England published in anno. Dom. 1637* (1645; STC T2092A), p. 5; William Wood, *New Englands prospect* (1634; STC 25957), pp. 19, 25.

7 A book of receipts and expenditures of William Petre, 1597–1610, Folger Shakespeare Library, MS V.a.334, ff. 79r, 96r, 123v; Barten Holyday, *Technogamia* (1618; STC 13617); Susan E. Whyman, *Sociability and Power in Late Stuart England: The Cultural Worlds of the Verneys, 1660–1720* (Oxford: Oxford University Press, 2002), p. 51; *By the King a proclamation for the better encouragement, and advancement of the trade of the East-Indie Companie* (1632; STC 8985).

8 *The king of Denmarkes welcome* (1606; STC 5194), p. 11; Francis Lenton, *The young gallants whirligigg* (1629; STC 15467), p. 12.

9 Appleby, *Fur, Fashion and Transatlantic Trade*, pp. 37–40; Carlos and Lewis, *Commerce by a Frozen Sea*, p. 18; *The great frost* (1608; STC 11403).

10 I. H., *The house of correction* (1619; STC 12572), sig. Br; John Cooke, *Greenes Tu quoque, or, The cittie gallant* (1614; STC 5673), sig. Kv.

11 Petition of Robert Lewis and Richard Blower, 18 July 1636, National Archives, SP 16/323, f. 26v; W. Noel Sainsbury (ed.), *Calendar of State Papers: Colonial, Vol. I* (London: Her Majesty's Stationery Office, 1860), pp. 112–14.

12 Wood, *New Englands prospect*, p. 26.

13 Ferdinando Gorges, *America painted to the life* (1628; Wing G1300), pp. 37, 208.

14 William Bradford, *Of Plymouth Plantation, 1620–1647: The Complete Text*, ed. Samuel Eliot Morison (New York, NY: Knopf, 1952), pp. 80, 94, 176, 260.

15 Betty Booth Donohue, *Bradford's Indian Book: Being the True Roote & Rise of American Letters as Revealed by the Native Text Embedded in 'Of Plimoth Plantation'* (Gainesville, FL: University of Florida Press, 2011), pp. 75–6.

16 Bradford, *Of Plymouth Plantation*, pp. 205–6.

17 Thomas Morton, *New English Canaan* (1637; STC 18202), pp. 41, 97, 153–4; see the On the Wampum Trail project, www.wampumtrail. wordpress.com [accessed 4 April 2024].

18 Wood, *New Englands prospect*, pp. 61, 70, 90.

19 Richard White, *The Middle Ground: Indians, Empires, and Republics in the Great Lakes Region, 1650–1815* (Cambridge: Cambridge University Press, 1991).

20 Carlos and Lewis, *Commerce by a Frozen Sea*, pp. 37–9.

21 Wood, *New Englands prospect*, pp. 61, 70, 90; Dawn Dove, 'In Order to Understand Thanksgiving, One Must Understand the Sacredness of the Gift', in Siobhan Senier (ed.), *Dawnland Voices: An Anthology of Indigenous Writing from New England* (Lincoln, NE: University of Nebraska Press, 2014), p. 526.

22 Leanne Betasamosake Simpson, *A Short History of the Blockade*, pp. 1–4; Dove, 'In Order to Understand Thanksgiving', p. 526.

23 John Pory to Dudley Carleton, 30 September 1619, in Lyon Gardiner Tyler (ed.), *Narratives of Early Virginia, 1606–1625* (New York, NY: Scribner, 1907), p. 285.

LOVELOCKED

1 Thomas Dekker, *The guls horne-booke* (1609; STC 6500).

2 William Prynne, *The unlovelinesse of love-lockes* (1628; STC 20477), 'To the Christian Reader', sigs. A4r, A4v.

3 Robert Greene, *A quip for an upstart courtier* (1592; STC 12300), sig. D3v.

4 *Haec-vir* (1620; STC 12599), sig. Cr; Prynne, *The unlovelinesse of love-lockes*, sig. B2v.

5 Prynne, *The unlovelinesse of love-lockes*, pp. 4–6.

6 Samuel Purchas, *Purchas his pilgrimes* (1617; STC 20507), p. 954.

7 Henry Spelman 'Relation of Virginia', in Henry S. Burrage (ed.), *Early English and French Voyages* (New York, NY: Scribner, 1906), pp. 52–3.

8 Linwood 'Little Bear' Custalow and Angela 'Silver Star' Daniel, *The True Story of Pocahontas: The Other Side of History* (Golden, CO: Fulcrum, 2007), p. 75.

9 Francis Higginson, *New-Englands plantation* (1630; STC 13450), sig. C4r.

10 William Prynne, *Histrio-mastix* (1633; STC 20464a), p. 201 and index.

11 Quoted in Lauren Working, *The Making of an Imperial Polity: Civility and America in the Jacobean Metropolis* (Cambridge: Cambridge University Press, 2020), p. 164.

12 Quoted in Working, *The Making of an Imperial Polity*, p. 77.

13 John Smith, *The generall historie of Virginia, New England, and the Summer Isles* (1624; STC 22790), p. 146.

14 Quoted in Working, *The Making of an Imperial Polity*, pp. 77–8.

15 Prynne, *The unlovelinesse of love-lockes*, p. 36.

16 William Davenant, *Madagascar with other poems* (1638; STC 6304), p. 8.

17 'Prince Rupert's Voyage to the West Indies', 1648, British Library, Add. MS 30307, f. 16v.

18 Master Ralph Rokeby to Robert Cecil, 4 January 1570, National Archives, SP 63/30, f. 8v; [Meeting] At Greenwich, 17 July 1590, National Archives, PRO, PC 2/17, f. 754r; *By the Lord Deputie and Councell whereas for prevention of such disorders, ryots and rebellions within this realme* (1625; STC 14190.5).

19 'Commonplace book: poetical and legal', Huntington Library, California, mssHM 46323, *c.*1623–40[?], f. 11v.

20 Robert Hayman, *Quodlibets* (1628; STC 12974), p. 58.
21 Quoted in Barbara Donagan, 'A Courtier's Progress: Greed and Consistency in the Life of the Earl of Holland', *The Historical Journal*, 19:2 (1976), pp. 317–53, at p. 322.

PRICKLY PEARS AND DANBY'S GATE

 1 Alden T. Vaughan, *Transatlantic Encounters: American Indians in Britain, 1500–1776* (Cambridge: Cambridge University Press, 2006), pp. 101–2.
 2 Nicholas Rogers, 'Caribbean Borderland: Empire, Ethnicity, and the Exotic on the Mosquito Coast', *Eighteenth-Century Life*, 26:3 (2002), pp. 117–38.
 3 Quoted in Lauren Working, *The Making of an Imperial Polity: Civility and America in the Jacobean Metropolis* (Cambridge: Cambridge University Press, 2020), p. 47.
 4 Quoted in Jill Francis, '"A ffitt place for any Gentlemen"? Gardens, Gardeners, and Gardening in England and Wales, 1560–1660' (unpublished PhD thesis, University of Birmingham, 2011), p. 119.
 5 *The essayes or counsels, civil and morall, of Francis Lo[rd] Verulam* (1625; STC 1148), pp. 266, 270–5.
 6 George Percy, 'Observations', in Lyon Gardiner Tyler (ed.), *Narratives of Early Virginia, 1606–1625* (New York, NY: Scribner, 1907), pp. 6–7, 15–16.
 7 'From the Archives: Strawberry Thanksgiving', 19 June 2021, Tomaquag Museum, www.tomaquagmuseum.org/belongingsblog/2021/6/18/from-the-archives-strawberry-thanksgiving [accessed 20 June 2024].
 8 *The essayes or counsels*, p. 266.
 9 William Wood, *New Englands prospect* (1634; STC 25957), pp. 71–2.
10 Christine DeLucia, *Memory Lands: King Philip's War and the Place of Violence in the Northeast* (New Haven, CT: Yale University Press, 2018), pp. xv, 3.
11 Betty Booth Donohue, *Bradford's Indian Book: Being the True Roote & Rise of American Letters as Revealed by the Native Text Embedded in 'Of Plimoth Plantation'* (Gainesville, FL: University of Florida Press, 2011), pp. xii, 5.
12 Stephen Harris, 'Seventeenth-Century Plant Lists and Herbarium Collections: A Case Study from the Oxford Physic Garden', *Journal of the History of Collections*, 30:1 (2018), pp. 1–14, at pp. 1–3; 'Between Two Worlds: The Danby Gate to the Physic Garden in Oxford, 1632–3', *Cabinet*, www.cabinet.ox.ac.uk/between-two-worlds-danby-gate-physic-garden-oxford-1632-3 [accessed 24 June 2024].
13 Anne Daye, 'The Banqueting House, Whitehall: A Site Specific to Dance', *Historical Dance*, 4:1 (2004), pp. 3–22, at p. 16.

14 Thomas Carew, *Coelum Britanicum* (1634; STC 4618), pp. 2, 15, 26, 28.

15 Carew, *Coelum Britanicum*, p. 12.

16 José Barreiro (Taíno), 'Taíno *zemí* of Itiba Cahubaba', National Museum of the American Indian, www.americanindian.si.edu/exhibitions/ infinityofnations/meso-carib/127442.html [accessed 27 June 2024].

17 John Gerard, *The herball or Generall historie of plantes. Gathered by John Gerarde of London . . . and very much enlarged and amended by Thomas Johnson* (1633; STC 11751), 'To the courteous and well willing Readers'.

18 Gerard, *The herball*, pp. 83, 356, 1522.

19 Gerard, *The herball*, 'To the courteous and well willing Readers'.

20 Carew, *Coelum Britanicum*, p. 14.

21 Gerard, *The herball*, pp. 1599, 1621; George Charles Williamson, *George, Third Earl of Cumberland, 1558–1605, His Life and Voyages: A Study from Original Documents* (Cambridge: Cambridge University Press, 1920), pp. 61, 202; Samuel Purchas, *Purchas his pilgrimes* (1617; STC 20507), pp. 1152, 1141, 1163.

22 Gerard, *The herball*, pp. 1156, 1178.

23 Gerard, *The herball*, p. 1546.

24 John Parkinson, *Paradisi in sole paradisus terrestris* (1629; STC 19300), sig. 3v.

25 Parkinson, *Paradisi in sole*, pp. 70, 281, 364–6.

26 Parkinson, *Paradisi in sole*, pp. 194, 434, 295, 396, 450, 491.

27 Gerard, *The herball*, p. 1177; Parkinson, *Paradisi in sole*, p. 433.

28 Parkinson, *Paradisi in sole*, pp. 432–3.

29 *The lawes resolutions of womens rights* (1632; STC 7437), pp. 71–2.

30 Karen Kupperman, *Providence Island, 1630–1641: The Other Puritan Colony* (Cambridge: Cambridge University Press, 1993), pp. 24–5.

31 Kupperman, *Providence Island*, pp. 17, 26.

32 Kupperman, *Providence Island*, pp. 30–3.

33 Ned Blackhawk, *The Rediscovery of America: Native Peoples and the Unmaking of US History* (New Haven, CT: Yale University Press), pp. 50–6; Kerry Apps, 'Enslavement in the English Atlantic World, 1616–1641', (unpublished MA thesis, Cambridge University, 2022), p. 66.

34 Alison Games, '"The sanctuarye of our Rebell Negroes": The Atlantic Context of Local Resistance on Providence Island, 1630–41', *Slavery and Abolition*, 19:3 (1998), pp. 1–21, at pp. 7, 12, 16; Providence Island Company to Nathaniel Butler, 7 June 1639, in W. Noel Sainsbury (ed.), *Calendar of State Papers: Colonial, Vol. I* (London: Her Majesty's Stationery Office, 1860), p. 295.

35 Kupperman, *Providence Island*, pp. 85–6, 345; *Certaine inducements to well minded people* (1644; Wing C1701), pp. 1–7.

36 *Certaine inducements*, pp. 5, 10, 14.

37 Susan Dwyer Amussen, *Caribbean Exchanges: Slavery and the Transformation of English Society, 1640–1700* (Chapel Hill, NC: University of North Carolina Press, 2007), p. 9.

38 'The Voyage of Henry Colt', in Vincent T. Harlow (ed.), *Colonizing Expeditions to the West Indies and Guiana, 1623–1667* (London: Hakluyt Society, 1925), pp. 66–7.

39 Richard Ligon, *A true & exact history of the island of Barbados* (1657; Wing L2075), pp. 27, 40, 54–5.

40 Derek Walcott, *Collected Poems, 1948–1984* (New York, NY: Noonday, 1988), pp. 19–21.

41 John Donne, *Devotions upon emergent occasions* (1624; STC 7033a), pp. 415–16.

42 Susan M. Hill, *The Clay We Are Made Of: Haudenosaunee Land Tenure on the Grand River* (Winnipeg: University of Manitoba Press, 2017), pp. 14–18.

43 Robert Brenner, *Merchants and Revolution: Commercial Change, Political Conflict, and London's Overseas Traders, 1550–1653*, 2nd edn (London: Verso, 2003), pp. 113–14.

44 Johan Wedel, 'Human–Plant Interaction and Spiritual Healing among the Miskitu', *Anthropos*, 112:1 (2017), pp. 262–70, at pp. 264–6.

45 Donohue, *Bradford's Indian Book*, p. 21.

CHILLI RED IN AN ENGLISH STILL LIFE

1 Sam Segal, *A Fruitful Past: A Survey of the Fruit Still Lifes of the Northern and Southern Netherlands from Brueghel till Van Gogh*, tr. P. M. van Tongeren-Woodland (Amsterdam: Herzog Anton-Ulrich-Museum Braunschweig, 1983); Sam Segal, *A Prosperous Past: The Sumptuous Still Life in the Netherlands, 1600–1700*, ed. William B. Jordan (The Hague: SDU, 1998).

2 Mark Doty, *Still Life with Oysters and Lemon: On Objects and Intimacy* (Boston, MA: Beacon, 2001), pp. 5, 50.

3 Barrie Juniper, 'Sir Nathaniel Bacon II: The Vegetable World', *The British Art Journal*, 1:2 (2000), pp. 16–18.

4 John Pory to Dudley Carleton, 30 September 1619, in Lyon Gardiner Tyler (ed.), *Narratives of Early Virginia, 1606–1625* (New York, NY: Scribner, 1907), p. 284.

5 Thomas Blundevile, *M. Bludevile his exercises containing sixe treatises* (1594; STC 3146), p. 261.

6 Thomas Hariot, *A briefe and true report of the new found land of Virginia* (1590; STC 12786), p. 18.

7 Molly Harbour Bassett and Jeanette Fabrot Peterson, 'Colouring the Sacred in Sixteenth-Century Central Mexico', in Andrea Feeser, Maureen Daly Goggin, and Beth Fowkes Tobin (eds), *The Materiality of Colour: The Production, Circulation, and Application of Dyes and Pigments, 1400–1800* (Abingdon: Routledge, 2012), pp. 45–54, at p. 48. See also the work of Mexican artist Elena Osterwalder, who experiments with traditional Mesoamerican methods of cochineal dyeing and *amatl* bark paper-making.

8 Elena Phipps, *Red: The Art History of a Color* (New Haven, CT: Yale University Press, 2010); Barbara C. Anderson, 'Evidence of Cochineal's Use in Painting', *The Journal of Interdisciplinary History*, 45:3 (2015), pp. 337–66; see also the work of the Zapotec artist Porfirio Gutiérrez.

9 [John Parkinson], *Theatrum botanicum, The theater of plants* (1640; STC 19302), pp. 1498–9.

10 Robert Cecil to Lord Chancellor [Christopher] Hatton, 7 September 1591, in 'Letters from Sir Robert Cecil to Sir Christopher Hatton, 1590–1591', *Camden Fifth Series*, 22 (2003), pp. 248–9.

11 Rowland Whyte to Sir Robert Sidney, 11 February 1597, in Arthur Collins (ed.), *Letters and Memorials of State, in the reigns of Queen Mary, Queen Elizabeth, King James, King Charles the First . . . Written and Collected by Sir Henry Sydney* (London: T. Osborne, 1746), p. 89. 'Relation of Richard Wyan', in John Bruce (ed.), *Calendar of State Papers: Domestic, Charles I, 1635* (London: His Majesty's Stationery Office, 1865), pp. 610–13; Richard Carmarden to Robert Cecil, 7 November 1597, in R. A. Roberts (ed.), *Calendar of the Cecil Papers in Hatfield House: Vol. 7, 1597* (London: Her Majesty's Stationery Office, 1899), pp. 5–15.

12 Thomas Gage, *The English-American* (1648; Wing G109), pp. 100–1.

13 *The Poems of Andrew Marvell*, ed. Nigel Smith (Edinburgh: Pearson, 2007), pp. 133–4.

14 John Smith, *The generall historie of Virginia, New England, and the Summer Isles* (1624; STC 22790), p. 171.

15 Edmund Waller, *A panegyrick to my Lord Protector* (1655; Wing W506), p. 4.

16 Segal, *A Fruitful Past*, p. 3.

EPILOGUE

1 John Williams, *A sermon of apparel* (London, 1620; STC 25728.5), pp. 15–16, 18.

2 Thomas Dekker, *The pleasant comedie of old Fortunatus* (1600; STC 6517), sig. B3v.

3 Joseph Addison, 'The Adventures of a Shilling', *Spectator*, 249 (1710).

4 Edmund Waller, 'Upon the Present War with Spain', in [S. Carrington], *The history of the life and death of His Most Serene Highness, Oliver, late Lord Protector* (1659; Wing C643), p. 195.

5 Samuel Daniel, 'The Epistle to Prince Henry', in John Pitcher (ed.), *Samuel Daniel: The Brotherton Manuscript: A Study in Authorship* (Leeds: University of Leeds, 1981), p. 131.

6 Walter Hamond, *A paradox* (1640; STC 12735), sigs. E2r–v; Thomas Howell, *H. his devises* (1581; STC 13875), sig. Gr.

7 John Beaumont, *The metamorphosis of tabacco* (1602; STC 1695), sigs. Dv–Ev.

8 Henry Fitzgeffrey, *Certaine elegies* (1618; STC 10945.3), sigs. Fr, F4v.

9 Quoted in Gregory Martin, *Rubens in London: Art and Diplomacy* (London: Harvey Miller, 2011), p. 30.

10 Gerald Vizenor, *The Heirs of Columbus* (Hanover, CT: Wesleyan University Press, 1991), p. 98.

11 Vizenor, *The Heirs of Columbus*, pp. 152, 103, 108.

12 'Romance, n.', *Oxford English Dictionary*.

13 Glicéria Tupinambá, 'An Indigenous Woman Troubling the Museum's Colonialist Legacy: Conversation with Glicéria Tupinambá' [interviewed by Bruno Brulon Soares], *Museum International*, 74 (2022), pp. 1–23, at pp. 21–2.

14 Betty Booth Donohue, *Bradford's Indian Book: Being the True Roote & Rise of American Letters as Revealed by the Native Text Embedded in 'Of Plimoth Plantation'* (Gainesville, FL: University of Florida Press, 2011), pp. xvi, xviii; Nisha Ramayya, '"Rehearsal for the World-Building Outside of Colonialism": A Conversation with Leanne Betasamosake Simpson and Billy-Ray Belcourt', *Wasafiri*, 37:3 (2022), pp. 50–6, at p. 52.

List of Illustrations

Anthony van Dyck, *Self-Portrait with a Sunflower, c.* 1632–3. Duke of Westminster Collection/Wikicommons, CC0 1.0 Universal (photo: Odecalchi).

Inca feathered bag by unknown maker(s), feathers on cotton, coca leaves, circa fifteenth to sixteenth century. The Metropolitan Museum of Art.

Studio of Nicholas Hilliard, *Anne of Denmark, c.* 1605, gouache on vellum laid into card. Yale Center for British Art, Paul Mellon Collection, B1974.2.50.

John White, *Arnaq and Nutaaq, c.* 1585–93. Pen and brown ink and watercolour over graphite, touched with white. © The Trustees of the British Museum.

Caribou parka from Greenland by unknown maker(s), circa nineteenth century. © The Trustees of the British Museum.

The Allegory of America published by Philip Galle, part of the 'The Four Continents' series [after Marcus Gheeraerts the Elder], *c.* 1590–1600. The Metropolitan Museum of Art.

Eastern Bluebird [?] and Twohee [after John White], *c.* 1585-93. © The Trustees of the British Museum.

Nicholas Hilliard, *Portrait of a Young Man, Probably Robert Devereux, Second Earl of Essex,* 1588. The Metropolitan Museum of Art.

Thomas Hariot's *A Brief and True Report of the New Found Land of Virginia* (1590), engraved by Theodor de Bry. Private collection/Wikicommons CC BY-SA 3.0 (photo: Livinncary).

Terra cotta tobacco pipe made by Robert Cotton in Jamestown, *c.* 1608–24. Courtesy of Jamestown Rediscovery Foundation (Preservation Virginia).

'The Founding of Tenochtitlan' in the Codex Mendoza, *c.* 1541. © Bodleian Libraries, University of Oxford/Bridgeman Images.

Unknown English artist, *Elizabeth I,* 1588. Woburn Abbey/Wikicommons CC0 1.0 Universal (photo: Shakko).

Hand-coloured engraving of Cartagena by Baptista Boazio ['Maps and Views Illustrating Sir Francis Drake's West Indian Voyage, 1585–6'], 1589. Jay I. Kislak Collection. Library of Congress, Washington DC.

Pearl fishing boat and divers depicted in the 'Histoire naturelle des Indes' ['Drake Manuscript'], *c.* 1586. © The Morgan Library & Museum. MA 3900. Bequest of Clara S. Peck, 1983.

A piece of eight coin minted in Potosí before 1617. Reproduced from the original held by the Department of Special Collections of the Hesburgh Libraries of Notre Dame.

Copper-gold Muisca bird pendant by unknown maker(s), circa tenth to sixteenth century. The Metropolitan Museum of Art.

Pair of silver flagons with maritime imagery, 1597-8. The Metropolitan Museum of Art.

Andrés Sánchez Gallque, *Portrait of Don Francisco de Arobe and Sons Pedro and Domingo,* 1599. Museo del Prado/Wikicommons CC0 1.0 Universal (photo: Outisnn).

Unknown English artist, *Walter Ralegh,* 1588. © National Portrait Gallery, London.

Drilled pearls from the Jamestown site, 1608–1610. Courtesy of Jamestown Rediscovery Foundation (Preservation Virginia).

Clay tobacco pipe fragments, circa early seventeenth century. From author's own collection. Image: Lauren Working.

Henry Peacham, *Minerva Britanna* (1612), STC 19511 Copy 1 [image 67037], p. 199. Folger Shakespeare Library, Washington, DC.

Detail of a headdress of blue and red macaw feathers and small green (parrot?) feathers on a cotton band, by unknown maker(s), circa pre-1829. Courtesy of the Pitt Rivers Museum.

Salamander brooch from the Cheapside Hoard, circa late sixteenth to early seventeenth century. © London Museum / Cheapside Hoard Collection.

Watch case (reverse), *c.* 1620. The Metropolitan Museum of Art.

Michael Van Meer, 'Album Amicorum', *c.* 1615–1616. The University of Edinburgh.

Caribou skin shirt from North America (Canada?), circa early seventeenth century. © Ashmolean Museum/Bridgeman Images.

Portrait of Three Elizabethan Children by an unknown artist, *c.* 1580. Private Collection/Wikicommons CC0 1.0 Universal (photo: PKM).

Samuel Cooper, *Portrait of Margaret Lemon, c.* 1635–37. © Frits Lugt Collection, Fondation Custodia, Paris.

John Gerard, *A Herball* (1597), STC 11750 Copy 3 [image 62099], p. 781. Folger Shakespeare Library, Washington DC.

Pumpkin (cucurbit) seeds, circa late sixteenth century, found at the Rose Playhouse. Courtesy of MOLA/Andy Chopping.

Cookmaid with Still Life of Vegetables and Fruit, c. 1620–25, Nathaniel Bacon. Photo: Tate.

Daniel Mytens, *Charles I*, 1631. © National Portrait Gallery, London.

Detail from the printed version of the codex in Samuel Purchas, *Purchas his Pilgrimes*, vol. III (1625). Courtesy of Winchester College Fellows' Library.

Index

Sierra Leone, 90, 127

silver: Addison's coin, 302–3; allusions in art and literature, 7; boxes, 299; decline in purity, 9; earrings, 67; as East India Company currency, 86, 92, 97; English corruption equals Spanish, 97; hampers Spain, 22–3; Heath on, 94–5; James I bans Spanish coins, 92; mannerist designs, 93; mercury use, 85; mining in Drake manuscript, 60; Parnassus lacks, 83; Philip II's betrothal gift, 85–6; Philips works in mines, 90–1; pieces of eight, 86, 292; piracy, 2, 8, 9, 16, 86–90, 228; Potosí mine, 84–5; Providence Island rumours, 282; reworking in England, 92–3; and slavery, 90, 96–7, 282; trade, 8–9; Tudor, composition of, 93–4; vs manufacture, 95–6; in watercolours, 50–1, 61

Simpson, Leanne Betasamosake, 249, 308

Sireniacs (fraternity), 195–6

Skicowaros (Abénaki man), 176

skins: bear, 216; caribou, 27, 30, 31, 40, 41, 45, 216; deer, 18, 48, 61, 170, 216, 217; jaguar, 82, 308; muskrat, 231, 239–40, 245; otter, 75, 177, 219, 231, 245; raccoon, 216; sable, 151; seal, 29–30, 31, 38–9, 40–1, 44, 45; *see also* beavers

slavery/enslavement: on Barbados, 284; and Donne, 21; in Drake manuscript, 59; in mines, 90, 96–7, 203–4; Pequots, 282; in Potosí, 84; on Providence Island, 282; reliance on, in colonies, 16;

Restoration rise, 265; Spanish buy from Hawkins, 90; and sugar boom, 22; tobacco plantations, 124–5, 186, 198; voyages to Africa, 16; *see also cimarróns*; pearl divers

Smith, John, 69, 70, 139, 177–8, 256, 257; *The Generall Historie of Virginia, New-England, and the Summer Isles*, 54, 208–10, 213, 257

Smith, Thomas, 222

Somers Isles, 204; *see also* Bermuda

Somers Isles Company, 15, 124, 205–6

Somodonco (Chivor), 149–50, 160

Soto, Hernando de, 56

Southampton, Henry Wriothesley, 3rd Earl of, 140, 176, 181, 198, 222

Spain: absence in Ralegh-sponsored art, 55–6; Anglo-Spanish treaty (1604), 92, 156; Armada (1588), 52, 66, 122, 154–5; Black Legend, 19–20, 80, 95, 156; Buckingham's piracy, 228; *cimarróns* threat, 60, 87; colonial enrichment, 12–13; colonises Florida, 56–7; in Davenant opera, 142–3; and emeralds, 149–52, 153–5, 160; English blame for mining brutality, 97; goldsmiths, 104; influence on cabinets, 226; pearl trade, 113, 114, 116, 117–18; San Tomé attacked, 108; silver hampers, 22–3; smoking habits, 183; Spanish Inquisition, 91; Spanish Match, 195, 229; 'Spanish money', 86; spying on Ralegh's colonial plans, 65; tobacco